W9-DBE-227

# Atlas of Infertility Surgery

Second Edition

**Grant W. Patton, Jr.,** M.D., F.A.C.O.G.
Director, Southeastern Fertility Center; Assistant
Clinical Professor of Obstetrics and Gynecology,
Medical University of South Carolina, Charleston

**Robert W. Kistner,** M.D., F.A.C.S., F.A.C.O.G.
Assistant Professor of Obstetrics and Gynecology,
Harvard Medical School; Associate Chief of Staff,
Brigham and Women's Hospital; Consultant in
Gynecology, New England Baptist Hospital, Boston

with illustrations by

Robert Galla and Edith S. Tagrin
Department of Medical Illustration,
Massachusetts General Hospital, Boston

**Little, Brown and Company**   **Boston/Toronto**

Library of Congress Catalog Card No. 83-80297

ISBN 0-316-69387-1

Printed in the United States of America

HAL

To the continuation of the tradition of surgery for the infertile woman initiated by John Rock, M.D., and William Mulligan, M.D.

# Contents

# Preface

Since the first edition of the *Atlas of Infertility Surgery*, two changes have had a profound influence on the development of infertility surgery. The first, a sociologic change, has been the marked increase in patients whose tubal damage and infertile status relates to a prior inflammatory insult rather than to endometriosis. This increase reflects a sweeping change in American sexual attitudes as sexual intercourse outside of marriage has become socially acceptable and an epidemic of venereal disease—owing to the gonococcus, *Chlamydia*, *Trichomonas*, and herpes organisms—has become rampant.

The second change, microsurgery, has fortuitously permitted the infertility surgeon to deal with this influx of tubal pathology in a new and innovative manner. The introduction of the operating microscope into the field of infertility surgery occurred in the late 1970s and dramatically changed the surgical approach to the diseased oviduct. This instrument allowed the gynecologist to inspect tubal anatomy in the operating room at magnifications that permitted the separation of normal and diseased tubal mucosa with great accuracy. This improved visualization led to the development of new surgical approaches to fimbrial and cornual disease. Tubal reanastomosis performed for reversal of prior tubal sterilization or for removal of tubal pathology became commonplace as the need for uterotubal implantation declined. Coincident with these changes in surgical technique was a significant elevation of postoperative pregnancy rates. The advent of microsurgery of the female oviduct has been a truly exciting surgical advance. It has provided hope for those increasing numbers of female patients with tubal pathology and confidence for the surgeon confronted with these difficult patients that the most adequate surgical repair has been performed.

The second edition of the *Atlas of Infertility Surgery* has been completely rewritten to present the microsurgical approach to infertility surgery. A new chapter, Essential Elements of Microsurgical Technique, has been added to assist in understanding the microscope and includes a discussion of optical principles, types of microscopes, microsurgical instruments, sutures, and needles. A section on the principles of electrosurgery should assist the surgeon in selecting the proper generator and microelectrode.

The authors are indebted to Joseph H. Bellina, M.D., Ph.D., for his chapter on the use of carbon dioxide laser in infertility surgery, a new and exciting advance. Applications of this new cutting technique have been included in the appropriate sections of oviductal surgery.

During the years since the first edition, diagnostic laparoscopy has evolved, and operative laparoscopy has become a viable surgical alternative. Hysteroscopy, not discussed in the first edition, has become an important diagnostic tool in evaluating the interior of the uterus, and surgical procedures performed during hysteroscopy are encouraging. Use of the laser during these endoscopic procedures is a promising development and has been described by a pioneer in this field, James F. Daniell, M.D.

The authors thank Jerome Feist for reviewing the section on microsurgical principles and Lou A. Wetterman for assisting with the section on endoscopic principles. The assistance of Zeiss and Wolf instrument companies in providing instructive photographs is appreciated.

We thank the operating room personnel at St. Francis Xavier Hospital for their patience in helping the surgeon grow through the levels of microsurgical technique. We are also indebted to Carolyn Keating for her persistence in organizing this material and to Margie Moxley for her many hours of typing.

G. W. P.
R. W. K.

# Introduction

It is estimated that 15 to 20 percent of married couples in the United States are unable to bear a child. Since few babies are available for adoption, active pursuit of the cause of sterility and aggressive treatment are considerably more commonplace today than previously. Three sociological changes have altered the practice of infertility in the United States since 1975. The first involves the female who has entered a profession or pursued a career and has therefore postponed pregnancy until her late twenties or early thirties. No longer is it unusual to find a woman in her midthirties about to have her first child. Secondly, the liberation of the sexual mores and the availability of contraceptive techniques have permitted the American female to experience sexual intercourse prior to and outside of marriage, often involving different sexual partners. This sweeping change has contributed to the third factor, namely the marked increase in the incidence of pelvic infection in the middle-class American female. This third change has been discussed at length in Chapter 7. Remarkably, one million cases of gonorrhea were reported in the United States during 1978, and it has been estimated that the number was actually closer to two million, that is, one case of gonorrhea for every 100 Americans. Although gonococcal salpingitis occurs in approximately one in five of these female patients, this organism is responsible for only half the cases of pelvic inflammatory disease (PID). It has been estimated that 17 percent of women who have an attack of acute salpingitis will become sterile because of postinfection tubal occlusion.

Observed and estimated studies on the number of months required for conception in the absence of use of contraception clearly indicate that 25 percent of women will be pregnant within the first month, 63 percent in six months, 75 percent in nine months, 80 percent in one year and 90 percent in 18 months. Thereafter, irrespective of the age of wife or husband, or the frequency of coital exposure, the longer the couple have been married the greater is the progressive decline in conception rate. In these latter cases, undiscovered medical factors exist. These are the cases that will benefit from a complete investigation by the infertility specialist. One should not delay, however, in the patient who is over 30 years of age and who complains of her infertile status. It is recommended that these patients be evaluated after twelve months of unprotected intercourse. It has been estimated that the major causes of infertility are as follows: male factor, 30 to 35 percent; ovulation problems, 15 to 20 percent; tubal factor, 20 to 30 percent; and cervical factor, 5 percent; unexplained infertility occurs in 10 to 15 percent of these patients.

A complete infertility evaluation must be carried out and an accurate diagnosis made prior to definitive therapy. Present diagnostic techniques are presented in Chapters 1 and 2. Numerous medical advances have increased the physician's therapeutic armamentarium since the first edition. These include the increased use of ovulatory agents (Clomiphene, Pergonal, and Parlodel) and management of hormone deficiencies of the corpus luteum. Specific timing of ovulation by ultrasound, initially utilized by those interested in in vitro fertilization, has now been found useful in the routine use of Clomid, Pergonal, and artificial insemination. Increased interest in sperm evaluation and sperm antibody production has been associated with improved treatment of the male factor. The diagnostic techniques of laparoscopy and hysteroscopy have also permitted more accurate diagnosis of pelvic and uterine abnormalities before surgical intervention.

Before considering a patient for surgical treatment of her infertility, an extensive interview with the patient and her husband should take place. This interview has three goals: (1) to review diagnostic studies and clearly identify the etiologic factor involved, (2) to discuss in detail the surgical technique to be utilized; and (3) to discuss management of postoperative pregnancy results.

During this interview, all prior infertility tests should be discussed and incomplete studies scheduled to be repeated, if necessary. Such an interview permits the surgeon to review laparoscopic, hysteroscopic, and hysterosalpingographic findings with the couple to clarify the exact nature of the tubal or uterine pathology. The surgical procedure to be performed should then be outlined at length, perhaps with the use of slides. This author (G.W.P.) has found that a short slide presentation made in the consulting room is helpful in demonstrating the operating microscope, the principles of magnification, and other factors in a manner that the couple can easily understand. Lastly, the results of surgery should be discussed. This includes the overall pregnancy expectation and length of time to achieve a pregnancy. Most patients do not realize that pregnancy success is often considered during a 24 to 36 month postoperative interval. Future follow-up by laparoscopy or hysterosalpingography should be mentioned at this time and discussed further immediately following surgery.

An interesting change has occurred in the attitude of the patient and the physician toward infertility surgery. Previously, surgery was thought of only as a last resort following many years of sterility; today, many gynecologists, particularly younger ones who are well trained in the diagnosis of infertility, are more likely to refer a patient with a uterine anomaly or fimbrial disease for definitive surgical correction. This changed attitude is also related to refinement in surgical technique, such as microsurgery, and to markedly improved pregnancy results. In vitro fertilization (IVF) has now become the treatment of last resort. Most patients are interested in the role of IVF during their treatment program, and even in those individuals in whom a microsurgical technique is deemed preferable, this author (G.W.P.) has found it beneficial to discuss the technique of in vitro fertilization and its anticipated pregnancy result.

# 1 Infertility Investigation Before Surgery

An infertility study should have a definite plan with a predictable end point. Such a standardized regimen usually can be concluded in five or six office visits spaced at approximately one-month intervals, and the couple should be so informed at the first visit. Today more and more infertile couples are seeking help in achieving conception, and perhaps because of widespread media coverage, they seem to be coming for help earlier. In this situation, the traditional injunction to wait and see should give way to the concept that any couple who have cohabited normally and have not conceived within a year are entitled to a full infertility workup.

On the premise that infertility is often a syndrome of multiple origins, an adequate investigation requires studies of all reasonable etiologies in *both* husband and wife. Thus, the finding of a single causative factor, such as oligo-ovulation in the wife, does not rule out the possibility of other causes as well, such as oligospermia in the husband; nor does it rule out the possibility that more than one factor is operative in one or both partners. Although statistical data are only approximate, there is evidence that fully 35 percent of all infertility problems are of multiple origins [1]. The variety of possible causes listed in Table 1-1 underscores the need for systematic investigation in both husband and wife, and only on this basis can therapy be undertaken with maximum expectation of success.

A well organized program can best be pursued by dividing the investigation into two phases, one using the resources available to the physician in the office, and the other using those of the hospital. Hospital admission should be utilized to complete the workup with a minimum of expense, inconvenience, and delay, for time is an important consideration. Generally, the patients have already spent a year or so in attempting to conceive. When they seek professional help, they hope their problem can be solved quickly.

**Study of the Male Partner**

Evaluation of the male factor is important before infertility surgery. A detailed discussion of the investigation of this area is not within the scope of this book, however the infertility surgeon should be able to assess these studies. Several excellent and well organized approaches are available to the reader and these have been listed in the references [1, 6]. An outline of diagnostic procedures for the husband is given in Table 1-2, and regard-

**Table 1-1.** Etiologic interpretation of cause of infertility as related to husband, wife, and the couple as a unit

| Female factors | Male factors |
|---|---|
| General | General |
|   Dietary disturbances |   Fatigue |
|   Severe anemias |   Excess smoking, alcohol |
|   Anxiety, fear, etc. |   Excess coitus |
|     (hypothalamus) |   Fear, impotence, etc. |
| Developmental | Developmental |
|   Uterine absence, hypo- |   Undescended testis |
|     plasia |   Testicular germinal |
|   Uterine anomalies |     aplasia |
|   Gonadal dysgenesis |   Hypospadias |
| Endocrine |   Klinefelter's syndrome |
|   Pituitary failure | Endocrine |
|   Thyroid disturbances |   Pituitary failure |
|   Adrenal hyperplasia |   Thyroid deficiency |
|   Ovarian failure, poly- |   Adrenal hyperplasia |
|     cystic disease | Genital disease |
| Genital disease |   Orchitis, mumps |
|   Pelvic inflammation, |   Venereal disease |
|     tuberculosis |   Prostatitis |
|   Tubal obstructions | |
|   Endometriosis | |
|   Myomas and polyps | |
|   Cervicitis | |
|   Vaginitis | |
| Male-female factors | |
|   Marital maladjustments | |
|   Sex problems | |
|   Ignorance (timing, douching, sperm leakage, etc.) | |
|   Low fertility index | |
|   Immunologic incompatibility | |

Source: Behrman, S. J., and Kistner, R. W. A Rational Approach to the Evaluation of Infertility. In S. J. Behrman and R. W. Kistner (eds.), *Progress in Infertility* (2nd ed.). Boston: Little, Brown, 1975.

**Table 1-2.** Diagnostic procedures—male partner

Initial interview
  History; include inquiry about exposure to DES and environmental toxins
  Physical examination; check for possible varicocele
Semen analysis (stained slide for morphology, mucus penetration test, and hamster egg assay when indicated)
Laboratory studies as indicated
  Blood count
  Urinalysis
  Prostatic secretions (smear and culture)
  Androgen profile; gonadotropins
  Karyotyping when indicated
Sperm antibody study when indicated
Testicular biopsy and vasogram

less of whether these procedures are performed by the infertility specialist or an andrologist, a systematic approach must be adopted. It would be pertinent to note at the initial interview whether the male had been exposed to diethylstilbestrol (DES) in utero. Recent studies [3] show that DES-exposed males appear to have a higher incidence of epididymal cysts and other structural genitourinary abnormalities.

The practice of stating that a male exhibits normal fertility on the basis of a sperm count is no longer valid. A detailed personal history and physical examination should be followed by a complete semen analysis that includes evaluation of sperm motility and morphology as well as measurement of numbers of sperm and semen volume. A stained slide is used to evaluate morphology. Identification of immature forms, white blood cells, and a stress pattern is important. More than one specimen should be evaluated when an abnormality is identified. The basic evaluation of the initial semen specimen also includes a mucus penetration assay. Finally, in instances where a male's fertility is questionable, oocyte penetration by the hamster assay provides useful information.

## Study of the Female Patient

The routine diagnostic procedures for the evaluation of female infertility are given in Table 1-3, and optimal times for such studies are shown in Figure 1-1. A detailed history should outline the menstrual pattern, including age of onset, duration and frequency of flow, amount of bleeding, presence or absence of pain, and any gross irregularity. In addition, the physician should inquire about premarital and postmarital coitus, especially with relation to frequency and timing with ovulation. Other points of importance include use or nonuse of contraceptives, intravaginal lubricants, or douches; history of pelvic infections, past surgery, accidents or illnesses; present and past occupations, and use of cigarettes and alcohol. A history of maternal use of diethylstilbestrol during pregnancy involving the patient suggests the possibility of a uterine malformation in this individual. This may be an etiologic factor in patients with habitual abortion.

**Table 1-3.** Diagnostic procedures—female partner

Initial interview with husband and wife; physical examination of wife

Laboratory studies, as indicated by history and physical
   LH, FSH
   Prolactin
   $T_3$, $T_4$, Free $T_7$
   Androgen profile
   Serology
   Complete blood count with sedimentation rate

Basal body temperature chart times one cycle

Postcoital test

Hysterosalpingogram

Endometrial biopsy and serum progesterone

Ultrasonic evaluation of ovary for follicular development

Sperm agglutination studies

Diagnostic laparoscopy and hysteroscopy

**Figure 1-1.** Composite figure of major areas of investigation in cases of infertility. Large arrows indicate optimal day for each specific investigation. (From S. J. Behrman and R. W. Kistner, A Rational Approach to the Evaluation of Infertility. In S. J. Behrman and R. W. Kistner (eds.), *Progress in Infertility* (2nd ed.). Boston: Little, Brown, 1975.)

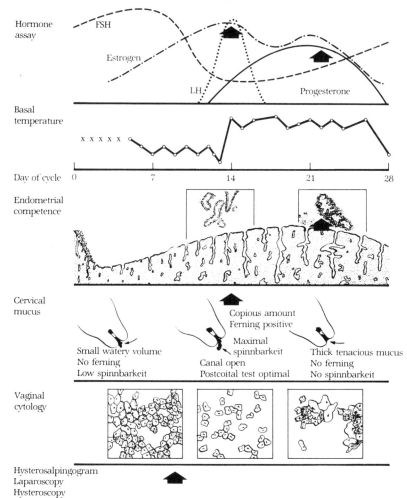

When previous abdominal operations have been performed, it is advantageous to secure copies of the operative description and the pathology reports. Surgery performed during childhood for a ruptured appendix suggests peritubal adhesions as a possible etiological factor. Rarely, an operation described by the patient as "conservative" has, in fact, been a bilateral salpingectomy. Extensive, and expensive, investigation is thus immediately avoided.

During the physical examination the physician should pay particular attention to external body contour, hair distribution, fat deposits, and breast development. The breasts should be thoroughly examined for nipple abnormality, dominant masses, or nipple discharge frequently associated with prolactin elevation and oligo-ovulation. Stigmata of hypothyroidism should be looked for. A thorough pelvic examination should be conducted in which the size, shape, and position of the internal and external genitalia are noted, and particular search is made for signs of infection. An enlarged clitoris and male distribution of pubic hair should warn the examiner to look for other evidences of masculinization due to adrenal or ovarian tumors. If purulent material can be expressed from the urethral meatus or periurethral glands, it should be stained and cultured for gonococci. Specific vaginal infections, such as those caused by *Trichomonas* and *Candida* (*Monilia*), may be important factors in infertility. The finding of a vaginal septum or double cervix demands that the uterus and oviducts be investigated radiologically for other congenital abnormalities.

The cervix should be carefully evaluated and mucus-sperm interaction detailed as discussed later. Uterine enlargement may suggest myomas. A fixed, retroverted uterus with nodularity in the uterosacral ligaments alerts the examiner to the diagnosis of pelvic endometriosis. Adnexal thickening may suggest previous inflammatory disease. The caveat to remember is that physical examination does not establish a diagnosis of endometriosis or inflammatory disease, and judgement must be withheld until adequate evaluation, including endoscopy, has been performed.

The laboratory procedures indicated by the initial history and physical examination may include (1) a complete blood count and determination of erythrocyte sedimentation rate, (2) a blood type and rubella titer, and (3) assays of thyroid function, such as triiodothyronine ($T_3$) and thyroxine ($T_4$) when indicated. The thyroid function tests should be obtained before performing Schiller's test, because a false high value will be present for 6 to 8 weeks after Schiller's solution (potassium iodide plus iodine) is applied to the cervix. If endocrine abnormalities or increased hirsuitism is evident or if there is menstrual irregularity (oligo-ovulation) the following tests are indicated: (1) serum prolactin; (2) a serum adrenal androgen profile, including dihydroepiandrosterone (DHEA) and androstenedione; (3) serum testosterone; (4) serum follicle-stimulating hormone (FSH) and luteinizing hormone (LH); and (5) pituitary tomogram or CAT scan, if the prolactin is significantly elevated. In patients with primary amenorrhea or prolonged secondary amenorrhea, nuclear sex determinations, and a karyotype are obtained.

It has been mentioned that diagnostic procedures should be completed during a reasonable interval and prognostic advice then given the couple [2]. These procedures require proper timing and interpretation and can be discussed under the general headings of sperm-mucus interaction, ovulation factors, and uterine and tubal factors.

*Sperm-Mucus Interaction*
Evaluation of the male factor discussed above included a detailed semen analysis. Functional capability of the sperm suggested by evaluating motility was further considered in the mucus penetration assay and occasionally by means of the hamster test.

The postcoital test provides important information regarding the interaction of sperm and cervical mucus and is usually performed early in an infertility evaluation. Abnormal aspects of sperm motility within the mucus suggest influence of a chronic cervical infection, a vaginal infection (i.e., *Monilia*), and sperm antibodies. Marked variation in the mucus itself may be seen and appropriate therapy suggested.

TECHNIQUE

The postcoital test should be performed just before ovulation. Correlation with changes in basal body temperature is extremely helpful as is correlation of presumed ovulation with subsequent confirmation by serum progesterone or endometrial biopsy. Figure 1-2A illustrates a plastic suction cannula with a narrow tip that provides atraumatic access to the endocervical canal (Milex Corp., Chicago, Ill.). A syringe is attached to the open end, and gentle suction is used to obtain a specimen. Removal of mucus is then performed by inserting the stylet and spreading the specimen on a microscope slide for evaluation. A tuberculin syringe has been found to be useful during quantitative evaluation of cervical mucus (Figure 1-2B).

Visual observation of the color and presence of cellular material is useful as is the volume of mucus obtained. At the time of ovulation, the mucus forms a thin, continuous thread as it is pulled apart—a phenomenon called *spinnbarkeit*. This physical characteristic is a function of increasing levels of estrogen and disappears after the appearance of progesterone. When allowed to dry on a slide, such mucus crystallizes into a fernlike pattern—the *arborization phenomenon*. This phenomenon also disappears after ovulation, as a result of progesterone secretion. When the cervical mucus is examined under the high-dry magnification, the number of cellular elements (leukocytes) and spermatozoa per high-power field are noted. The motility and quality of progression of the spermatozoa are similarly observed.

**Figure 1-2.** Instruments used during mucus evaluation. **A.** Tuberculin syringe used to quantitate amount of mucus. **B.** A plastic cannula (Milex Corp., Chicago, Ill.) with syringe attached.

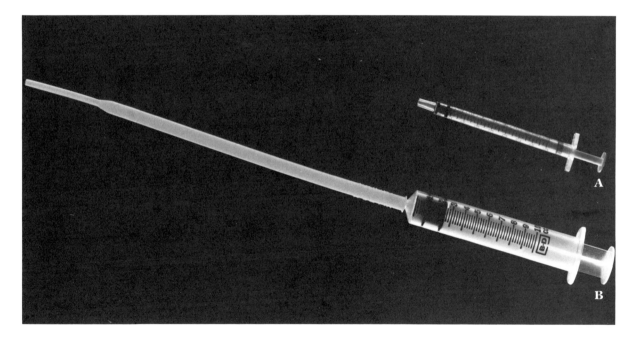

**Table 1-4.** Cervical mucus score

| | |
|---|---|
| Amount | 0 = 0 |
| | 1 = 0.1 ml |
| | 2 = 0.2 ml |
| | 3 = 0.3 ml or greater |
| Viscosity | 0 = thick, highly viscous |
| | 1 = intermediate (viscous) |
| | 2 = mildly viscous |
| | 3 = normal midcycle (ovulatory) |
| Ferning | 0 = none |
| | 1 = atypical fern formation |
| | 2 = primary and secondary stems |
| | 3 = tertiary and quarternary stems |
| Spinnbarkeit | 0 = <1 cm |
| | 1 = 1–4 cm |
| | 2 = 5–8 cm |
| | 3 = ≥9 cm |
| Cellularity | 0 = ≥11 cells/HPF |
| | 1 = 6–10 cells/HPF |
| | 2 = 1–5 cells/HPF |
| | 3 = 0 cells/HPF |
| Total score: | |

Source: Adapted from M. A. Belsey et al. (eds.). Laboratory Manual for the Examination of Human Semen-Cervical Mucus Interaction. Singapore: Press Concern, 1980. P. 42.

INTERPRETATION

Increased use of this test in association with in vitro fertilization has led to a quantitative score. Accurate timing of the procedure is important. Under optimal conditions the postcoital test may be scored as shown in Table 1-4.

In general, there is a positive correlation between the postcoital test and the quality of the semen and cervical mucus; however, a good postcoital test may be found even if the sperm count is subnormal, and conversely a poor postcoital test may occur in the presence of a normal count. The physician should remember that the postcoital test reflects not only the cervical environment of spermatozoa but also the ovarian function controlling it. As such, it is of great value in evaluation of the hormonal milieu present at that time. Georgianna Jones, M.D., has used examination of mucus and vaginal smear to determine the biological shift associated with impending ovulation in patients undergoing in-vitro fertilization. Mucus evaluation does not appear to be useful during high dose personal therapy, however.

Treatment of abnormal mucus associated with low grade cervicitis has been rewarding. Low dose estrogen may improve the quality and amount of mucus seen in patients receiving Clomid. Sperm antibody titers have been successfully treated with Prednisone. It is recommended that these forms of therapy coincide with surgery. The authors have not considered sperm antibodies to be a contraindication to surgery.

## Ovulation Factors

Evaluation of ovulation should be carried out before infertility surgery. A basal body temperature graph is of great value and, as noted earlier, may be correlated with cervical mucus to establish impending ovulation. Confirmation of ovulation with serum progesterone is useful; however, accurate determination of endometrial development can only be obtained by an endometrial biopsy. Establishment of the quality of the luteal phase requires this test, although occasional luteinized follicles may produce changes similar to normal ovulation.

Endometrial biopsy is an office procedure that produces only minor discomfort and does not require anesthesia. The timing of the procedure is important, the optimum time being the twenty-second day of the menses. The bleeding may then be correctly interpreted as being menstrual or anovulatory in type, and the chances of disrupting a normal pregnancy are minimal. Some pathologists prefer the intact, well differentiated late secretory endometrium of day 27 or 28 to the fragmented tissue obtained after menstruation has begun. In women with regular cycles this can be timed rather precisely. Pregnancies have been observed to occur frequently in the cycle during which the endometrial biopsy is obtained. It has been suggested that the trauma of the biopsy elicits a "deciduoma effect," which actually promotes implantation at that site. Figure 1-3 illustrates the various endometrial morphologic changes that occur during a normal cycle.

**Figure 1-3.** Morphologic criteria used to assess the menstrual date of the endometrium. (From R. W. Noyes, A. T. Hertig, and J. Rock, Dating the endometrial biopsy. *Fertil. Steril.* 4:10, 1953.)

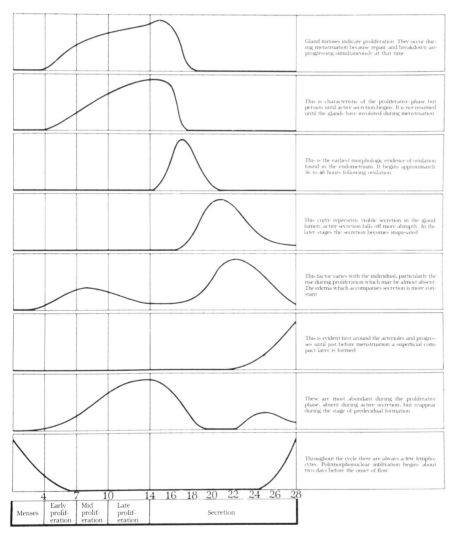

A pelvic examination should precede the biopsy so that the position and size of the uterus can be ascertained. The cervix is exposed with a speculum and cleansed with a povidone-iodine solution (Betadine Solution). Slight traction is placed on the cervix with a tenaculum. Although we do prefer the Duncan curet (Fig. 1-4) because of its relatively small size, any of the various types of curet will give adequate samples. We routinely obtain samples from both the anterior and the posterior surface of the endometrial cavity, using a firm but gentle stroke from the fundus to the cervix. The most representative samples are obtained from high in the corpus. The tissue is immediately fixed in Bouin's fluid. Care should be taken not to traumatize the tissue in transferring it from the curet to the fixative.

**Figure 1-4.** Endometrial biopsy. **A.** Cutting edge of the Duncan curet. This instrument can be introduced easily through an undilated, nulliparous cervical os without undue discomfort. **B.** Proper technique of endometrial biopsy with the Duncan curet. Samples are taken from both the anterior and the posterior surfaces of the cavity. (From R. W. Kistner, *Gynecology: Principles and Practice* (3rd ed.). Chicago: Year Book, 1979.)

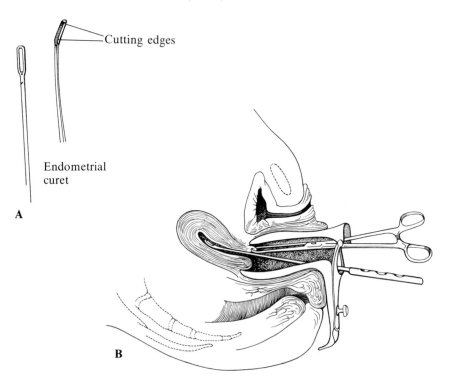

Cutting edges

Endometrial
curet

A

B

Although exact dating of the endometrium during the secretory phase of the cycle is practiced by many gynecologic pathologists, it is not absolutely necessary, and adequate interpretation or presumption of ovulation may be made in most patients. If the endometrial biopsy reveals abnormal tissue of any variety, a thorough curettage should be done for adequate diagnosis and to rule out malignancy.

Noyes and associates [7] have suggested certain essentials for obtaining and interpreting the endometrial biopsy: (1) Chart the basal body temperature (BBT) and perform the biopsy during a BBT cycle. (2) Perform the biopsy after two or three BBT cycles have been charted and during at least two cycles. (3) Do the biopsy on the sixth and ninth postovulatory days; be certain to get fundal surfaces. (4) Try to obtain superficial endometrium—do not go too deep. (5) Fix the tissue in Bouin's solution. (6) Date the endometrium, but date the most advanced area. (7) Look at your own slides.

Absence of ovulation should be adequately studied before infertility surgery, and a specific diagnosis should be made. Although demonstration of successful ovulation with agents such as Parlodel or clomiphene sulfate is not critical, a clear indication of the presumed success of this therapy is necessary. An abnormality of the luteal phase requiring replacement therapy with progesterone suppositories or other drugs should be delayed until surgical treatment has been completed.

### Tubal and Uterine Factors

Hysterosalpingography and endoscopy are the tests used today to evaluate the uterus and oviducts. These procedures should be regarded as complementary rather than competitive since each provides specific useful information. This author (G.W.P.) performs a hysterosalpingogram in almost all patients before endoscopy. This practice permits discussion of normal or abnormal findings with the infertile couple and better prepares them for the findings of endoscopic evaluation. Hysteroscopy and laparoscopy are frequently performed concurrently in an ambulatory surgical unit as described in Chapter 3.

Hysterosalpingography was originally introduced for evaluation of tubal factors in infertility; however, the indications for its use have been markedly increased. Hysterography permits evaluation of the functional behavior of the uterus as well as the size and configuration of the uterine cavity in both normal and abnormal conditions (Fig. 1-5). The recognition of congenital malformations as well as of uterine hypoplasia or synechiae is facilitated by hysterography (Fig. 1-6). Furthermore, it is a valuable method for the detection of submucous myomas, particularly in those patients in whom the uterus is not enlarged so that the clinical diagnosis may be difficult or impossible (Fig. 1-7). Endometrial hyperplasia, endometrial polyps, and adenomyosis (Fig. 1-8) may be recognized by their characteristic patterns on the hysterogram. Hysterography is a valuable method for detecting many of the causes of habitual abortion, and it provides evidence of the etiologic factor in nearly half of these patients. The usual causes are uterine myomas and congenital uterine malformations, some of which may be due to prior exposure to diethylstilbestrol in utero. Functional abnormalities, such as excess uterine irritability, may frequently be evident by this method. Widening of the lower uterine segment and internal cervical os may be demonstrated in patients with cervical incompetence (Fig. 1-9).

The most important application of salpingography is in the diagnosis of abnormalities of the oviducts in patients with infertility. Rozin [9] believes that repeated salpingographic procedures may be used to control the results of treatment of infertility due to tubal factors. He has shown that salpingography, by itself, has been of therapeutic benefit in cases of infertility and points out that it is not uncommon for previously infertile women to become pregnant shortly after salpingographic examination.

**Figure 1-5.** Hysterosalpingograms showing **(A)** uterus and oviducts in a normal patient; **(B)** free passage of the dye from the oviducts into the peritoneal cavity; and **(C)** a dilated and convoluted tube on the right and accumulation of dye in sacculations at the tubal fimbriae on the left in a patient with chronic pelvic inflammatory disease and bilateral hydrosalpinges. (From R. W. Kistner, *Gynecology: Principles and Practice* (3rd ed.). Chicago: Year Book, 1979.)

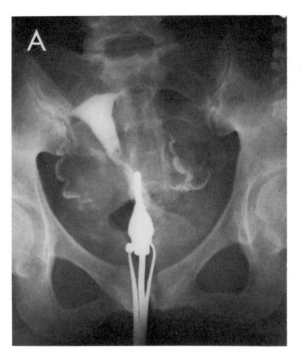

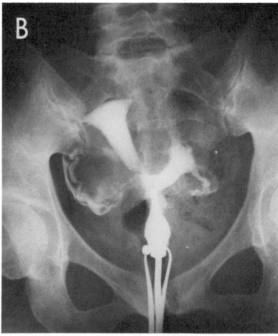

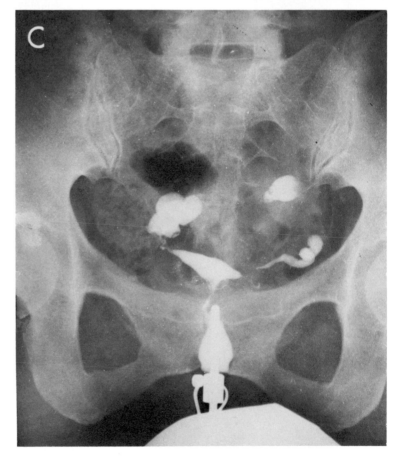

**Figure 1-6.** Hysterogram showing distortion of endometrial cavity due to submucous leiomyomas. (Courtesy of John Twaddle, M.D.)

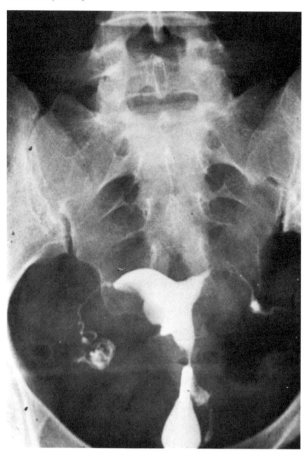

**Figure 1-7.** Hysterogram showing complete bicornuate uterus. (Courtesy of John Twaddle, M.D.)

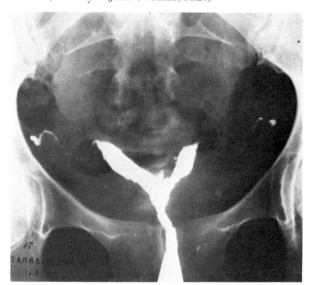

**Figure 1-8. A.** Hysterogram showing adenomyosis in a 20-year-old infertile female. The diagnosis was verified by biopsy at the time of hysterotomy. **B.** Same patient. Uterus anteverted to show extensive spread of dye into areas of adenomyosis of the posterior uterine wall. (From R. W. Kistner, *Gynecology: Principles and Practice* (3rd ed.). Chicago: Year Book, 1979.)

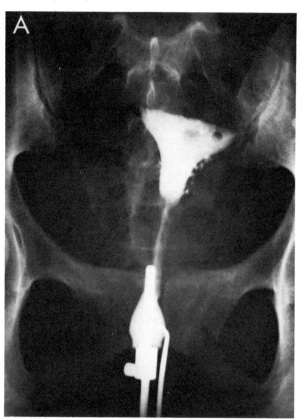

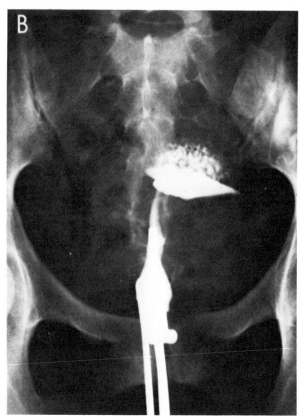

**Figure 1-9.** Hysterogram showing widened lower uterine segment in a patient with cervical incompetence. (Courtesy of John Twaddle, M.D.)

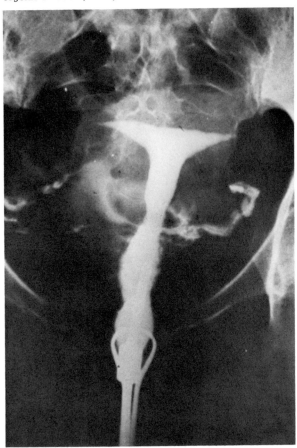

CONTRAST MEDIA

Accurate diagnosis in hysterosalpingography depends to a large extent on the contrast media employed and the technique with which they are used. Ever since the introduction of oily solutions there has been a constant search for alternative substances because of the disadvantages which have been attributed to the oily media.

Two decades ago the most popular contrast medium was Lipiodol, an iodized oil containing 40 percent iodine in combination with poppy-seed oil. However, oil solutions are absorbed very slowly from the pelvis, and when large amounts are injected a residual may persist in the pelvic cavity for several months. In the presence of a hydrosalpinx, absorption is delayed for an even longer period of time.

Oil solutions have a viscosity suitable for lining the uterine and tubal surfaces, resulting in a sharp, distinct radiographic shadow. Because of the slow absorption of these solutions, excellent radiograms may be obtained both during the procedure and after an interval of several weeks. Oil media are of special value in cases of delayed tubal patency or in patients with peritubal adhesions.

Numerous investigators [1, 5, 8] have objected to the use of oil solutions, citing examples of foreign-body reactions, with adhesions, salpingitis, and parametritis. In addition, oil-retention cysts, foreign-body granulomas, and psammoma bodies have been described. Several investigators [9, 11] have noted that when Lipiodol was injected in excessive amounts, it resulted in a peritoneal focus consisting of oil, fibrin, and leukocytes.

Although pain is seldom observed when oil is introduced and, when present, is usually transient, large amounts of oil entering the peritoneal cavity may occasionally cause severe cramping abdominal pain. Similarly, when large amounts of oil are injected under high pressure in the presence of tubal obstruction, intravascular dissemination may occur, with the possibility of oil pulmonary embolism.

**Figure 1-10.** Hysterogram showing intravasation of dye into uterine and infundibulopelvic veins. Both oviducts were closed at the isthmic portion. (Courtesy of John Twaddle, M.D.)

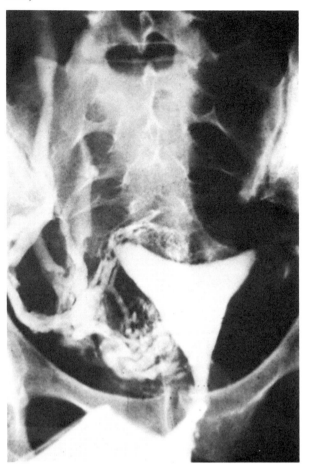

Intravasation of oily media (Fig. 1-10) can be a serious complication, especially when large amounts of the medium are injected. Embolic transport of larger amounts to the pulmonary capillaries is indicated by a rapid pulse rate, dyspnea, and a feeling of oppression in the chest. X-ray films of the lungs reveal granular shadows. Intravasation of water-soluble contrast media is not associated with the dangers that accompany intravasation of oil solutions.

Water-soluble media are of low viscosity but are not always well tolerated and tend to produce pelvic pain. Unfortunately, they are rapidly absorbed and do not have the advantage of permitting delayed control films, which occasionally are indispensable for the accurate diagnosis of tubal patency or occlusion. Water-soluble media are not reliable for the demonstration of gross intrauterine lesions, such as submucous uterine myomas or polyps, because of their rapid absorption. They are, however, very suitable for the demonstration of various pathologic conditions of the tubes and of delicate changes in the uterine mucosa. They are also of value in certain patients in whom the tubes are not demonstrable by the use of the more viscous oil media.

The amount of water-soluble medium necessary for obtaining a diagnosis of tubal patency is greater than with an oily medium, but the use of large amounts of this solution is not usually associated with tissue reactions or the dangers of intravasation. Table 1-5 summarizes the differences between the oily and the aqueous media.

**Table 1-5.** Comparison of oily and water-soluble contrast media

| Parameter | Oily | Water-soluble |
| --- | --- | --- |
| Viscosity | High | Low to moderate |
| Radiopacity | Very good | Moderate to satisfactory |
| Absorption | Very slow; delayed for many months when large amounts are injected | Prompt excretion through the kidneys after 20–60 minutes; in hydrosalpinx the medium is only slowly absorbed and may persist for up to 28 hr |
| Toxicity | Not observed unless decomposed oil is used | Rare |
| Allergic reactions | Not observed | Occasionally observed |
| Peritoneal reactions | Only when large amounts injected; not observed when small quantities are injected | Observed, mostly transient |
| Pain | Not observed when small amounts are injected under low pressure | Nearly always present; may be transient or persist for many hours |
| Dangers | Intravasation, pulmonary embolism | None |

Source: Rozin, S. *Uterosalpingography in Gynecology.* Springfield, Ill.: Thomas, 1965.

One of the major hazards of hysterosalpingography is that of reactivation of chronic pelvic inflammatory disease. This may occur following the use of either oily or water-soluble media and should not be attributed to the medium used. Rather, such reactions are the result of the mechanical procedure and may occur after carbon dioxide insufflation, cervical dilatation or cauterization, or endometrial biopsy. For this reason, in patients who give a history of pelvic inflammatory disease, hysterosalpingography is not performed until the white blood cell count and erythrocyte sedimentation rate are within normal range. In addition, antibiotic protection is given both before and after the procedure. Figure 1-11 shows bilateral hydrosalpinges with tubal closure.

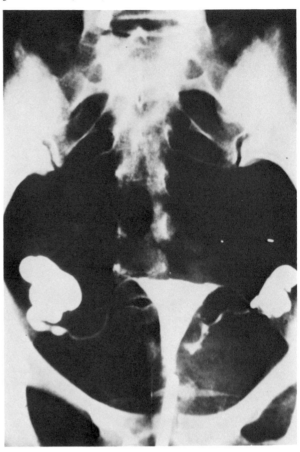

**Figure 1-11.** Hysterogram showing normal proximal oviducts but bilateral terminal hydrosalpinges. (Courtesy of John Twaddle, M.D.)

TECHNIQUE

The most suitable time for hysterosalpingography is the sixth or seventh day following the cessation of menstruation. During the first two to three days following the menses, the procedure is unsafe because of incomplete regeneration of the surface epithelium and the increased possibility of diffusion of the contrast medium into the uterine veins. During the week preceding menstruation, edema and thickening of the endometrium may produce a functional closure of the tubal ostia.

A detailed menstrual history should be obtained before hysterosalpingography is performed. Abnormalities of the cycle or diminution of the last menstrual period suggest the possibility of intrauterine or ectopic pregnancy, and further investigation should be carried out before performing this test. In patients having prolonged amenorrhea, the possibility of pregnancy should be entertained because ovulation and gestation occasionally occur in amenorrheic women.

Hysterosalpingography is contraindicated in the presence of any pelvic infection. Therefore, the vagina and cervix should be inspected to exclude the presence of a purulent discharge, and a thorough pelvic examination should be performed to determine the size and position of the uterus. At the same time, the adnexal structures should be palpated.

The following sterile instruments should be arranged in a row on a table covered with a sterile cloth:

1. Two Graves specula (one medium and one large)
2. Two long tissue forceps
3. Two curved cervical tenacula
4. One Jarcho self-retaining rubber-tipped acorn cannula, a Mälmstrom vacuum uterine cannula, or a small disposable plastic cannula
5. One 10-ml syringe, preferably of the Luer-Lok type
6. Several cotton pledgets
7. Vaginal tampons
8. Sterile gloves

Because the patient is likely to be tense and nervous, gentle technique is most important. The procedure should be explained and an effort made to divert her attention, thus enabling her to relax.

The procedure must be performed under sterile conditions since the contrast medium, after passing through the genital tract, may otherwise introduce infection into the peritoneal cavity.

Following the pelvic examination, a speculum is gently inserted into the vagina, and the cervix is exposed and washed with aqueous benzalkonium chloride (Zephiran). The cervix is then very gently grasped with a tenaculum placed transversely at 12 o'clock. At this point the patient is told that she will feel a slight pinch or stinging sensation. Traction is then placed on the tenaculum in the axis of the vagina, thus straightening the uterus and eliminating kinking at the internal cervical os.

The length of the cannula introduced into the cervical canal is of extreme importance. If the cannula beyond the acorn is too long, it may directly traumatize the uterine mucosa. If the uterus is small and traction on the cervix has not straightened the cervix-corpus angle, it is very easy to perforate the posterior wall of the uterus. In addition, the contact of the cannula against the uterine wall induces strong muscular contractions. However, if the cannula is too short, free passage of the medium into the uterine cavity will not occur, particularly in patients with a narrow internal os or a kinked cervical canal. For most patients, the length of the cannula or plastic tip should be 3 to 3.5 cm beyond the acorn. This will reach approximately 0.5 cm beyond the internal os.

Before the cannula is introduced through the cervical canal, it should be checked for patency by injecting the medium through it, thus expelling all air. As the cannula is inserted, the patient should be told that slight cramping pain may occur. To prevent reflux of the medium, the cannula is inserted firmly into the cervix and fixed to the tenaculum with the self-retaining device. The vaginal speculum is then withdrawn before the x-ray films are taken.

The Mälmstrom uterine cannula obviates the use of a tenaculum, because it produces a vacuum effect on the external cervical os. The acorn tip of the cannula is inserted and the cervix is grasped in a glass or plastic suction cup; then the vacuum is exerted. This cannula is of particular value for demonstrating the incompetent cervical os, but it is rather difficult to apply when the cervix is small or located high in the vaginal vault without the usual amount of protrusion into the vagina. After the equipment is in place, a plain film of the pelvis should be taken to visualize any radiopaque structures in the pelvis.

**Figure 1-12.** Hysterogram showing partial fimbrial occlusion of the elevated right oviduct. Complete left fimbrial occlusion was present. Three radiologic findings associated with partial fimbrial occlusion are dilatation of the distal ampullary segment, preservation of rugae, and a narrow stream or jet stream of dye (often seen at fluoroscopy) squirting from the constricted fimbrial opening.

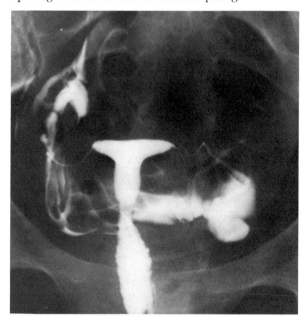

It is recommended that the pressure during the injection of the medium not exceed 200 mmHg, because excessive pressure may produce spasm of the uterus and oviducts as well as accidental intravasation. However, for an experienced clinician, the use of manometric control is not necessary. It is important that each single injection of contrast medium not exceed 2 to 3 ml, and after each injection an x-ray film should be taken, exposed, and studied.

*Fluoroscopic Control.* Most hysterographic studies today are performed under fluoroscopic control, and immediate evaluation of uterine and tubal contour is therefore possible. Completion of the study is accomplished during a single interval, and subsequent delayed films are rarely necessary. Conventional spot film fluoroscopy is used in most radiology departments and is quite satisfactory for infertility evaluation. A more recent x-ray technique that utilizes 105 mm photographic film permits multiple rapid sequence photographs during hysterosalpingography. The image on the photograph is taken from the television monitor, however, and the pictures are smaller and provide less detail of tubal architecture than does the conventional spot film technique.

The basic fluoroscopic technique of hysterosalpingography requires the assistance of an x-ray technician or radiologist. A water soluble contrast medium should be injected slowly without undue pressure. Early films of uterine and tubal architecture are essential. A uterine defect may be hidden by the presence of an excessive amount of dye. At times, the gynecologist will need to aspirate dye from the endometrial cavity to verify the presence of an intrauterine defect, such as a submucous fibroid. Likewise, the presence of rugae in the ampullary tubal segments should be carefully discerned. The diagnosis of partial fimbrial occlusion has recently been described by Patton (Fig. 1-12) and may be made when a careful examination has been performed. Three observations that support this diagnosis are the presence of rugae, mild ampullary dilatation, and the observation of a jet stream of dye that appears to pass through a small fimbrial opening.

It is a simple matter to record the image seen on the fluoroscopy monitor on either one-half inch or three-quarter inch video tape. The cassette recorder used during video recording of diagnostic laparoscopic procedures or microsurgical procedures using the Zeiss operating microscope may be employed for this purpose. This recorder is easily attached to either the conventional spot film x-ray machine or the 105 mm photographic monitor. Video recordings are particularly useful in a teaching environment; it is exceedingly helpful to review the hysterographic study with residents and students following the procedure. The simplicity of this technique should be stressed.

INTERPRETATION

The following summary by Parekh and Arronet [8] indicates the most common causes of false-positive and false-negative salpingographic findings:

A. Causes of false-positive findings (tubes are open)
   1. Foley catheter blocking uterine cavity or tip of cannula impinging on myometrium (avoidable)
   2. Widening of cervical canal with stenosis of internal os (unavoidable)
   3. Admixture of air or blood with the dye producing spasm (avoidable)
   4. Cornual spasm due to procedure (avoidable)
   5. Localized uterine contraction or synechiae (unavoidable)
   6. Differences in tubal diameter or structure producing apparent unilateral closure (unavoidable)
   7. Too little contrast medium or omission of delayed film (avoidable)
   8. Large uterine cavity (avoidable)
   9. Extravasation of dye into myometrium (unavoidable)
   10. Peritubal adhesions or narrow fimbrial opening (unavoidable)
   11. Pocketed spill near fimbriae may be mistaken for hydrosalpinx, or vice versa (avoidable)
   12. In tuberculous salpingitis, the tobacco-pouch appearance of the fimbriae may give the impression of pocketed spill (avoidable)
B. Causes of false-negative findings (tubes are closed, or phimotic tubes)
   1. Free spillage from a pinpoint opening of an otherwise phimotic fimbria may suggest normal fimbrial function
   2. Extravasation of dye through uterine or ovarian vasculature may be misinterpreted as tubal patency
   3. Localized constriction in a tortuous hydrosalpinx may suggest pocketed spill
   4. Free pelvic dissemination of dye from a unilateral phimotic tube may give the impression of bilateral spill

## References

1. Behrman, S. J., and Kistner, R. W. (eds.). *Progress in Infertility* (2nd ed.). Boston: Little, Brown, 1975.
2. Behrman, S. J., and Kistner, R. W. A Rational Approach to the Evaluation of Infertility. In S. J. Behrman and R. W. Kistner (eds.), *Progress in Infertility* (2nd ed.). Boston: Little, Brown, 1975.
3. Gill, W. B., Schumacker, G. F. B., Hubby, M. M., and Blough, R. R. Male Genital Tract Changes in Humans Following Intrauterine Exposure to Diethylstilbestrol. In A. L. Herbst and H. A. Bern (eds.), *Developmental Effects of Diethylstilbestrol in Pregnancy.* New York: Thieme-Stratton, 1981.
4. Jones, G. S. Prognosis for the infertile couple. *Obstet. Gynecol. Surv.* 20:646, 1965.
5. Kistner, R. W. *Gynecology: Principles and Practice* (3rd ed.). Chicago: Year Book, 1979.
6. MacLeod, J., and Gold, R. Z. The male factor in fertility and infertility. *Fertil. Steril.* 4:10, 1953.
7. Noyes, R. W., Hertig, A. T., and Rock, J. Dating the endometrial biopsy. *Fertil. Steril.* 1:3, 1950.
8. Parekh, M. C., and Arronet, G. H. Diagnostic procedures and methods in the assessment of female pelvic organs, with special reference to infertility. *Clin. Obstet. Gynecol.* 15:1, 1972.
9. Rozin, S. *Uterosalpingography in Gynecology.* Springfield, Ill.: Thomas, 1965.
10. Rubin, I. C. Non-operative determination of patency of fallopian tubes in sterility. *J.A.M.A.* 74:1017, 1920.
11. Siegler, A. M. Dangers of hysterosalpingography. *Obstet. Gynecol. Surv.* 22:284, 1967.

He that hath seen hath more reason to believe, than he that hath not.

STEPTOE, 1973

The ability to see and to manipulate the uterus, fallopian tubes, and ovaries during a diagnostic procedure has made laparoscopy an essential part of infertility evaluation. Over a decade ago Frangenheim (1967) stated

All in all it may be said, on the basis of years of experience by many authors, that laparoscopy in cases of sterility diagnosis is superior to all other methods of examination and it should therefore be included as an integral part of the gynecological investigation [26].

This ability to contemplate tuboovarian anatomy without a need for haste has provided the gynecologist with a magnificent diagnostic tool. The viewer, peering through the laparoscope, sees only those entities that he has learned to recognize, however. Fine adhesions and endometrial implants hidden behind the ovary go unnoticed by the novice; cornual occlusion of the fallopian tube may be erroneously diagnosed and fimbrial agglutination missed. Laparoscopy, as with culdoscopy before it, requires practice and constant refinement of one's ability and instruments. It is not enough for the gynecologist accustomed to performing laparoscopic tubal sterilization to employ this same technique for diagnostic purposes. The rapid sterilization procedure performed with a single-puncture operating laparoscope is replaced by a two-puncture technique in which all areas of the pelvis are carefully examined.

All patients having surgery for infertility should have had diagnostic laparoscopy. Moreover, increasing numbers of infertility patients with ovulatory problems undergo this procedure, and a diagnosis of "unexplained" infertility cannot be made without having visualized the pelvis endoscopically. In fact, the incidence of unexplained infertility appears to diminish dramatically when careful examination of the pelvis is performed [19]. Endoscopic evaluation of the pelvis is now considered to be an essential diagnostic procedure in the evaluation of the infertile female.

## History

A brief perusal of the history of laparoscopy, or peritoneoscopy as it has been termed in Europe, in the twentieth century is quite interesting, because most Americans did not become acquainted with this technique until the 1970s. This review of the early part of the century reveals that an outstanding report of 500 laparoscopic procedures performed in the medical department at the University of Southern California was published by Ruddock in 1937 [66]. Called peritoneoscopy by Ruddock after Orndoff (1920), 215 male and 285 female patients were evaluated. This procedure was carried out under local anesthesia in patients with "ordinary atmospheric air" and, remarkably, "patients do not complain of any other sensation except one of fullness" [66]. Biopsy procedures were carried out on liver and multiple intraperitoneal tumors in 39 patients. Also, remarkably, 229 of these patients had ascites. There were only eight accidents of minor degree and one death in this series. "The death occurred because of insufficient coagulation of the (liver) biopsy wound. Many biopsies have been taken since, but thorough coagulation of the (liver) wound is done in all cases whether bleeding is noted or not" [66].

The concluding words of Ruddock [66] sound quite modern: "Peritoneoscopy is a minor procedure under local anesthesia, with practically no discomfort and small economic features in contrast to a diagnostic laparotomy." These words obviously went unheard by the American gynecologist until the studies of Fear and Cohen were published in 1967.

A chronology of the history of laparoscopy [20, 69] has been modified from Fear (1967) and Steptoe (1965).

1901    Kelling visualized the peritoneal cavity of a dog with a modified cystoscope. He called this procedure *celioscopy*.

1901    Vann Ott described *ventroscopy*, inserting a speculum through a small incision in the upper abdominal wall.

1910    Jacobaeus performed the first clinically successful laparoscopic procedure and used the term *laparoscopy*.

1911    Bernheim at Johns Hopkins University introduced a one-half inch proctoscope into a small abdominal incision to visualize the gallbladder and the liver.

1912    Norderdoff introduced the concept of pneumoperitoneum and the Trendelenburg position.

1920s   Widespread use of laparoscopy in Europe and Scandinavia.

1925    First English paper on laparoscopy by Rendle Short.

1928    First high-quality instrument (Kalk-Germany).

1937    Ruddock, first large series on laparoscopy in the United States; tubal sterilization through laparoscopy by Anderson (United States).

1942    Uterine suspension via laparoscope by Donaldson (United States).

1944    In Palmar, France, extensive use of biopsy forceps through laparoscope; two-puncture technique similar to that used in 1960s.

1952    Remote light source of high intensity.

1955    Improved lens system and modern instruments available.

1956    Color photography through laparoscope.

1959    Closed circuit television through laparoscope.

1961    Frangenheim published in German the first text on laparoscopy; others published in French and Italian.

1964    First international symposium on laparoscopy.

1967    First English text, published by Steptoe; first modern reports on diagnostic laparoscopy in America by Fear and Cohen.

1970    Laparoscopy in the infertile patient, Peterson and Behrman.

Culdoscopy became popular in the United States after 1944 and was the primary form of endoscopic evaluation of the infertile female during the 1950s and 1960s in this country. The most recognized authorities in the field of infertility also were outstanding culdoscopists. These included Decker, Clyman, Kelly, Rock, Digman, Riva, and Kistner. At the present time, only Diamond actively practices culdoscopy as an integral part of infertility evaluation, and he uses that technique extensively for postoperative evaluation [18]. The first edition of *Atlas of Infertility Surgery* described in detail the technique of culdoscopy as practiced at the Boston Hospital for Women (now part of the Brigham & Women's Hospital).

In the March 1968 edition of *American Journal of Obstetrics and Gynecology* two papers appeared that heralded the beginning of diagnostic laparoscopy in the United States [8, 25]. Although Cohen has been acclaimed as the father of diagnostic laparoscopy in the United States, his report appeared after that of Robert Fear in the March edition. In his report Fear described a two-puncture diagnostic technique similar to that practiced in Europe; however, a Wolf laparoscope was employed. Manipulation of the pelvic organs and lysis of adhesions were performed by Fear with the second puncture probe and scissors. A centimeter rule, biopsy forceps, and coagulating tips also were used. Fear listed the operative procedure performed by him as follows:

| Aspirations | 1. Ascitic fluid, pus, cyst fluid |
| | 2. Extended postcoital (PK) test |
| | |
| Surgical procedures | 1. Lysis of adhesions |
| | 2. Puncture of cysts |
| | 3. Tubal sterilization (clip, diathermy) |
| | 4. Electrocoagulation of implants |
| | 5. Uterine suspension |

Fear said, "Certainly infertility is one of the prime problems that lends itself to laparoscopic investigation" [25]. This report included 137 laparoscopic procedures of which 27 were performed for infertility evaluation. Thirteen others were performed for ovulatory abnormalities. In seven patients with prolonged infertility of unknown origin, clear cut pathology was discovered at the time of laparoscope. The laparoscopic findings in the entire group are listed below:

| | PATIENTS | PERCENT |
| --- | --- | --- |
| Normal | 6 | 22 |
| Pelvic inflammatory disease (PID) | 17 | 63 |
| Endometriosis | 3 | 11 |
| Other | 1 | 4 |

Dr. Melvin Cohen is credited with the initiation of interest in diagnostic laparoscopy in the United States. His report "Culdoscopy versus Peritoneoscopy" was published in 1968 [8]. In 1967, his experience with 102 peritoneoscopies was reported; a two-puncture technique modified from Palmer and described earlier by Frangenheim and Steptoe was employed. In fact, this was virtually the same technique employed by Fear in the report quoted above. Seventy-eight of Cohen's patients underwent laparoscopy because of sterility. Findings at laparoscopy were as follows:

| | PATIENTS | PERCENT |
| --- | --- | --- |
| Normal | 29 | 37 |
| Endometriosis | 15 | 19 |
| Adhesions | 18 | 23 |
| Chronic PID | 4 | |
| Hydrosalpinx | 3 | 10 |
| Cornual occlusion | 1 | |
| Other | 8 | 10 |

Cohen published excellent color photographs with his 1968 report and described a technique for 16mm photography. Operative procedures, including lysis of adhesions and ovarian biopsy, were also performed.

A third report, by Peterson and Behrman in 1970 [61], established the role of laparoscopy in infertility evaluation in the United States. These authors performed 538 laparoscopies during a two-year interval, and 276 of these were to evaluate the infertile female. Again, the technique was similar to that described by Steptoe and Cohen. One modification, also employed by Fear, included the use of the 180-degree 10mm Wolf laparoscope, although the standard two-puncture technique was employed. Laparoscopic investigation of 204 patients with the diagnosis of "unexplained infertility" was conducted.

Indications for laparoscopy in the above study were as follows:

| | |
| --- | --- |
| 1. Unexplained infertility | 204 |
| 2. Ovulation disorders | 50 |
| 3. Tuboplasty evaluation | 12 |
| 4. Adenexal mass | 10 |

Results of laparoscopy in those patients with "unexplained infertility" were as follows:

| | PATIENTS | PERCENT |
| --- | --- | --- |
| Normal | 86 | 40 |
| Endometriosis | 68 | 33 |
| Pelvic adhesions | 36 | 20 |
| Tubal occlusion | 10 | 5 |
| Sclerocystic ovary | 4 | 2 |

The impact of these surgeons' work was great, and it resulted in a dramatic change in American medicine; in the decade of the 1970s laparoscopy became an essential part of every infertility evaluation. The inclusion of this endoscopic technique in the diagnostic armamentarium of the gynecologist was probably advanced more by the need for tubal sterilization than for reasons of infertility or other diagnostic problems during the early 1970s, however. One cannot overlook the persistence of Wheeless in advocating laparoscopic cauterization for sterilization [89, 90] and the subsequent widespread acceptance of the Falope ring designed by Yoon [91]. The Hulka clip did not gain widespread use [54], although the bipolar forceps of Rioux [64] and, recently, Kleppinger [76] became useful tools in laparoscopic sterilization. As the decade of the 1970s drew to a close, however, several medical centers adopted the "mini lap" for safer and simpler tubal sterilization [67].

Although less emphasis may be placed on laparoscopic sterilization in the next decade, increased emphasis will be placed on operative laparoscopy for problems other than sterilization. The role of diagnostic laparoscopy by the general surgeon and oncologist will be expanded. The use of operative laparoscopy by a two- or three-puncture technique as performed by Ruddock and others in the 1930s and refined in the 1950s and 1960s by Palmer, Frangenheim, Semm, and Steptoe will undoubtedly become more widespread. Recent studies by Swolin, Gomel, and Semm have suggested that this technique may even replace laparotomy in the treatment of other types of gynecologic pathology, including ovarian cysts and uterine leiomyomata [33, 71, 83]. Recent use of the carbon dioxide laser during operative laparoscopy seems certain to change the field dramatically [14, 15].

## Laparoscopy in Infertility Evaluation

### Indications and Timing

Whenever possible, the gynecologist should begin the infertility evaluation in consultation with both husband and wife, and the overall plan of evaluation and common causes of infertility should be discussed. This initial contact provides both physician and patient with an important understanding of each other's hopes and fears and provides a framework for future discussion of pathologic processes that may be uncovered. It is one author's (G.W.P.) practice to initially evaluate sperm and ovulatory factors and perform a hysterosalpingogram. Diagnostic laparoscopy, therefore, follows the first visit by a two- or three-month interval. One of the authors (R.W.K.), in response to treating previously evaluated patients who have usually traveled long distances, has tended to admit these patients to the hospital early in the investigative phase. Early hospital admission has also been the practice of Frangenheim and others [3, 26]. During this time a hysterosalpingogram and, when indicated, endocrine evaluation are performed. Diagnostic laparoscopy is usually carried out on the day following admission. Naturally, repeat sperm evaluation of the husband can take place during that 48-hour visit.

Certainly there are instances of infertility evaluation when diagnostic laparoscopy is delayed or even unnecessary. Specific patterns of tubal disease (such as fimbrial occlusion) are obvious on hysterosalpingogram and may occasionally lead the surgeon directly to laparotomy (see discussion on p. 18). Likewise, request for reversal of sterilization will not always involve a preliminary diagnostic laparoscopy if careful review of the operative and pathologic reports reveals resection of a small tubal segment and a typical Pomeroy-type ligation. The infertility surgeon must err on the side of performing normal laparoscopic procedures, however, because an unnecessary laparotomy is not acceptable.

Some of the indications for diagnostic laparoscopy during a sterility evaluation are as follows:

1. Unexplained infertility, all tests normal
2. Evidence of tubal occlusion, or adhesion formation on hysterosalpingogram (HSG)
3. Clinical evidence of endometriosis
4. Failure to conceive after three cycles of artificial insemination with a donor (AID)
5. Failure to conceive within 6 months to 1 year following infertility surgery
6. Suspected uterine anomaly

In general, the important point to emphasize is that diagnostic laparoscopy should be given prime consideration during evaluation of infertile couples. In cases of apparent tubal disease, perhaps indicated by history of tubal infection, severe pain associated with use of an intrauterine device (IUD), a ruptured appendix, or prior ectopic pregnancy, the likelihood of tuboovarian adhesions is very high, and in these patients laparoscopy should be performed early in the investigative phase. However, patients who are oligoovulatory or who have an abnormal sperm factor would not undergo diagnostic laparoscopy if the HSG were normal, until treatment with Clomid or other drugs had begun. It is significant that, if surgery on the male is considered, diagnostic laparoscopy might also be included to establish the normal condition of the female. In the author's (G.W.P.) practice, diagnostic laparoscopy is not always performed prior to varicocele or vas reversal surgery, but this procedure is discussed with the couple prior to urologic surgery. The same pattern obtains with the couple undergoing AID. If the history, clinical examination, and HSG are normal, a diagnostic laparoscopy should be performed after three cycles of artificial insemination if pregnancy has not ensued. If any doubt exists regarding the status of the pelvic organs, diagnostic laparoscopy should be performed at that time.

The freedom to perform diagnostic laparoscopy whenever the infertility specialist feels it is indicated is essential. Certainly the "one day" surgical centers and the ability of a working wife to undergo laparoscopy on Friday and return to work on Monday have been important factors in achieving this freedom. Low complication rates and the high yield of pathologic entities are also important factors.

## Diagnostic Laparoscopy

### Technique of Laparoscopy

Diagnostic laparoscopy should employ a two-puncture technique. As mentioned earlier, it is remarkable how similar the present technique is to that of Ruddock (1937) [66]. Palmer developed the present technique during the 1940s, and Frangenheim, Semm, and Steptoe refined this approach during the 1950s and 1960s. An excellent description of the two-puncture technique using carbon dioxide is given in Steptoe's text (1967), in the report by Fear (1968) and in Semm's *Atlas of Gynecologic Laparoscopy and Hysteroscopy* [25, 69, 79]. This author's (G.W.P.) technique was learned during 1970–1972 interval at the Boston Hospital for Women (now part of the Brigham and Women's Hospital) from Dr. John Leventhal, a student of Melvin Cohen during the late 1960s. This technique was described in detail by Leventhal in the first edition of the *Atlas of Infertility Surgery*, 1975 [44].

In brief, the surgeon usually performs laparoscopy while standing on the patient's left side. The patient's left arm should be placed next to her hip or across her chest. This permits the surgeon to stand more comfortably at the patient's left side while viewing the pelvis, which is essential during operative laparoscopy or laparoscopic photography. The length of the instruments used requires the surgeon to stand in the area adjacent to the patient's left shoulder.

As described by others [8, 25, 78, 89] a modified lithotomy position with the patient's legs partially extended is employed. Knee supports are a welcome addition, providing stability of the legs during the procedure. They are essential if local anesthesia is to be employed. The table is then placed in 10 to 15-degree Trendelenburg position, which may be increased to 30 degrees if necessary.

A Cohen-Fear endocervical cannula, a Semm-type suction cervical cannula, or a Humi endocervical cannula can be used to manipulate the uterus and perform transcervical tubal lavage. The latter has been termed tubal lavage by the Boston group, hydrotubation by others and, more recently, chromopertubation [12, 36, 72]. It is useful to attach K-50 or K-52 plastic extension tubing with stopcock to the end of the endocervical cannula for placement in the area of the patient's left groin, thereby permitting either the surgeon or assistant to inject the indigo carmine or methylene blue dye.

A Verres needle and, later, the metal trocar and sheath are inserted through a periumbilical incision made on the inner fold of the umbilical skin. After viewing the anterior abdominal wall and bladder, a second-puncture (6 mm or 3 mm) trocar is inserted through a second incision. Many sites of insertion are possible for the second trocar, and each surgeon will develop a personal preference as to the best location. Naturally, the location will depend on the organ to be manipulated. In general, during diagnostic laparoscopy this author (G.W.P.) uses a second puncture in the midline at the level of the pubic hairline. This avoids injury to the deep epigastric vessels. During operative laparoscopy it is preferable to have the second puncture in either the left or right lower quadrant, because two lower abdominal punctures frequently are necessary during a "three-puncture" operative procedure. Details of insertion of the Verres needle and trocars have been published by Semm and by others [44, 69].

The choice of a telescope for evaluation of the female pelvis includes the diagnostic laparoscopes of diameters 5, 7, 8, and 10 mm (Fig. 2-1, Table 2-1). As is shown, the lens system and, thus, the field of view increase as the telescope diameter increases. The amount of light available also increases with increased lens size. These telescopes employ lens systems that provide an angle of view of 180, 165, and 130 degrees. Although most American laparoscopists use the 180 degree lens (straight ahead), Steptoe, Frangenheim, and others prefer a 130- or 165-degree fore-oblique telescope lens [27, 69, 80]. As will be shown later, these oblique lens angles increase the operative field seen during rotation of the laparoscope, but they are difficult to master and require extensive practice (see Fig. 2-11). By comparison, the culdoscope employs a 90-degree lens system that also requires extensive practice for optimum interpretation.

**Figure 2-1.** Three types of telescopes are shown. **A.** A diagnostic telescope with a 50 degree angle of view. **B.** The most popular straight diagnostic telescope with an angle of view of 180 degrees. **C.** An operating laparoscope with an angle of view of 10 degrees. The insert shows a close-up view of the bipolar forceps placed through the operating channel. (Courtesy of R. Wolf Co.)

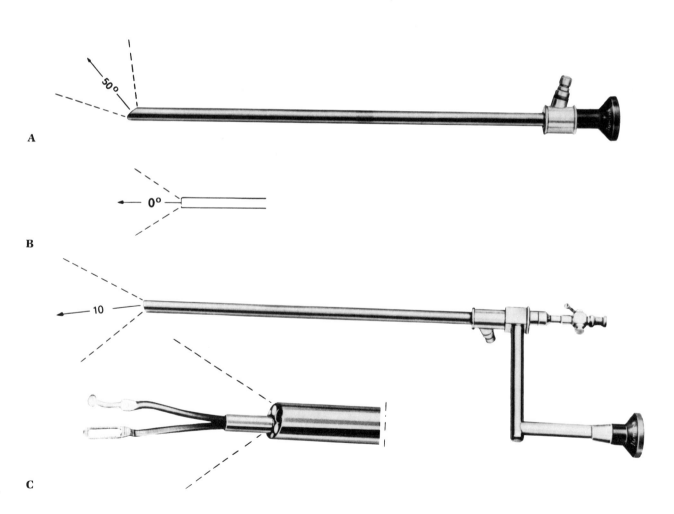

**Table 2-1.** Types of laparoscopes

| Diameter (mm) | Angle of view (degrees) | Channel (mm) |
|---|---|---|
| Diagnostic telescopes* | | |
| 5 | 180, 130, 160 | |
| 7 | 180, 130 | |
| 8 | 180, 130 | |
| 10 | 180, 130 | |
| Operating telescopes | | |
| 10 | 180, 170 | 3 |
| 12 | 180, 170 | 6 |

*Figures apply specifically to Wolf Instruments but are applicable in general to all other telescopes.

Operating laparoscopes are currently sold in diameters of 10 and 12 mm (Table 2-1). The 10 mm operative laparoscope has a 3 mm operating channel and is useful when the small (3 mm) operative instruments are employed. This author (G.W.P.) has found it convenient to switch from the 10 mm diagnostic laparoscope to the 10 mm operating laparoscope, thereby using the same trocar sleeve when it seems useful to lyse adhesions encountered during a routine diagnostic evaluation. The smaller 3 mm instruments have also been used routinely during a 3-puncture operative procedure. The 12 mm operating laparoscope commonly used during laparoscopic tubal sterilization procedures has a 6 mm operating channel. As was noted earlier, the most commonly used second-puncture sleeve is designed for the use of 5 mm instruments and, thus, the long instruments may be used interchangeably through these two openings. In general, however, the use of long instruments through the second puncture trochar has been awkward.

During a diagnostic laparoscopic procedure, this author (G.W.P.) uses a 6 mm second-puncture trocar with flap valve passed through a suprapubic incision. This permits use of the 5 mm probe with centimeter markings, suction cannula, and other instruments for manipulation of the fallopian tubes and ovaries. In general, although the 3-mm instruments are preferred during operative laparoscopy, the larger 5 mm instruments have been found easier to use through the second puncture site.

Inspection of the pelvis must be as complete as possible. Veils of omental adhesions should be swept aside or a small opening made in an avascular site of the omentum to visualize the fallopian tubes. Frequently, omental adhesions will cover only the uterine fundus and do not interfere with tuboovarian function. Descriptions of investigative technique have been published previously [69, 79].

Tubal lavage (chromopertubation) should be performed with dilute indigo carmine dye. Occasionally, focal areas of tubal dilatation may be difficult to differentiate from normal variations. The fimbria should be inspected closely, using the probe to elevate both ovary and tube; thin, filmy adhesions are then obvious. The possibility of "convoluted" tubes should be considered. Occlusion of one oviduct by compressing the isthmic segment against the side of the uterus with a probe eliminates many cases of suspected cornual occlusion. True cornual occlusion is identified by bulging of the cornual area synchronously with pressure and release of the plunger on the syringe containing indigo carmine dye (Shirodkar's sign). Implants of endometriosis should be looked for on the undersurface of the ovaries and uterosacral ligaments and biopsied if necessary. Cauterization of endometriotic implants has not been carried out routinely by the authors, although, occasionally, individual sites have been coagulated by use of the insulated probe or forceps. Areas of endometriosis on the rectosigmoid or overlying the ureter should not be fulgurated.

Laparoscopic findings should be recorded in detail immediately following the procedure. A complete description of all areas surveyed should be included. It is not sufficient to state "the fallopian tubes appeared normal." A preferable operative note would be "the right fallopian tube appeared normal, there were no adhesions between it and the ovary, the fimbrial elements were normal and, at tubal lavage, dye passed easily into and effused from the tube without difficulty." Such description will permit a subsequent investigator to determine that, indeed, "the fallopian tubes are normal." A drawing assists in accurate interpretation and is used by such noted laparoscopists as Steptoe, Cohen, and Swolin (Figure 2-2).

Details of the two-puncture diagnostic technique discussed above are included in Figures 2-3 through 2-5.

**Figure 2-2.** Laparoscopy report form. (From M. R. Cohen, Laparoscopy and Infertility. In J. M. Phillips (ed.), *Laparoscopy*. Baltimore: Williams & Wilkins, 1977. P. 199.)

Name

Surgeon                                      Assistant          LMP          Patient no.        Admission no.
                                                                                                Date
Preoperative diagnosis                                                                          Cycle day

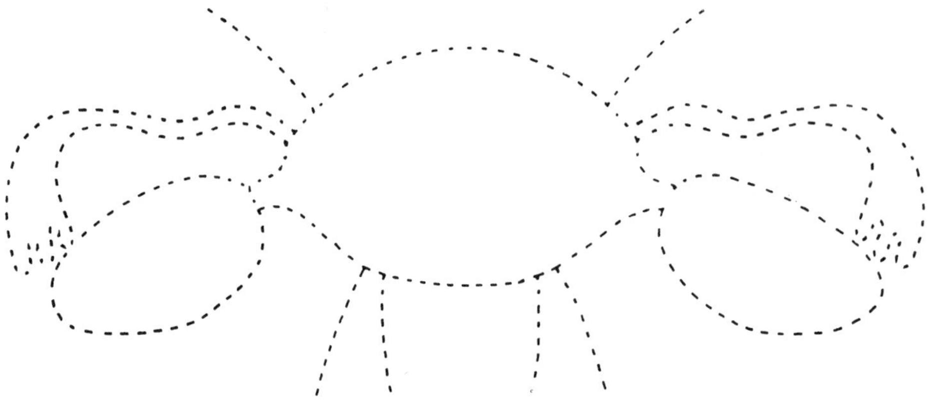

| Peritoneum: | | | | |
|---|---|---|---|---|
| Uterus: | Size | Shape | Color | |
| Abnormalities | | | | |
| Pathology | | | | |
| Uterosacral ligament | | | | |
| Right Ovary: | Size | Shape | Color | Blood vessels |
| Surface: | Smooth | Wrinkled | Tunic | Follicles |
| Luteal tissue | | | | |
| Abnormalities | | | | |
| Utero-ovarian ligament | | | | |
| Left Ovary: | Size | Shape | Color | Blood vessels |
| Surface: | Smooth | Wrinkled | Tunic | Follicles |
| Luteal tissue | | | | |
| Abnormalities | | | | |
| Utero-ovarian ligament | | | | |
| Right Tube: | Length | Color | Surface | |
| Fimbria | Patency | Movement | Peristalsis | |
| Left Tube: | Length | Color | Surface | |
| Fimbria | Patency | Movement | Peristalsis | |
| Photographs: | Voltage | Exposure | Film no. | Technical difficulty |
| Morbidity: | | | | |
| Therapy: | | | | |
| Response: | | | | |
| Pathology: | | | | |

**Figure 2-3.** A diagnostic laparoscopic procedure should involve two punctures. A 7, 8, or 10 mm 180-degree diagnostic telescope placed through a periumbilical incision produces a panoramic field of view. Manipulation of the fallopian tube and ovary will be performed through the 3 mm or 6 mm second-puncture trochar sleeve. In this drawing, a Semm suction cannula has been placed in the endocervical canal for uterine manipulation and tubal lavage.

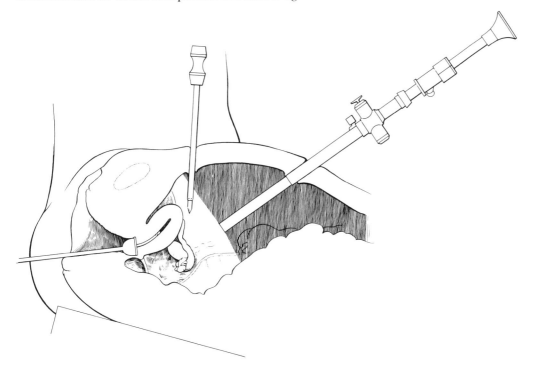

**Figure 2-4.** A blunt graduated probe inserted through the second-puncture site permits elevation of the ovary and inspection of the inferior surface, a common site of adhesion formation and endometriosis. The centimeter markings permit accurate measurement of ovarian cysts, and, more important, of segments of distal oviducts present in the patient who is seeking reversal of a prior tubal sterilization procedure.

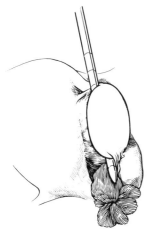

**Figure 2-5.** Elevation of the oviduct during tubal lavage is accomplished by use of the second-puncture probe. The fimbria should be carefully inspected because partial fimbrial agglutination may be overlooked.

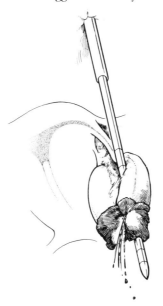

*Operative Laparoscopy*

Operative laparoscopy appears to be one of the most significant new procedures in female infertility, offering the possibility of an innovative surgical approach to abnormalities of tuboovarian anatomy previously treated only by laparotomy. How convenient it would be to cut tubal adhesions, coagulate implants of endometriosis, or open an occluded fallopian tube using a technique that would enable the patient to reduce her recovery time from 3 weeks to 3 days. This surgical approach has been championed by Swolin, Gomel, and Semm, although the Americans—Ruddock, and, later Fear and Cohen—were advocates of this approach in the late 1960s [8, 25, 33, 66, 72, 83]. Use of the carbon dioxide laser for this purpose is discussed later in this chapter by Dr. Daniell.

The summary of surgical procedures performed by Fear through the laparoscope appears quite modern. These procedures have been updated and are listed as follows:

| | |
|---|---|
| Aspiration | 1. Ascitic fluid, pus, cyst fluid |
| | 2. Extended PK test |
| Surgical Procedures | 1. Lysis of adhesions |
| | 2. Puncture of cyst |
| | 3. Tubal sterilization |
| | 4. Electrocoagulation of implants |
| | 5. Uterine suspension |
| Recent Additions | 6. Salpingostomy (Gomel) |
| | 7. Myomectomy (Semm) |
| | 8. Marsupialization of ovarian cyst (Kleppinger) |
| | 9. Ovarian biopsy, wedge resection (B. Cohen) |
| | 10. Aspiration of ova (Steptoe) |

Two general types of operative procedure may accompany laparoscopy. The first are those operative techniques that are easily performed at the time of a diagnostic laparoscopy. These include aspiration of a cyst or aspiration of fluid for culture, ovarian biopsy, coagulation of endometrial implants and lysis of very small tuboovarian adhesions. All can easily be performed with the two-puncture technique simply by inserting an ancillary instrument through the 6 mm second-puncture sleeve. Instruments, including the Palmer biopsy tong, hollow probe, insulated probe, and scissors are useful.

In contrast to the first group of operative procedures that can be performed easily during a two-puncture diagnostic procedure are those operative procedures that require better stabilization of an anatomic structure by a "three-puncture" technique. Extensive omental adhesions or thin tuboovarian adhesions may be cut safely only with adequate exposure and visualization. Ovarian cysts may be extensively biopsied and essentially marsupialized (fenestrated) [45]. Recently Semm [71] has performed myomectomy by a laparoscopic technique and Gomel [35] has performed salpingostomy in at least eight patients by a laparoscopic technique. Those procedures require manipulation from two and, sometimes, three points of entry. Coagulation of small vessels is performed by either monopolar or bipolar high frequency electrosurgical units (see Chap. 5) or by a low-frequency thermocoagulator. Stabilization of a structure is the most difficult aspect of operative laparoscopy. Yuzpe [92] has described retroversion of the uterus and placement of the ovary across the fundus at the time of ovarian biopsy. Semm [70] has championed a suction cannula to hold the fallopian tube during manipulation. The operative laparoscopic approach has also been used to perform oocyte retrieval [81].

*Three-puncture Technique*

When attempting a significant operative procedure by means of the laparoscope it is necessary to utilize two lower-puncture sites of entry as well as the midperiumbilical incision (Fig. 2-6). The surgeon will find it convenient to use one of the lower-puncture instruments to stabilize the fallopian tube or ovary during manipulation. It is also helpful to have an instrument that permits irrigation and suctioning during the act of cutting. Lastly, it is necessary to be able to cut and coagulate while the fallopian tube or omental adhesions is carefully held and the site irrigated. This author (G.W.P.) has used two lower punctures (3 mm or 5 mm) and the 10 mm 170-degree Wolf operating laparoscope with a 3-mm channel inserted through a periumbilical incision. As shown in Figure 2-7, the author prefers to cut and coagulate with the smaller 3 mm instruments inserted through the operating channel of the laparoscope. One could also pass the scissors through one of the lower-puncture trochar sleeves and cut from this perspective. In fact, irrigation and suctioning could be performed through the channel of the operating laparoscope. Regardless of the approach used, the surgeon himself must manipulate all instruments for cutting and coagulation. This type of procedure requires extensive practice and, of course, the proper instruments, all of which must be in perfect working order. Application of the three-puncture technique to lysis of a tubal adhesion and to ovarian biopsy has been shown in Figures 2-7 and 2-8.

**Figure 2-6.** The three-puncture technique of laparoscopic surgery employs two lower-abdominal puncture sites and the insertion of the operating telescope through a periumbilical incision. A Semm cannula or Humi intrauterine cannula permits excellent mobility of the uterus.

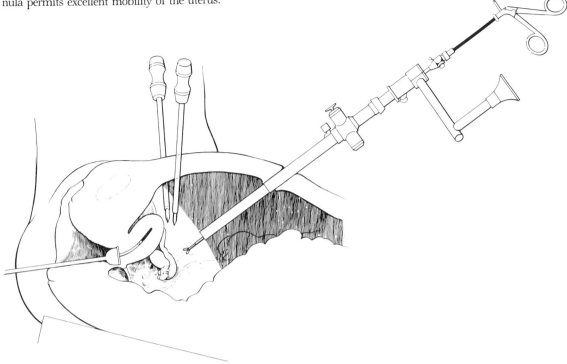

**Figure 2-7.** Tension on a peritubal adhesion is obtained by use of the two lower-puncture instruments. In this drawing, a blunt forceps is used to hold the fallopian tube, and a probe is inserted along the line of the adhesion. A 3 mm scissor has been inserted through the operating channel of the 10 mm operating telescope and will be used to cut the adhesion. By using the operating channel, visualization of the area to be cut is maintained at all times. Electrocoagulation by means of the monopolar scissor or bipolar forceps is possible when indicated.

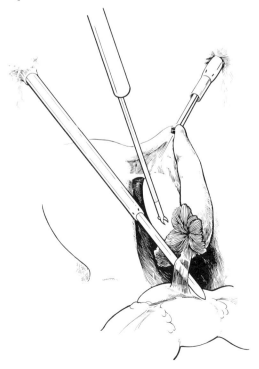

**Figure 2-8.** Extensive ovarian biopsy, excision of endometriosis, or fenestration of an ovarian cyst requires the three-puncture technique. A Palmer forceps may be used to stabilize the ovary and a probe passed through the second lower puncture used to elevate the ovary or to irrigate the area being cut. An ovarian biopsy punch, scissor, or biopsy tong may be used to remove a segment of the ovary.

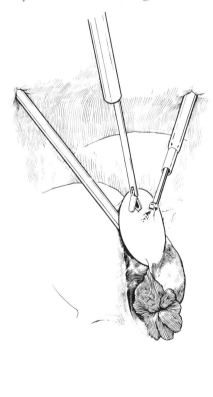

*Understanding the Laparoscope*

Most endoscopists perform diagnostic laparoscopy and culdoscopy without considering the type of optical lenses in a particular telescope. Moreover, if additional light is needed, the nurse is asked to turn the rheostat to the maximum level for "full illumination." In contrast to the operating microscope, magnification or the size of available field of the laparoscope cannot be altered,* or so it seems, because magnification and demagnification do take place during a laparoscopic procedure. Having worked diligently to focus the operating microscope one might also wonder why the laparoscope lens is always in focus. Similar to the microscope, laparoscopic photography and television require more than simply increasing the amount of light to maximum intensity. As with the operating microscope, the camera reflects the quality of the image and brightness available during a diagnostic procedure. If laparoscopy photographs are scrutinized for clarity, the characteristics of the lens and the amount of illumination are immediately apparent.

The modern laparoscope came into use during the 1950s and 1960s. Marked improvement in lens systems

---

*The exception to this is the Lent zoom laparoscope, Wolf Instrument Co.

occurred concurrently with the introduction of "cold" fiberoptical lighting. Although the fibers are not really cold, their ability to transfer light from a proximal light source to the telescope by means of fiberoptics cable was a major advance. Dr. Henry Hopkins, a British physicist, deserves credit for introducing the "rod lens system," which is discussed below [69].

ANGLE OF VIEW

The most commonly used diagnostic laparoscope in the United States has an angle of view of 180 degrees, which is straight ahead. Recently this terminology was standardized among endoscopy manufacturers; the view straight ahead is now referred to as 0 degrees. This direct view permits the novice to quickly become oriented when viewing the pelvis and is very close to the angle of view in operating laparoscopes (170 degrees) that are commonly used for tubal sterilization. It has, therefore, become a simple matter for the surgeon to use diagnostic and operating laparoscopes interchangeably (Fig. 2-9).

---

**Figure 2-9.** The direction of vision employed in a particular telescope is referred to as the angle of view. A right-angle view (90 degrees) is commonly used in the culdoscope. The laparoscope is available in fore-oblique angles of 130 to 165 degrees (50 to 15 degrees) and in the straight ahead, 180-degree (0-degree) view. (Courtesy of R. Wolf Co.)

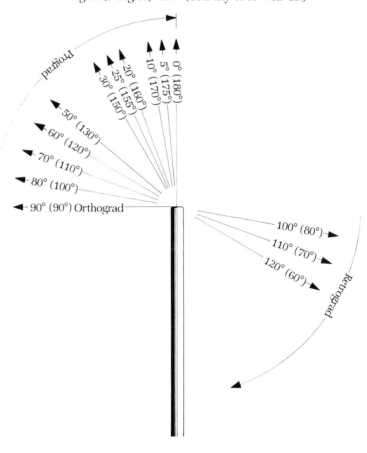

**Figure 2-10. A.** The angle of view may be straight ahead (180 degrees) or fore-oblique (135 degrees). (Courtesy of Eder Instrument Co.) **B.** The field of view includes the field seen in an angle of 55 degrees ±5 degrees. **C.** The complete field of view shown in this drawing is a three-dimensional area visualized by the telescope. (Parts **B** and **C** from L. A. Wetterman, From Endoscopy to Arthroscopy. In R. L. O'Connor (ed.), *Arthroscopy*. Philadelphia: Lippincott, 1977.)

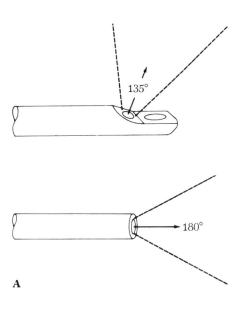

**A**

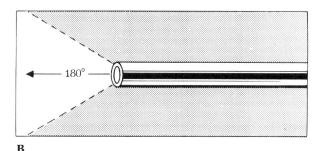

**B**

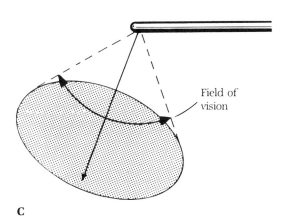

Field of vision

**C**

Frangenheim, Steptoe, and others have used a fore-oblique lens system during diagnostic laparoscopy [27, 80]. Many surgeons will recall the 90-degree or right-angle lens employed in the culdoscope. Orientation was at times difficult with this lens and certainly one missed the panoramic view of the 165-degree or 180-degree laparoscope. A fore-oblique lens system refers to two general lens angles, both greater than 90 degrees. The first, termed *forward-oblique*, is actually a 165-degree angle and the second, *lateral-oblique*, is 130 degrees. Significant differences exist in the technique of use and views between the three angles, and these are discussed further in the following sections (Fig. 2-10A).

FIELD OF VIEW

The field of view of a laparoscope refers to the area visualized through a particular lens system (Fig. 2-10B). It is determined in part by the angle of the lens system employed in a laparoscope. To relate this idea to the use of a camera lens system, recall that as the photographer attempts to expand the field above 70 degrees in the area of a wide angle lens, some degree of distortion occurs at the periphery of the field. Laparoscope manufacturers take great pride in describing the absence of distortion in their lens systems. Most laparoscopes, therefore, utilize a 50 to 60-degree field of view (Fig. 2-10B). The complete visual field of a laparoscope is a three dimensional area determined by the angle of view and the field of view (Fig. 2-10C).

Prescott [62] has expanded the concept of a complete visual field to include the field seen directly through a particular lens system in addition to the field achieved by rotating the laparoscope in a complete circle (Fig. 2-11). The advantage of the fore-oblique lens system is that rotation of the laparoscope greatly enlarges the areas of the pelvis that can be visualized. Although this concept is applicable to both the 160-degree and 130-degree lens, this author (G.W.P.) has not found useful a 130-degree lens. Steptoe apparently used this lateral-oblique lens very successfully for a number of years [80] in gynecologic laparoscopy, but the author has found it awkward. This is the lens system most often employed in gastrointestinal laparoscopy, a type of endoscopy in which a straight-ahead view is not helpful.

**Figure 2-11.** A comparison of fields of view through three different endoscopes. In each part the largest circle to the left indicates the field of view covered by rotating the endoscope. All have a 60-degree field of view. Rotation of a 180-degree endoscope about its own axis does not change the field of view **(A).** Rotation of a 160-degree endoscope **(B)** causes a scanning effect that increases by nearly three times the area viewed while keeping constantly in view a 20-degree area (small circle) centered on the axis. Such an endoscope is termed fore-oblique. Rotation of a 130-degree endoscope **(C)** scans an area nearly seven times the area of the 180-degree endoscope but never sees what is in a 40-degree area (hatched circle) directly ahead of it. It should be noted that in no case does the image rotate. (From R. Prescott, Optical principles of endoscopy. *J. Med. Primatol.* 5:136, 1976.)

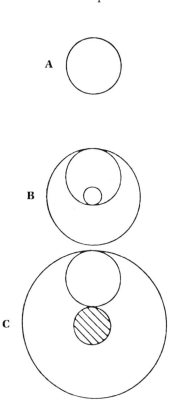

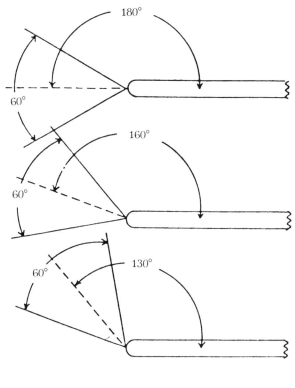

The lens system used in modern laparoscopes has three basic components: the objective lens, the relay lens, and the ocular (Fig. 2-12). Characteristics of the objective lens and ocular are discussed in chapter 5. A prism is used with the ocular lens to reorient the image, which had previously been inverted by the objective lens. A second prism would be used on a telescope with an oblique lens but is obviously not necessary with a 180-degree direct view.

As was noted in the discussion of optical principles of the operating microscope, there is variation in focal distance and magnification with change in either the objective lens or the ocular. It is not possible (with one exception*) to vary the lens system in a laparoscope. The surgeon must therefore select a lens that is comfortable.

---

*Lent's zoom laparoscope—Wolf Instrument Co.

---

**Figure 2-12.** Light is transmitted through a flexible fiberoptic light cable from a light projector to the tip of an endoscope where it provides illumination for visual examination and observation of body cavities. (From L. A. Wetterman, From Endoscopy to Arthroscopy. In R. L. O'Connor (ed.), *Arthroscopy.* Philadelphia: Lippincott, 1977.)

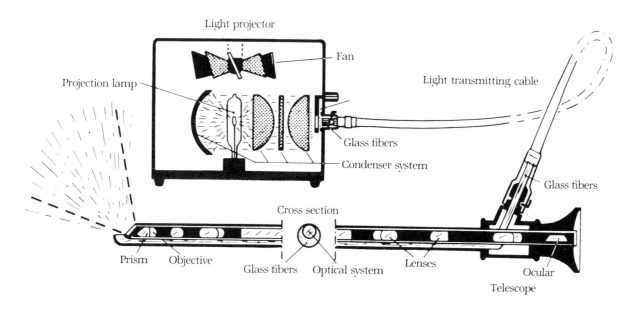

A dramatic advance in this area occurred during the 1950s when Dr. Henry Hopkins found that rod lens systems would transport the image from the objective to the ocular lens with markedly improved precision and clarity, as well as a marked increase in light transmission and expansion of field. The small bead lenses with large air spaces used in earlier telescopes were replaced by the long rod lenses with short air spaces. The rod lens systems are employed on all modern endoscopes, although only Storz utilizes the trade name Hopkins*. Wolf utilizes a rod lens system as well as computerized calculation of lens specifications. The differences between modern endoscopes will therefore relate primarily to the type of relay lens employed in the particular telescope.

*Storz had a license agreement with Dr. Hopkins to market the lens designed by him; however, this patent expired in 1970.

The surgeon might ask whether a laparoscope lens magnifies the area being seen. All are familiar with the difficulty encountered when estimating the size of an object in the pelvis during laparoscopy and the need to use a centimeter ruler to estimate the size accurately. Interestingly, as in so many other areas of gynecology, it was the Swedish professor, A. Sjovall, who discussed this difficulty in a short report in 1963 [75]. Dr. Sjovall demonstrated that "at laparoscopy there is the optical difficulty that magnification varies with the distance between the distal lens of the laparoscope and the objective being viewed in the abdominal cavity." This surgeon published a graph in which this principle was illustrated (Fig. 2-13).

**Figure 2-13.** Variation in magnification at distances from the end of the telescope. Notice with this particular laparoscope a magnification of 1× at 3.5 cm. Objects at shorter distances appeared larger and objects at longer distances appeared smaller than unity. (From A. Sjovall, Size measuring at laparoscopy. *Acta Obstet. Gynecol. Scand.* 42:279, 1963.)

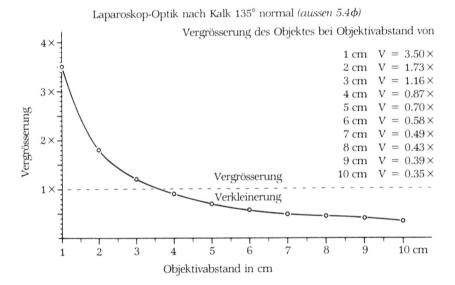

Laparoskop-Optik nach Kalk 135° normal *(aussen 5.4φ)*

Vergrösserung des Objektes bei Objektivabstand von

| | |
|---|---|
| 1 cm | V = 3.50× |
| 2 cm | V = 1.73× |
| 3 cm | V = 1.16× |
| 4 cm | V = 0.87× |
| 5 cm | V = 0.70× |
| 6 cm | V = 0.58× |
| 7 cm | V = 0.49× |
| 8 cm | V = 0.43× |
| 9 cm | V = 0.39× |
| 10 cm | V = 0.35× |

Vergrösserung
Verkleinerung

Vergrösserung

Objektivabstand in cm

This same type of calculation can be made with a Wolf 10 mm straight 180-degree laparoscope. Sjovall introduced the concept of using a centimeter ruler, termed *measuring needle*, to measure ovarian size, because it was so difficult to ascertain actual size during a diagnostic procedure [75].

*Focus.* After struggling to maintain the proper focus with an operating microscope, it is a relief to look through the lens system of a laparoscope and to find objects at both short and long distances in sharp focus. Perhaps it will help to understand this principle if one again relates this lens system to that used in a 35 mm camera.

The image seen through the laparoscope is formed at infinity. In fact, the objective lens system of the laparoscope can be thought of as having a very large depth of field, which is achieved in photography by decreasing the size of the aperture (F-stop) of the camera lens. As the size of the aperture decreases, the depth of field increases. Most 35-mm cameras have lenses with F-numbers, at least F/2.8. The F-number of a standard telescope is F/50 or greater; therefore the depth of field is almost infinite, and no focusing is necessary. The Wolf laparoscope lens in the standard telescope is adjusted to be in focus at a distance of 50 cm from the tip of the objective lens to the object. Because most cameras cannot be focused at this short distance, a dioptric lens has been incorporated into the laparoscope-camera adapter, permitting the camera lens to focus at a shorter distance than is designed for this lens. In the case of the 100 mm 2.8 Zuiko lens used on the Olympus camera, a minimum focal distance of 1 m is normal; however, with addition of the dioptric lens, a setting of 1.5 m is required for optimal focus. In practice, it is possible to focus the camera lens at either 1.5 m or infinity for excellent results.

*Lighting.* The surgeon understands that fiberoptical lighting is essential in modern laparoscopy but may not realize that each cable contains about 250,000 small glass fiber threads. Few surgeons understand how the light rays travel along these threads. The explanation is as exciting as it is simple and will aid the surgeon in evaluating the quality and maintenance of his fiber light-cables.

The components of a lighting system for laparoscopy, therefore, include the light source, which supplies illumination by means of a tungsten or halogen-tungsten bulb. The light is conveyed to the laparoscope by means of a fiberoptics cable and conveyed to the distal end of the laparoscope by additional fiberoptical strands or quartz rods that run along the outer circumference of the lens system. One seldom thinks of any portion of this system other than the cable, unless, of course, the bulb burns out.

Endoscopic lighting in the years prior to 1950 was achieved by means of a small incandescent bulb placed at the distal end of the telescope. Many recall the great care necessary in adjusting the rheostat of the light source to prevent blowing out the bulb. Both culdoscopy and peritoneoscopy used this type of lighting prior to the introduction of quartz rod and fiberoptical transmission systems.

In 1952, Fourestier, Gladu, and Vulmiere introduced a new approach that "revolutionized endoscopic techniques" (Steptoe, 1965). These investigators developed a technique of transmitting intense light along a quartz rod to the end of a telescope. This ability to reflect light rays through a glass rod without significant loss of light intensity and without the transmission of heat markedly improved visual clarity and removed a major source of danger that had been associated with electric and heat injuries. The improved lighting also permitted photography through the telescope for the first time. Still photography became commonplace and endoscopic color films were produced. In 1955, a closed circuit television program was first produced with this equipment [9]. During the 1950s and early 1960s, Frangenheim pioneered the advance of peritoneoscopy both by improving the lens system of a telescope that bore his name, as well as by stressing safety and experience as essential qualities for the operating technique [26].

The quartz rod apparatus was inconvenient, however, because it used a glass rod that ran along the outer edge of the laparoscope. The bulb used for illumination was placed in a light box adjacent to the eyepiece of the telescope, and ventilation tubing ran from the light box to a power unit three feet away. Obviously, this bulky arrangement was a far cry from modern laparoscopic equipment. An additional inconvenience of the quartz rod was its fragility; obviously, long cords containing this type of rod were impractical. We owe the convenience of the modern system of laparoscopy in part to the introduction of the fiber light cable a few years after the quartz rod. This transmission system permitted removal of the light box and fan to approximately 180 cm from the proximal end of the telescope.

Each fiber light cable used by the laparoscopist consists of bundles of hairlike glass fibers (about 250,000 in a 5 mm-diameter cord). Occasionally the outer rubber coating will tear or "explode," and many of the fibers will be seen sticking out and glowing like stars in the night. This cable transmits the light rays from the light source to the proximal end of the laparoscope as "cold light," because reflection at the light box removes most of the infrared rays that are responsible for heat. In fact, each of these hairlike threads is a small glass fiber equal to the length of the cord, which is usually 180 cm. The glass fibers are usually 0.050 to 0.076 mm in diameter and are composed of two types of optical glass. The inner core is responsible for conveying light rays (or visual images) along the length of the fiber. This glass thread is surrounded by a thin layer of glass with a lower refractive index that acts like a covering insulation and is called *cladding*. The glass core transmits the light, and the cladding prevents the reflected light ray from leaving the inner fiber. Light travels through this glass fiber by a series of reflections along straight paths. Once light enters the fiber, it is reflected along the path of the fiber without loss of illumination until it reaches the end. The outer layer of glass prevents loss of light at each angle of reflection. This principle also applies to transmission of visual images along these fibers, and it has recently been employed in the transmission of laser beams (Fig. 2-14).

A fiber light cable is composed of bundles, each of which contains about 5,000 individual glass fibers. The bundles are gathered together in groups and constitute the larger cable. Small spaces are present between these bundles, however, and are responsible for the loss of light at the junction between the light cord and the telescope. It was originally estimated that a good quality light guide would transmit about 40 percent of the light available [62]; however, reduction of this space by modern technology has reduced this loss substantially. Quint estimated that approximately two-thirds of the light was lost at the junction between the fiberoptics cord and the laparoscope [63]. However, more recent studies place this loss at about 50 percent. Quint felt that the major factors causing this loss were the following: (1) the impossibility of lining up the ends of the fiber filaments at the end of the fiber bundle with those of the endoscope; (2) loss of the physical contact between the fiber elements; and (3) a decollimation effect that oc-

**Figure 2-14.** The basic process of light transmission through optical glass fiber. The inner glass core must be coated with a thin film of glass of a lower refraction index to prevent light from leaking through its sides. (From L. A. Wetterman, From Endoscopy to Arthroscopy. In R. L. O'Connor (ed.), *Arthroscopy*. Philadelphia: Lippincott, 1977.)

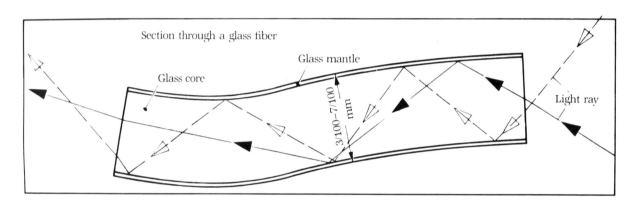

curs when the light emitting from the fiber bundle increases its angular spread by about 20 degrees from what it was at the input end of the fiber. He comments that "while these losses are not of overall importance in visualizing through the large bore instruments used in pelvic endoscopy, they are of paramount importance for photographic and television transmission" [63]. Recently, Prescott (1976) has stated that the fiberoptic cable will transmit about 65 percent of the light focused on the ends of it, with an additional loss of 3 percent per foot. This investigator stated that "there is a minimum light loss of about one-third at the endoscope light-guide junction." Prescott felt that the two prime determinants of the amount of light at the tip of an endoscope were: (1) the area of the fiberoptics bundle; and (2) the intrinsic brightness of the light source itself (Fig. 2-15). Certainly the quality of the light cord is very significant and the junction of the light cord and telescope crucial.

Some endoscopes have an integral light guide system in which the fiberoptic light cord is continuous with the fiber cables that run along the shaft of the laparoscope. In this system, there is no break at the junction of light cord and telescope. This may cause problems with maintenance, however, because the light guide is usually exposed to much abuse, and replacement of a separate light guide is a major effort in this system.

Laparoscopic equipment in use today employs a proximal illumination system that includes a light box containing one or two 150-watt projection lamp systems. It is necessary that a cooling fan be supplied to alleviate the rapid heating of the box that contains this lamp.

**Figure 2-15.** Fiberoptic light guide **(C)** is illuminated by the light of the tungsten halogen (or arc) lamp **(A)** concentrated on one of its ends by the reflector **(B)**. Transmitted light is coupled into the fiberoptic light guide of the endoscope **(D)** and emitted **(E)** to illuminate the field of view of the endoscope. (From R. Prescott, Optical principles of endoscopy, *J. Med. Primatol.* 5:136, 1976.)

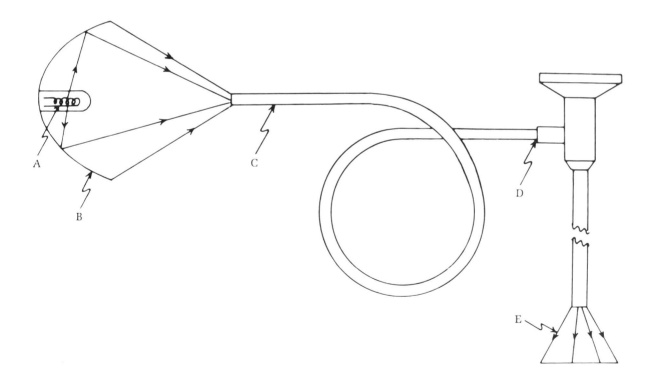

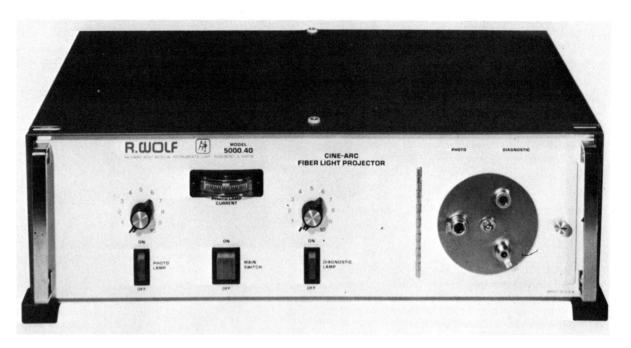

**Figure 2-16.** This solid-state Cine-Arc fiber light projector provides excellent illumination for cine, television, or 35-mm photography. A dimmer system permits the reduction of illumination to standby and eliminates the need to wait for reignition. (Courtesy of R. Wolf Co.)

Although earlier systems used a single lamp, most modern systems use two tungsten filament lamps; this is a great convenience when emergency conditions arise, such as failure of the lamp during a surgical procedure in which hemorrhage has occurred. The backup lamp is immediately available by simply pushing a switch (Fig. 2-16).

Other illumination sources, such as arc lamps, which produce a whiter, high intensity light, are considerably more expensive. Only when photographic requirements prevail are the expensive arc lamp and its supplies warranted. As we have noted above, it has been estimated by Quint that a loss of about 30 percent of light occurs during the process in which light is reflected onto the fiberoptic bundle. Quint has also estimated that a typical 150-watt lamp filament delivers approximately 10 percent of its original light capability to the distal end of the fiber bundle [63].

PHOTOGRAPHY

Excellent 35 mm photographs can be taken through the laparoscope. Almost any 35 mm single-lens reflex (SLR) camera can be adapted to this unit. This author (G.W.P.) has employed an Olympus OM-2 SLR camera with automatic film advance, termed *Winder I.* The ability to advance the film without breaking concentration or moving the laparoscope is essential. A clear-glass viewing screen is available and must be used to see clearly through the camera viewing area. A 55 mm, 100 mm, or 105 mm lens can be used; however, the author prefers the 100 mm 2.8 Zuiko lens used by Olympus. Regardless of the lens employed, the surgeon must purchase an adapter to hold the telescope firmly against the lens; and, in fact, in most cases the adapter contains a lens system that shortens the focal distance of the camera lens. Wolf, Eder, and Storz instrument companies manufacture separate lens adapters that may be used with their telescopes. Kodak 400 ASA or 200 ASA Ektachrome films have been found useful. Various light sources that are available will be discussed in a later section.

Without question, the distal laparoscope flash produces the best picture obtainable. It has been estimated that approximately 3,000 of these instruments are in use throughout Europe and a lesser number in the United States. It is significant to recall that the photographs of Cohen, Semm, and Frangenheim were taken with a distal flash system incorporated into a 130-degree lens system. The author has used the distal strobe 130-degree laparoscope and feels that this technique provides excellent photographs that are very useful in selected circumstances.

**Figure 2-17.** The proximal electronic flash generator has been found useful for 35 mm photography with an Olympus OM-2 camera equipped with Winder I (not shown) for automatic film advance. (Courtesy of R. Wolf Co.)

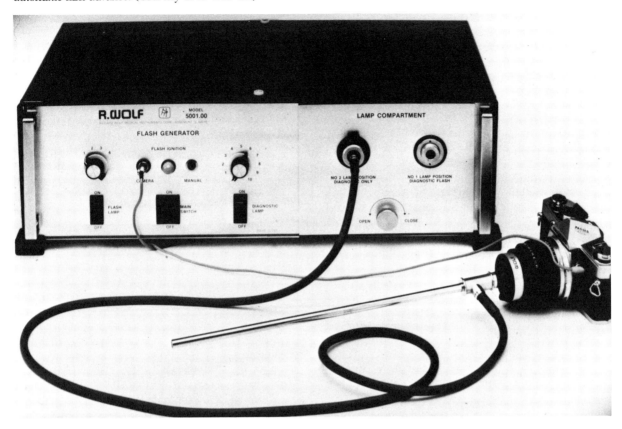

Of more practical value in routine use are the proximal flash units (Fig. 2-17; see also Fig. 2-16). The 10 mm diagnostic laparoscope with continuous fiber light cable may be used with the Wolf 3001 proximal flash generator or the 5005 arc light generator for excellent results (see Fig. 2-17). If a continuous cable is not employed, a significant amount of light is lost in this system owing to the fiber-light laparoscope junction. Broken fibers resulting from abuse of the light cord are also a significant problem. This author (G.W.P.) has found this a disappointing technique when a separate cable was used.

Eder Instrument Company has marketed a strobe flash attachment that can be placed on the hot shoe of the Olympus camera at the proximal end of the laparoscope. Cohen has obtained excellent photographs with this technique, and the author has also used this flash successfully. A proximal flash generator has also been marketed by Storz and, apparently, it has been used extensively by Semm.

Finally, one can use the 1,000-watt light source or a separate constant-light inserted through a second-puncture site, particularly when utilizing the new 35 mm cameras that automatically select the necessary light. Ektachrome daylight high speed film should be used with this technique to eliminate the bluish white color.

*Video and Photographic Recording.* The use of a video camera during diagnostic laparoscopy has become almost commonplace. A solid-state video camera* that can be decontaminated in Cidex is now available and can be shared by the laparoscopist and the arthroscopist. A new Sony video camera that provides 400 lines per inch appears to be the state of the art in this field. Video recording on a ¾ inch commercial tape or a ½ inch tape by a video recorder is now practical during diagnostic laparoscopy and laparoscopic egg retrieval associated with in vitro fertilization. At this writing almost all centers performing in vitro fertilization in the United States record egg retrieval on a video tape. The components of a video system include the following: a video camera that attaches to the laparoscope either directly or by means of a beam splitter, a video recorder, and a video monitor.

*Syn-Optics, Stryker Instrument Co., Kalamazoo, Mich.

The technique of laparoscopy may undergo a change as the use of video monitoring increases. The arthroscopist performs both diagnostic and operative procedures by viewing the inner aspects of the knee on a video monitor. This approach is certainly applicable to diagnostic and operative laparoscopy, and, in fact, egg retrieval can be easily performed by viewing the ovary and aspiration needle on the video screen rather than looking directly through the telescope. This author (G.W.P.) has utilized this approach during diagnostic laparoscopy as well as egg retrieval and feels that it is a technical advance.

Super 8 or 16 mm photography is possible through the diagnostic laparoscope; however, these two procedures require significant additional equipment. Photography is not as useful to the surgeon and assistant as is the use of video since it is not possible to monitor the field being photographed. The quality of the image presented on 16 mm film is, however, superior to a video image at this time. It is recommended that the 16 mm photographic technique be used when a documentary film is being prepared. The reader may consult additional references for further information [9, 46, 77, 93].

*Results of Laparoscopy in the Infertile Patient*
The significance of endoscopic evaluation of the infertile female is uncontested. The realization that 30 to 35 percent of infertility is related to tubal dysfunction [3] places great emphasis on evaluation of this factor. Initial evaluation with carbon dioxide insufflation (Rubin's test) gave way to salpingography with radiopaque material (oil base or water base). Although this x-ray technique represented a significant improvement over tubal insufflation in evaluating tubal patency and uterine contour, the error remained significant, and the information it provided regarding tubal adhesions and endometriosis was minimal. Infertility specialists, including Frangenheim and Kistner [3, 27], therefore, became strong advocates of early endoscopy as a part of infertility evaluation. Although one of these surgeons performed peritoneoscopy and the other culdoscopy, both felt endoscopy provided the greatest information regarding tubal function. Repeated comparisons of laparoscopy and hysterosalpingography appeared to substantiate this belief.

Most large series of laparoscopic procedures in the United States reported during the 1970s have included significant numbers of patients who have undergone tubal sterilization. In a comparison that involved two community hospitals, Edgerton reported 4,157 cases at St. Luke's Hospital, Davenport, Iowa, 12 percent of which were performed for diagnostic purposes [21]. Kleppinger reported 3,113 laparoscopic procedures at Reading Community Hospital in Reading, Pennsylvania; again remarkably enough, 12 percent were performed for diagnostic purposes [21]. At both centers, approxi-

**Table 2-2.** Laparoscopic findings in infertile patients*

| Author | Year of study | Number of patients | Laparoscopy Normal (%) | Abnormal (%) |
|---|---|---|---|---|
| Steptoe | 1965 | 74 | 26 | 74 |
| Fear | 1968 | 27 | 22 | 78 |
| Cohen | 1968 | 78 | 37 | 63 |
| Neuwirth | 1969 | 56 | 39 | 61 |
| Peterson | 1970 | 204 | 40 | 60 |
| Swolin | 1972 | 143 | 33 | 67 |
| Maathius | 1972 | 207 | 43 | 57 |
| Gabos | 1976 | 117 | 61 | 39 |
| Gomel | 1977 | 300 | 39 | 61 |
| Hutchins | 1977 | 409 | 70.4 | 29.6 |
| Duignan | 1972 | 675 | 59 | 41 |
| Liston | 1972 | 197 | 46 | 54 |
| Peterson | 1970 | 204 | 42 | 58 |
| Goldenberg | 1976 | 108 | 31 | 69 |
| Patton | 1983 | 637 | 74 | 26 |

*Other studies reviewed but not listed.

mately one in eight laparoscopic procedures performed was for diagnostic purposes, a figure that is probably typical of the overall experience in the United States. Corson, in 1972 [13], found that in 1,545 laparoscopic procedures at the University of Pennsylvania Medical Center, 40 percent (618) were diagnostic but only 247 were for infertility evaluation. Overall, at the University of Pennsylvania Medical Center, 16 percent of the laparoscopic procedures performed were for infertility evaluation.

In contrast to these large series of sterilization procedures, only Duignan [20] (1972) has reported a comparable series of diagnostic procedures. In 1,000 consecutive diagnostic laparoscopic procedures, 68 percent were performed for infertility evaluation. Most series in which diagnostic laparoscopy has been performed in infertility patients are much smaller, as is noted in Table 2-2. Review of numerous series of diagnostic laparoscopic procedures reveals that the incidence of infertility evaluation varies considerably [10, 13, 25, 78]. Fear and Cohen performed, respectively, 20 and 27 percent of their procedures for infertility evaluation, in contrast to Steptoe who, in an early report [78] stated that 59 percent underwent infertility evaluation. In this large series, Duignan noted that 68 percent of his patients were evaluated for sterility. Clearly, the proportion of patients undergoing infertility evaluation depends to a large extent on the interest and reputation of the individual surgeon.

The percentage of infertility patients who undergo diagnostic laparoscopy is not as well substantiated. It can be estimated, however, that at least one-half of the

**Table 2-3.** Laparoscopic findings in patients with normal hysterosalpingograms

| Author | Year of study | Number of patients | Normal hysterosalpingogram, total series (%) | Abnormal laparoscopy, normal hysterosalpingogram (%) | False-negative (%)[a] |
|---|---|---|---|---|---|
| Swolin | 1972 | 143 | 32 | 30 | 10[b] |
| Maathius | 1972 | 207 | 44 | 41 | 18 |
| Gomel | 1977 | 300 | 46 | 30 | 14 |
| Gabos | 1976 | 117 | 54 | 24 | 21 |
| Hutchins | 1977 | 409 | 73 | 13 | 10 |
| Goldenberg | 1976 | 108 | 59 | 58 | 34 |
| Duignan | 1972 | 273 | 69 | 23 | 16 |

[a]Calculated by dividing the number of patients with abnormal laparoscopic findings in the group that had a normal hysterosalpingogram by the number of patients in this entire series.
[b]There were 24 additional cases in which the abnormality found at hysterosalpingogram did not agree with the abnormality found at laparoscopy.

**Table 2-4.** Laparoscopic findings in patients with abnormal hysterosalpingograms

| Author | Year of study | Number of patients | Abnormal hysterosalpingogram, total series (%) | Normal laparoscopy, abnormal hysterosalpingogram (%) | False-positives (%)* |
|---|---|---|---|---|---|
| Swolin | 1972 | 143 | 67 | 15 | 11 |
| Maathius | 1972 | 207 | 56 | 30 | 17 |
| Gomel | 1977 | 300 | 54 | 12 | 7 |
| Gabos | 1976 | 117 | 46 | 43 | 20 |
| Hutchins | 1977 | 409 | 27 | 27 | 7 |
| Goldenberg | 1976 | 108 | 41 | 16 | 7 |
| Duignan | 1972 | 273 | 31 | 33 | 10 |

*Calculated by dividing the number of patients with normal laparoscopic findings in the group with an abnormal hysterosalpingogram by the number of patients in the total series.

infertility couples who complete an infertility evaluation have had laparoscopy. Certainly this number would be higher if one considered all those patients who remained infertile at the completion of evaluation, because in that instance, almost all patients would have had laparoscopy. As was noted, even those patients whose husbands are azoospermic may undergo laparoscopy if artificial insemination is unsuccessful in three or more cycles.

*Laparoscopy and Hysterosalpingography*
The findings in 15 series of infertile patients who had undergone diagnostic laparoscopy are presented in Table 2-2. The early studies of Steptoe [78], Cohen [8], Fear [25] and Peterson [61] have been commented on earlier in this chapter. One should recall, however, that the 204 patients reported by Peterson [61] all had normal hysterosalpingograms and were classified as having "unexplained infertility" prior to laparoscopy. The fact that 58 percent of these patients demonstrated pelvic pathology at laparoscopy was therefore quite significant. In addition, the observation that 60 percent of the abnormal findings involved endometriosis compared to 40 per-

cent of patients who demonstrated postinflammatory changes also relates to the selection process, which involved normal preoperative salpingography. Rarely does endometriosis represent this large a proportion of pathologic findings in unselected infertility patients.

In contrast to Peterson's review of patients with normal preoperative hysterosalpingography are the series of Swolin [84], Maathius [51], Gomel [34], Hutchins [38], Gabos [28], Duignan [20], and Goldenberg [31]. In these reports, the authors have compared groups of patients who have undergone both hysterosalpingography and laparoscopy. Interestingly, a comparison of these seven series is facilitated by the similarity in patient classification. Tables 2-3 and 2-4 review this data.

Normal hysterosalpingography was found in 32 to 73 percent of these patients (Table 2-3). The report by Hutchins [38] appears unique in finding an unusually high rate of normal hysterosalpingography, because he also found that 70 percent of his entire group of patients were normal at the time of laparoscopy. All other authors found fewer normal patients in this group. The mean number of patients with normal hysterosalpingograms in all seven series was 54 percent. Table 2-3 summarizes these reports and lists the percentage of patients with normal hysterosalpingography who were then found to have pathologic findings at laparoscopy. Again, Hutchins' figure was only 13 percent; however, pathologic findings occurred in 23 to 56 percent of the remaining six reports. The rate of false-negative findings at hysterosalpingography has been calculated for the entire group of patients and found to vary between 10 and 34 percent. A calculation of 23 to 58 percent would appear more accurate, however, because it would reflect the actual number of patients in whom the diagnosis would have been overlooked if one failed to perform laparoscopy on patients who had a normal hysterosalpingogram.

On the other hand, if one reviews all patients who had an abnormal hysterosalpingogram (see Table 2-4), it is apparent that many of these patients had normal tubal function. In the seven series, 27 to 67 percent of the patients studied had abnormal hysterosalpingography. The mean number of patients with abnormal hysterosalpingogram in these groups was 46 percent. Of interest is that more than one-half of all patients (60 to 70 percent) of the entire series (see Table 2-2) had abnormal findings at laparoscopy. Diagnostic laparoscopy in the patients with abnormal findings at the time of hysterosalpingography revealed normal tuboovarian anatomy in 15 to 43 percent of cases. The rate of false-positive findings was 7 to 20 percent, a much lower figure. Again, one must realize that the number of greater significance is the earlier one of 15 to 43 percent, which reflects the number of patients with abnormal hysterosalpingography who actually were found to have a normal pelvis.

The inability of hysterosalpingography to adequately diagnose tuboovarian adhesions is apparent from the studies noted in Tables 2-3 and 2-4. Gomel [34] has noted the difficulty in attempting to diagnose tubal adhesions by hysterosalpingography and has reported an erroneous diagnosis in 38/300 of patients with total tubal occlusion. Although one would consider this failure acceptable even under optimal circumstances, the diagnosis of adhesions is frequently missed by hysterosalpingography even when tubal occlusion is not present. El-Minawi [24] found that, of 151 cases found by laparoscopy to have adhesions, only 76 of these were suspected as a result of x-ray studies, for a failure rate of 50 percent. Equal difficulty is encountered in the diagnosis of endometriosis by hysterosalpingography. Little data is available on this subject; however, as was noted earlier, Peterson found endometriosis in 33 percent of patients with normal hysterosalpingography, and Moghissi also found a high incidence of endometriosis in his patients [55]. This author (G.W.P.) could find no report in which endometriosis had been accurately diagnosed by x-ray studies.

Of greater significance, however, is the observation that even patients with suspected bilateral tubal occlusion on x-ray studies may, in fact, be normal. This applies not only to cornual occlusion, which is widely recognized as secondary to "spasm" in many cases, but also to fimbrial occlusion. In an early study, Coltart (1970) [11] reviewed 36 patients who gave evidence of tubal occlusion following hysterosalpingography. Remarkably, 31 percent of these patients had bilateral patency at laparoscopy. Only 1/18 patients with cornual occlusion had bilateral patency; however, 7/14 patients thought to have fimbrial occlusion had patency at the time of laparoscopy. El-Minawi [24] found that 10/25 (40 percent) of patients with cornual occlusion had bilateral patency. The difficulty in attempting to diagnose cornual occlusion is discussed at length in Chapter 7. The probable role of tubal spasm, which is apparently eliminated by general anesthesia, or the lower viscosity of dilute indigo carmine compared to water-soluble sinographin or certainly the oil mixture of Lipiodal is a consideration.

More disturbing, however, is the observation by Coltart [11] that 7/14 (50 percent) with fimbrial occlusion had bilateral patency. In the study by El-Minawi [24], 30 patients with fimbrial occlusion at hysterosalpingography underwent laparoscopy. Twenty-four of these patients were classified as having fimbrial occlusion at laparoscopy; however, El-Minawi has noted that "12/24 of these patients had dense adhesions simulating tubal occlusion." Certainly this is consistent with Gomel's observation that 12/72 patients thought to have tubal occlusion at hysterosalpingography actually were normal at laparoscopy and did not require surgery. While this figure of 17 percent is significant, the incidence of cornual or fimbrial occlusion in this group was not given. Recall, however, that Coltart found patency in 11/33 patients with total occlusion at x-ray, and this was 50 percent in patients with fimbrial occlusion. Again, the incidence of adhesion formation in these patients was not given. Interesting aspects of the correlation between hysterosalpingography and laparoscopy have been reported by Keirse [41]. In 25 patients with patent tubes by hysterosalpingography 6 (24 percent) actually were found to have one tube occluded at laparoscopy. In contrast to the apparently normal patients were 25 patients with evidence of single or bilateral tubal occlusion at hysterosalpingography, 4 (16 percent) of whom had bilateral tubal patency at the time of laparoscopy. All 9 patients with bilateral occlusion at hysterosalpingography were found to have at least one tube occluded at laparoscopy. The correlation between hysterosalpingography and laparoscopy was very high in patients with cornual and isthmic occlusion in this study in which a water-soluble dye and an extremely gentle injection technique were used.

**Table 2-5.** Classification by anatomy

| Author | Year of study | Patients | % Abnormal | Pathology | | Adhesions and tubal occlusion (%) |
| | | | | Adhesions (%) | Tubal occlusion (%) | |
|---|---|---|---|---|---|---|
| Swolin | 1972 | 143 | 67 | 72 | 24 | 4 |
| Maathius | 1972 | 207 | 57 | 33 | 25 | 42 |
| Gomel | 1977 | 300 | 61 | 36 | 34 | 30 |
| Gabos | 1976 | 117[a] | 39 | 18 | 44 | 26 |
| Hutchins | 1977 | 409[b] | 30 | 31 | 55 | 13 |

[a] 6 cases of failed endoscopy included in total but not classified.
[b] Endometriosis in 21 cases.

**Table 2-6.** Classification by etiology

| Author | Year of study | Number of patients | % Normal | Prior infection (%) | Endometriosis (%) | Other (%) |
|---|---|---|---|---|---|---|
| Steptoe | 1965 | 74 | 26 | 74 | 0 | 0 |
| Fear | 1968 | 27 | 22 | 41 | 7 | 0 |
| Cohen | 1968 | 78 | 37 | 33 | 19 | 11 |
| Neuwirth | 1969 | 56 | 39 | 48 | 13 | 0 |
| Peterson | 1970 | 204 | 40 | 25 | 33 | 2 |
| Goldenberg | 1976 | 108 | 31 | 42 | 27 | 0 |
| Liston | 1972 | 197 | 46 | 36 | 6 | 12 |
| Patton | 1983 | 637 | 26 | 44 | 23 | 7 |

In summary, the authors wish to emphasize that hysterosalpingography and laparoscopy are complementary procedures, both of them useful in evaluation of tubal function. Hysterosalpingography is used as a diagnostic procedure during the early stage of a sterility evaluation by most investigators, including the authors. Although slightly more than one-half of these procedures will show normal results, all patients should undergo laparoscopy, whether they had normal or abnormal x-ray findings. If hysterosalpingography reveals abnormal findings, one is likely to find that 12 to 33 percent of these patients will, in fact, be normal. In the group of patients whose x-ray was normal, 25 to 85 percent will, in fact, have pathology not detected by the x-ray technique. It would appear, therefore, that a paradoxical situation exists in which laparoscopy is indicated irrespective of the x-ray findings. The authors feel this is not a paradox, but rather a change in the role of hysterosalpingography in evaluation of the infertile female. In brief, we feel that a hysterosalpingogram provides evidence of cornual patency, cornual occlusion, the presence of salpingitis isthmica nodosa in a patent cornual segment, or the presence of rugal markings in patients with fimbrial occlusion, as well as an accurate outline of the uterine contour. These are a few of the advantages of performing the hysterosalpingogram prior to the laparoscopic procedure, all of which help the surgeon evaluate the intrinsic tubal architecture when viewing the extrinsic surfaces endoscopically.

*Pathologic Findings at Laparoscopy*

In reviewing the reports listed in Table 2-2, it became apparent that the general types of pathology noted at laparoscopy during the 1970s were similar to those reported by Steptoe, Cohen, and Fear earlier in this chapter. In fact, these findings were also similar to early reports obtained at culdoscopy by Kistner [44]. These general categories are listed as follows:

1. Normal
2. Evidence of prior infection
   a. Pelvic adhesions
   b. Tubal occlusion—fimbrial or cornual
   c. Adhesions and tubal occlusion
3. Endometriosis
4. Other (fibroids, sterilization, ovarian and uterine pathology)

The presence of endometriosis has caused confusion in attempting to compare the abnormal reports listed in Table 2-2, because adhesion formation and, occasionally, tubal occlusion may occur as a result of endometriosis as well as prior pelvic infection. A classification of findings by etiology (pelvic infection and endometriosis), therefore, often conflicts with the anatomic classification that lists only adhesions and tubal occlusion. This comparison has been demonstrated by dividing patients from Table 2-2 into the two groups listed in Tables 2-5 and 2-6. The reports by Swolin, Maathius,

Gomel, and Gabos have excluded a discussion of endometriosis.

Patients in these studies have been classified in terms of pelvic adhesions and tubal occlusion only (Table 2-5). The three studies of Swolin [84], Maathius [51], and Gomel [34] appeared very similar in structure and patient selection. Abnormalities were found in 57 to 67 percent of these patients. The mean for all five groups was 51 percent. Patients with adhesions only varied from 18 to 71 percent; however, three studies revealed 31, 33, and 36 percent of patients with only adhesions, and the mean number for the entire group was 38 percent. From this, one would conclude that approximately one-third of patients found to be abnormal will have pelvic adhesions only. Tubal occlusion occurred in 24 to 55 percent of cases. Interestingly, Swolin reported the lowest figure, 24 percent, and the highest figure of patients with adhesions only, 72 percent. Possible explanations for this include placing patients with partial fimbrial occlusion in the group with adhesions. The combination of adhesions and tubal occlusion found so often by the author was reported in only 4 to 42 percent of these patients. The author has found filmy adhesions involving either the fallopian tube or the ovary in almost all patients with fimbrial occlusion and in a number with cornual occlusion (see Chap. 7).

In contrast, the eight authors listed in Table 2-6 have carefully divided patients on the basis of the etiologic factors of endometriosis, evidence of prior pelvic infection, and other causes, such as fibroids, uterine anomalies, or ovarian disease. One finds marked consistency in the percentage of normal patients, 22 to 46 percent. Two studies found 40 and 46 percent of patients to be normal; the remaining six studies reported fewer than 40 percent, for a mean in the entire group of 34 percent. The routine diagnostic laparoscopy performed during infertility evaluation may, therefore, be expected to reveal pelvic pathology in two-thirds of those patients. As we noted earlier, the study of Peterson [61] is unique in that all patients had normal preoperative hysterosalpingograms. Even in these patients with "unexplained infertility," 60 percent were found to be abnormal.

These types of pathology are listed in Table 2-6. Evidence of prior pelvic infection occurs more often than does endometriosis. This category includes all types of prior infection, which, of course, combines intrinsic tubal infection, that is prior salpingitis, and extrinsic disease, prior surgery. The report by Patton [60] involving 637 consecutive infertility patients noted abnormalities in 73 percent. One-third of the abnormalities involved endometriosis, whereas 58 percent of abnormal patients had some evidence of prior pelvic infection. Endometriosis was not found in the early study reported by Steptoe [78]. In contrast, Kistner [44] found that endometriosis and prior pelvic infection occurred in almost equal numbers. His report of 1,500 patients who had undergone culdoscopy showed that only 12 percent were normal. Endometriosis occurred in 36 percent of the entire group and 41 percent of the abnormal patients, in contrast to pelvic infection, which occurred in 37 percent of the entire group and 42 percent of the abnormal group.

Diagnostic laparoscopy permits the surgeon to survey the female pelvis and detect abnormalities in tubal anatomy, pelvic adhesions, endometriosis, or other unusual findings, including uterine anomalies. While inspecting the tuboovarian relationship and the results of tubal lavage, the surgeon must also evaluate the role of medical and surgical therapy for the pathology observed. The question of prognosis is crucial in the field of infertility surgery and is a forecast only the infertility surgeon can make. For this reason, the infertility surgeon should perform diagnostic laparoscopy in prospective surgical patients whenever possible. The ability to ascertain a second tubal block at the time of laparoscopy, that is, cornual or fimbrial, is highly significant. This condition precludes surgery in almost all cases. Likewise, the presence of extensive pelvic adhesions with a large hydrosalpinx results in a low pregnancy rate following surgery and is best unoperated. The evidence of Israel [39] in evaluating 115 patients was significant. In spite of eliminating 46 percent of these patients at the time of laparoscopy, the term-pregnancy rate in the remaining 54 percent who underwent infertility laparotomy was only 11 percent. In fact, there were only 15 uterine pregnancies and 7 tubal pregnancies in these 83 patients. Israel's comment that "the vast majority of surgical procedures were performed in the presence of significant tubal damage and associated pelvic adhesions" is further indication for careful and thoughtful preoperative laparoscopy. The fact that Israel also found "the presence of additional infertility factors" to be a significant element in the lower pregnancy rate again supports the concept of separating laparoscopy and definitive conservative infertility surgery.

## Laparoscopy and Endometriosis

Infertile patients found to have endometriosis at laparoscopy are shown in Table 2-6, and the role of endometriosis and its surgical treatment are discussed in Chapter 8. Fulguration of endometrial implants at the time of laparoscopy has not been extensively practiced in the United States until recently. Although Fear [25] and Cohen [8] reported in 1968 that they performed this operative procedure on their infertile patients, little enthusiasm for this approach to endometriosis developed during the 1970s. This was in spite of a strong support for surgical laparoscopy by Frangenheim [27] and Semm [69] in Germany. A recent report by Edwards [23], however, appears to demonstrate significantly improved pregnancy results following fulguration of implants in the early stages of endometriosis. Twenty-five patients with stage 1 and 2 endometriosis were treated by fulguration of implants at laparoscopy. A corrected pregnancy rate of 80 percent was achieved in stage 1 patients, and 71 percent of those with stage 2 disease conceived. Cohen [10] has also advocated fulguration of endometriotic implants at laparoscopy, but stated that "medical treatment is indicated following surgical laparoscopy for endometriosis." This combination of therapy creates great difficulty in evaluating the benefit of the surgical approach. Kistner [43], however, has been a strong proponent of treatment of endometriosis by either medical or conservative surgical therapy. The presence of adhesions or a moderate to large endometrioma has been considered indication for conservative laparotomy. Kistner has already reported pregnancy in 76 percent of 232 patients operated on who did not have adhesions, compared to 38 percent of 106 patients with adhesions (43).

At present, the role of a laparoscopic approach to the treatment of mild or moderate endometriosis has not been established. The simplicity of fulgurating small implants of endometriosis makes this approach appealing. The increased facility of the laparoscopic surgeons as well as improvement in the equipment certainly will lead to further evaluation of this approach during the 1980s.

## Unexplained Infertility

The diagnosis of "unexplained infertility" is one of exclusion. Previously thought to include 10 to 20 percent of all infertility couples, the incidence has gradually decreased [3]. As one might expect, the careful use of laparoscopy and extensive sperm antibody evaluation have resulted in reduced numbers of patients in this category. The report by Peterson [61] discussed earlier revealed that 60 percent of patients thought to be normal prior to laparoscopy actually had pelvic pathology; this discovery was a major advance in the field of infertility. Endometriosis was the most common finding, occurring in 33

percent of all patients and 58 percent of abnormal patients reported by Peterson. Pelvic infection was responsible for 39 percent of the abnormal cases. El-Minawi [24] also found pathology in about 60 percent of patients with unexplained infertility studied in Cairo; however, only 5 percent of this group had endometriosis, compared to 33 percent of Peterson's patients. Prior pelvic infection was responsible for most of the pathology in the group of Egyptian patients. Before in 1977, Drake [19a] studied 24 out of 229 couples thought to have unexplained infertility by laparoscopy. Diagnostic laparoscopy demonstrated abnormal pathology in 18 (75 percent) of these females. Unsuspected endometriosis was found in 11/26 (46 percent) and peritubal adhesions in 29 percent. In this total group of 229 couples, only 8 (3.5 percent) failed to demonstrate an abnormality associated with infertility. Treatment of the abnormalities found in these patients at laparoscopy resulted in a 60 percent term pregnancy rate [19].

## Results of Operative Laparoscopy

Indications for most operative procedures performed at the time of laparoscopy have not been clearly established. A list of operative procedures has been recently published by Semm [71, 72]:

1. Ovariolysis, salpingolysis, fimbrioplasty
2. Tubal sterilization
3. Intraabdominal adhesiolysis
4. Coagulation of endometrial foci
5. Biopsy of ovary
6. Resection of ovarian cysts
7. Conservative extrauterine pregnancy surgery

During the years 1971–1976, Semm apparently performed 3,300 operative laparoscopic procedures only 1,339 of which were associated with tubal ligation. In this group, 668 underwent a procedure associated with infertility. Semm [73], a strong proponent of low-frequency cautery termed *endocoagulation*, has argued against the use of high-frequency current during laparoscopic surgery. In the system used by Semm, coagulation occurs by direct contact between a hot instrument and the involved tissue by a technique that is essentially similar to hot-wire cautery.

Regardless of the form of coagulation employed, it is possible to cut fine adhesions that involve the fallopian tube or ovary at the time of laparoscopy with minimal apparent bleeding. Palmer [57] (1971) appears to have been one of the early proponents of laparoscopic surgery in the infertile female. This surgeon demonstrated the value of laparoscopic dilatation of phimosis of the distal fallopian tube and salpingolysis, reporting a pregnancy rate of 33 percent in patients treated. In 1975, Gomel [33] reported the value of salpingolysis and dilatation of distal fallopian tubes; of 29 patients who subsequently attempted to conceive, 14 gave birth to a living child, a pregnancy rate of 42 percent. Recently Semm [71] reported that between the years 1971–1976, 668 patients underwent operative laparoscopy by his endocoagulation technique. Infertile patients underwent ovariolysis, salpingolysis, fimbriolysis, and salpingostomy. Remarkably, 223 patients in this group had tubal occlusion preoperatively, and 77 percent had patent tubes after surgery. Postoperatively, 33.5 percent of these patients conceived.

Swolin [83] has attempted to prevent postoperative adhesion formation by performing laparoscopy 6 to 8 weeks following infertility surgery. This surgeon has found adhesions to be soft after this interval, and by using a blunt probe he was able to gently separate them. Although this approach is fascinating, Swolin did not offer statistical evidence of its value, and it does not appear to be used by other surgeons at this time. This author (G.W.P) has not employed this approach, although he feels it may have beneficial aspects.

Ovarian biopsy has been performed by Yuzpe and many others [92] and recently has been evaluated in detail [23, 81]. The value of ovarian biopsy in evaluation of gonadal function has been controversial. Extensive biopsies appear to simulate wedge resection and have been found valuable in anovulatory patients by Swolin [83], Cohen [8] and others [13]. The presence of ova in a patient with primary amenorrhea or presumed premature menopause is highly significant.

Certainly, one of the most controversial surgical approaches has been that of salpingostomy performed by operative laparoscopy, reported by Gomel [35]. Pregnancy occurred in 4 of 8 patients operated on as a "last effort" by Gomel. This author (G.W.P.) has attempted this procedure in three patients and found it totally unsatisfactory in two. In the third patient, an excellent cuff was achieved, although postoperative pregnancy has not yet occurred. Bleeding is a significant problem and coagulation worrisome in these patients. It is extremely difficult for a surgeon accustomed to approaching the closed fimbria under the operating microscope to change to a gross technique of cutting and coagulating widely, which is often necessary in operative laparoscopy. The operative laparoscopic technique appears to be useful only in those patients whose distal tubal disease is severe and fimbria almost totally absent. Unfortunately, pregnancy following surgery in such patients is unusual. Recent studies by Daniell [14, 15] show that the use of the carbon dioxide laser during laparoscopic salpingostomy procedures seems promising.

Lastly, aspiration of ova as described by Steptoe [81] and Edwards [23] has become a more commonplace procedure. The recent successful pregnancies in Norfolk, Virginia and at other American centers have established this approach. Low tubal ovum transfer [47] would also employ this technique and may present an alternative to in vitro fertilization.

In summary, the operative laparoscopic approach to abnormalities of the infertile female is in its infancy. Improved instrumentation and surgical technique will undoubtedly lead to increased use of this approach and, it is hoped, to improved pregnancy results. At present, neither Gomel nor Swolin has been able to achieve pregnancy results approaching those obtained by macrosurgical salpingolysis [5] or microsurgery. It may be possible, however, to perform lysis of adhesions or dilatation of the distal tube by operative laparoscopy, with an interval of 6 to 12 months before microsurgical laparotomy is carried out. At present there is no data to suggest that operative laparoscopy aggravates adhesions or tubal occlusion. Certainly this is a consideration if extensive coagulation is necessary, or if significant bleeding occurs at the time of the procedure. Recently the carbon dioxide laser has been used during operative laparoscopy with encouraging results. A review of this technique is presented at the end of this chapter.

## Hysteroscopy

The development and wide acceptance of laparoscopic visualization of the pelvis during infertility evaluation in the decade of the 1970s did not find a parallel in the realm of hysteroscopy, although endoscopic visualization of the interior of the uterine cavity has been found both fascinating and informative. Major problems with uterine distention as well as with instrumentation have recently been overcome, however, and there is likely to be increased use of this procedure in the 1980s for both diagnosis and therapy of intrauterine defects associated with adhesions, myomas, polyps, and congenital uterine defects. Physiologic studies of endometrial development and sperm migration are also possible, particularly with the introduction of the new microhysteroscope. In the field of temporary sterilization the successful insertion of plastic tubal plugs would produce a dramatic change in the gynecologist's approach to hysteroscopy.

The history of hysteroscopy dates to the turn of the twentieth century. Sugimoto [82] credits Pantaleoni [58] with the first inspection of the interior of the uterine cavity in a live subject in 1869. Bumm [7] (1895) also visualized the interior of the uterus using a male urethroscope and attempted to cauterize endometrial lesions, such as endometriosis and endometrial polyps but was often unsuccessful because of bleeding that obscured his view. Modification of the cystoscope by David [16] (1907) included an outer sheath, obdurator, and lens system with a distal light source, producing an instrument very similar to modern hysteroscopes, except for fiberoptic lighting. In fact, Sugimoto [82] has called David "the father of modern hysteroscopy." In the 1960s, proximal illumination by means of fiberoptical systems eliminated the need for distal bulbs and provided a safer and more intense lighting system. These systems are described in detail earlier in this chapter.

### Distention of Uterine Cavity

Two characteristics of the endometrial cavity noted by Rubin [65] prevented successful use of the hysteroscope during the first half of the twentieth century. Rubin noted that the failure of hysteroscopy was due to (1) the slitlike uterine cavity with uterine walls in opposition and (2) the readiness with which the endometrium bleeds on contact with any instrument. To overcome these two obstacles, a system of uterine distention as well as a method of irrigation were necessary. Both distention and irrigation were intrinsic to the technique of cystoscopy; these problems were not solved easily by hysteroscopists. Gauss [30] (1928) devised a method of injecting liquid under pressure to rinse the uterus. Schroeder [68] (1934) stated that adequate dilatation of the uterine cavity required a pressure of 650 mmHg of water, whereas a pressure higher than 950 mmHg of water caused leakage through the tubes into the uterine cavity.

Water and $CO_2$ distention were not notably successful and led to the design of the balloon-type hysteroscope. Silander [74] performed hysteroscopy through a transparent rubber balloon placed in the uterus and filled with water. However, the pressure of the balloon compressed the endometrium and distorted the view through the hysteroscope.

In 1970, Edström and Fernström [22] distended the uterine cavity by injecting a dextran solution through the hysteroscope; in 1972, Neuwirth and Levine [48] reported a series of 20 patients in whom 32 percent dextran 70 (Hyskon) had been used successfully. Hyskon has little effect on light transmission and has the great advantage of not mixing with blood or mucus. In fact, blood is concentrated into tiny droplets that flow laterally out of the line of vision. In addition, Hyskon distends the uterine cavity easily and quickly with little of the solution passing into the fallopian tubes. It is now readily available in 100 ml bottles. A minor disadvantage of Hyskon is that all hysteroscope instruments need to be carefully cleaned with warm water immediately after the procedure.

Lindemann [49] has strongly recommended the use of carbon dioxide for distention of the uterine cavity and has recently demonstrated the advantages of this technique for infertility evaluation. The extended sperm migration test discussed by this author (G.W.P.) is not possible when a liquid has been used to distend the uterine cavity. Early difficulty in obtaining a tight cervical seal and maintaining a constant, controlled pressure has been overcome with a new $CO_2$ insufflation device, termed the *Metromat*,* designed specifically for use with hysteroscopy. This technique requires more skill than does the use of Hyskon, because bleeding must be kept at an absolute minimum for successful inspection of the endometrial cavity. Irrigation of bleeding sites is not possible with this technique; however, it appears that adequate distention of the uterine cavity at pressures of 100 mmHg will stop the flow of blood from the endometrium and permit excellent visualization.

Finally, a third approach has been the use of 5 percent dextrose in distilled water to distend and irrigate the endometrial cavity during hysteroscopic evaluation. This author (G.W.P.) has not found visualization with this medium to be as good as that with Hyskon or carbon dioxide. The major advantages of distilled water are its low cost and availability, both of which make it useful during office hysteroscopy. Sugimoto [82] has discussed at length the use of this water medium.

*Wolf Instrument Co.

*Types of Hysteroscopes*

Numerous models of hysteroscopes are available from Wolf, Eder, Storz, and ACMI. Two basic designs are offered. The first, similar to the design of a cystoscope, includes an outer sheath, obdurator, removable fore-oblique telescope, and operating channel through which flexible instruments can be inserted to cut adhesions or to cannulate the tubal ostea (Fig. 2-18). The second design is similar to the operating laparoscope and provides a single telescope with offset viewing lens containing an operating (3 mm) channel for insertion of rigid

**Figure 2-18.** The most common hysteroscope, the cystoscope design. A flexible scissor is also shown. The carbon dioxide insufflation device (Metromat 2121) designed by Lindemann has been found useful. (Courtesy of R. Wolf Co.)

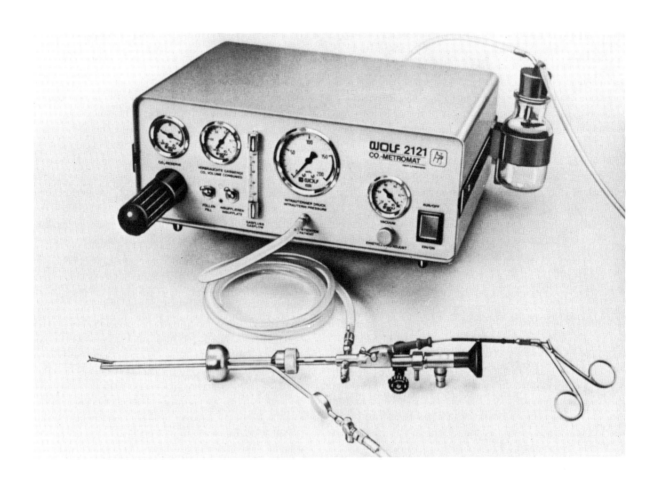

instruments (Fig. 2-19). The latter design is, of course, familiar to the gynecologist who performs tubal sterilization and operative laparoscopy. The former design is that generally used by the urologist and has been the model most often employed by early hysteroscopists.

These two hysteroscope designs offer a choice of angle of the telescope lens and rigidity or flexibility of the operating instruments. The cystoscope-type design (see Fig. 2-18) has a fore-oblique lens and flexible instruments, permitting the operator to visualize the lateral walls of the endometrial cavity and to direct a flexible instrument at an angle perpendicular to the axis of the sheath and telescope. Biopsy of the anterior and posterior uterine walls is, thus, possible, as is cannulation of the tubal ostea. Also, Lindemann [49] has designed a special sheath using a lever for manipulating flexible ancillary instruments, much like those available with most operating cystoscopes. In contrast to this, the second hysteroscope shown in Figure 2-19, is similar to the operating laparoscope in design and provides an offset lens and channel for the use of rigid instruments that facilitate the cutting of intrauterine adhesions and biopsy of the fundus. Insertion of catheters or other instruments into the tubal ostea would be more difficult with this instrument, as would an attempt to biopsy the anterior or posterior uterine walls. The 170 to 180-degree viewing angle of this telescope design is more familiar to the gynecologist and permits a panoramic view of the uterine cavity.

**Figure 2-19.** The operating hysteroscope shown below is similar in design to the operating laparoscope. Rigid instruments (also shown) are used with this telescope. (Courtesy of R. Wolf Co.)

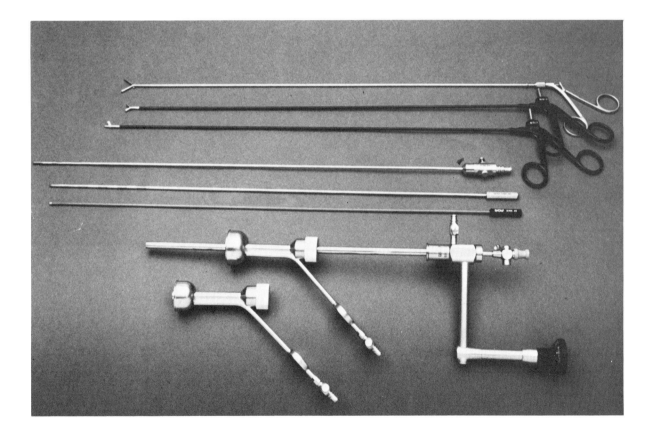

Recently, a third type of telescope termed a *microhysteroscope, microcolpohysteroscope* or *contact microcolpohysteroscope* has been introduced by Storz and Wolf instrument companies. In Paris, Jacques Hamou [37] developed and introduced a 4 mm microhysteroscope with a 30-degree oblique lens capable of varying magnifications from 1 to 150× (Fig. 2-20). Four different magnifications are possible with this telescope. Position 1 has a magnification of 1× and allows the conventional view of the endometrial cavity; position 2 provides 20× magnification for close inspection of the endocervical canal or endometrial lesions; positions 3 and 4 magnify of 60× and 150× when the distal end of the telescope (lens) is in contact with the mucosal lining. It is this feature that qualifies this instrument as a contact hysteroscope. Wolf has also introduced a 4 mm microhysteroscope capable of similar levels of magnification when brought into contact with the tissue being inspected. Use of the Wolf microhysteroscope with the hand-held sliding mechanism permits the control of the 4 mm 30-degree fore-oblique lens with a single hand. This small telescope diameter is suitable for office and outpatient use in inspecting the endocervical canal or endometrial cavity without cervical dilatation and, often, without the need for paracervical block.

**Figure 2-20.** The microcolpohysteroscope designed by Hamou. This telescope has a 30-degree lens angle and provides magnifications from 1× to 150×. (Courtesy of Storz Instrument Co.)

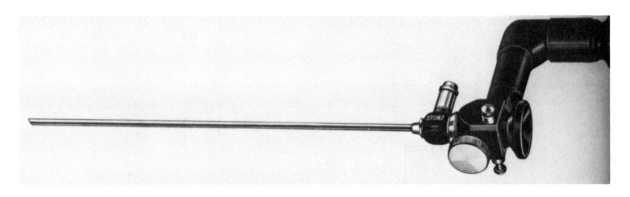

The predecessor of these microhysteroscopes was a simple contact hysteroscope introduced to the United States by Baggish [1]. This small diameter instrument (6 mm or 8 mm) collects room light in a light trap, permitting its use in an office procedure, presumably without dilatation of the endocervical canal (Fig. 2-21). The magnification of the eyepiece is $1.6\times$; however, an optical magnifying device is available that gives an additional $2\times$ magnification. This instrument was also developed in Paris and was designed by the Institut d'Optique de Paris. The hysteroscope itself is manufactured by the MTO Company, Paris, and distributed in the United States by Advanced Biomedical Instruments Company. Many of the original studies in Paris were carried out by Barbot [59].

This author (G.W.P.) prefers to dilate the endocervical canal and endometrial cavity with carbon dioxide, as described by Lindemann [49], and has found the new Wolf Metromat $CO_2$ insufflator to be exceedingly useful. All hysteroscopies performed prior to January 1982 utilized a 4 mm fore-oblique telescope with either a 5 mm diagnostic sheath or a 7 mm operating sheath. Recent preliminary studies with the microhysteroscope appear to indicate that this instrument will be the preferable telescope for future studies. Both the Wolf and Storz instruments appear to be excellent. However, it should be noted that the Hamou telescope is too short to be used with the obdurator that is available with the standard Storz hysteroscope; the Wolf microhysteroscope can be used interchangeably with the usual 4 mm fore-oblique telescope.

**Figure 2-21. A.** Contact hysteroscope shown with light trap near eyepiece, and attached camera with flash. **B.** Contact hysteroscope with light trap and holding device. (Courtesy of Storz Instrument Co.)

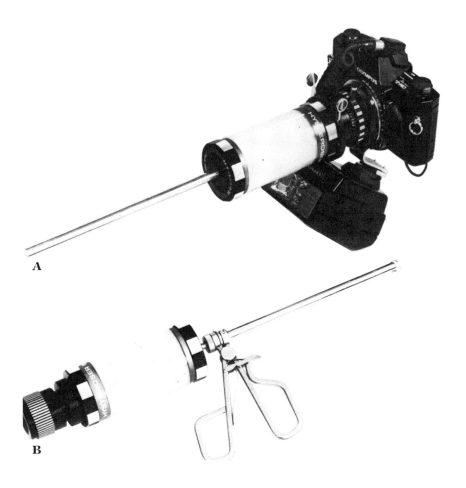

A

B

**Table 2-7.** Hysteroscopic classification
of Asherman's syndrome

| Classification | Involvement |
| --- | --- |
| Severe (N = 20) | More than ¾ of uterine cavity; agglutination of walls or thick bands; ostial areas and upper cavity occluded |
| Moderate (N = 24) | ¼ to ¾ of uterine cavity involved; no agglutination of walls—adhesions only; ostial areas and upper fundus only partially occluded |
| Minimal (N = 20) | Less than ¼ of uterine cavity involved; thin or filmy adhesions; ostial areas and upper fundus minimally involved or clear |

Source: C. M. March, R. Israel, and A. March, Hysteroscopic management of intrauterine adhesions. *Am. J. Obstet. Gynecol.* 130:653, 1978.

*Indications for Hysteroscopy*

The primary indication for hysteroscopy in the infertile patient at this time is for confirmation of a uterine defect seen during hysterosalpingography. Careful injection of water-soluble dye with fluoroscopic control will identify a filling defect typical of a submucous or intracavitary fibroid, an endometrial polyp, or intrauterine adhesions. Diagnostic hysteroscopy permits direct visualization of the lesion and enables the surgeon to confirm the presence of a fibroid and to differentiate this lesion from an endometrial polyp, thereby eliminating the occasional embarrassing situation of opening the uterus only to find a polyp or even a completely normal uterine cavity.

Identification of intrauterine adhesions is more accurately made by hysteroscopy than by the x-ray study, although the simplicity of hysterosalpingography and its low cost and ease of performance make it the primary diagnostic mode at the present time. A grading system proposed by March, Israel, and March [53] and by Valle [88] enables the hysteroscopist to classify intrauterine adhesions as minimal, moderate, or severe (Table 2-7). Prognosis for a successful posttherapy pregnancy and the possibility of recurrence of intrauterine adhesions are improved by using this system. It has also recently been demonstrated that hysteroscopic lysis of intrauterine adhesions under direct visualization may be the best form of treatment of Asherman's syndrome to date [52].

Other indications presently under study for hysteroscopy in the infertile patient include the following: (1) resection of an intraluminal or submucous fibroid [56], (2) resection of a uterine septum [17], (3) performing the extended sperm migration test [49], (4) evaluation of intramural tubal pregnancy [87] and catheterization of segment prior to tubal surgery [87], and (5) evaluation of endometrial development and directed endometrial biopsy.

The combination of diagnostic hysteroscopy and laparoscopy during evaluation of the infertile female has been found useful by this author (G.W.P.) and others [29, 86], permitting accurate definition of a uterine defect thought to be due to a submucous fibroid; an unusual uterine anomaly; or even endometrial adhesions. At times, this differentiation will be difficult and it has proved useful to be able to visualize the interior and exterior of the uterus at one time, as well as to biopsy through the hysteroscope an area thought to represent a submucous fibroid.

*Results of Studies*

Diagnostic laparoscopy is presently the most useful aspect of endoscopic visualization of the interior of the uterus. Operative procedures have been limited to the treatment of Asherman's syndrome and, sometimes, the removal of an intraluminal fibroid and excision of a thin uterine septum. In regard to the hysteroscopic lysis of adhesions, March and Israel [52] recently stated, "Division of adhesions under hysteroscopic control together with the adjunctive measures utilized is superior to all other methods of therapy for intrauterine adhesions and should replace them." Recent studies involving the use of the argon laser through the operating hysteroscope are presented at the end of this chapter.

Although an infrequent problem in the infertile patient, intrauterine adhesions (Asherman's syndrome) presents a significant diagnostic and therapeutic problem [88]. At present, intrauterine adhesions are usually diagnosed by hysterosalpingography, although hysteroscopy has been found to be a preferable method, because it permits accurate classification and surgical treatment. Although the presence of secondary amenorrhea was originally a criterion for the diagnosis of Asherman's syndrome, it has become clear that many patients with intrauterine adhesions may also experience hypomenorrhea or even normal menstrual flow. The classification of intrauterine adhesions proposed by March, Israel, and March has been given in Table 2-7.

A correlation between menstrual symptoms and the extent of adhesions found within the uterine cavity appears to exist. Amenorrhea was present in 41 of 64 patients with intrauterine adhesions studied by March, Israel, and March, but 9 of these patients had minimal adhesions [53]. Conversely, among 12 patients with normal menses, intrauterine adhesions were severe in 1, moderate in 3, and mild in 8 patients. In this study, there appeared to be little correlation between hysterosalpingographic findings and the extent of intrauterine adhesions found at hysteroscopy. These authors stated that ". . . although 23 of the 29 HSGs suggested extensive obliteration of the endometrial cavity, severe adhesions were present in only 9 of these 23 patients. In fact, 2 of the 23 patients had no intrauterine adhesions, despite nonvisualization of the endometrial cavity by HSG and a roentgenographic diagnosis of Asherman's syndrome." There were no patients in this study in whom hysteroscopic findings indicated adhesions more advanced than those suggested by HSG.

March and Israel [52] recently reported the results of hysteroscopic lysis of intrauterine adhesions in 38 infertile patients. Adhesions were severe in 11, moderate in 20, and minimal in 7 patients. All 38 patients underwent hysteroscopy prior to division of adhesions using miniature scissors. All patients were placed on postoperative estrogen treatment for 2 months and 32 of these patients had an intrauterine device (Lippes loop) placed in the endometrial cavity following surgery; three patients had a Foley catheter placed in the uterine cavity following lysis of adhesions; twenty-seven patients underwent postoperative hysteroscopy to verify the absence of adhesions, and in two of them a single residual adhesion was found and lysed at that time. These authors performed hysteroscopy as an outpatient procedure under intravenous meperidine or general anesthesia. A 7 mm hysteroscope and 32 percent dextran (Hyskon) [48] were used.

Prior to treatment of intrauterine adhesions, the 38 patients reported by March and Israel had been pregnant 103 times. All had been pregnant at least once; however, only 10 women had delivered living infants. Overall, 16.7 percent of pregnancies in these women had resulted in a living child. Following hysteroscopic lysis of intrauterine adhesions, the 38 women conceived 43 times and 79 percent of these pregnancies resulted in live births [52]. Remarkably, 33 of 34 women were delivered at term and one delivered prematurely, at 29 weeks. It is also of interest that only 7 women were delivered by cesarean section and of these only one involved abnormal placentation. There was no occurrence of placenta accreta, increta, or percreta.

These results are superior to those reported in the literature in which various techniques of lysis were used. One review of 369 pregnancies in patients treated for Asherman's syndrome revealed a term pregnancy rate of only 39 percent [40]. Placenta accreta occurred in 10 percent of these women and the cesarean section rate was high. Neuwirth [56] has stated that in his experience 25 percent of patients conceived following hysteroscopic lysis of intrauterine adhesions. In this study, only 14 of 45 patients conceived postoperatively and 5 of these were delivered by cesarean section.

Other forms of hysteroscopic treatment include removal of submucous fibroids and resection of a uterine septum. Neuwirth [56] pioneered the removal of submucous fibroids transcervically by the use of a hysteroscopic technique. In 1976, however, he reported the removal of pedunculated fibroids in five patients. Heavy vaginal bleeding was a major concern and led to the design of a Silastic balloon for control of postoperative hemorrhage. A modified cystoscope, termed *resecto-scope*, was used by Neuwirth during this procedure, which also employed electrocoagulation. Few other hysteroscopists have attempted this procedure, however [87].

Recently DeCherney [17] described resection of a uterine septum in 11 patients under hysteroscopic control, using electrosurgery. Among these patients who aborted habitually and were found to have a septate uterus, all were treated transcervically by resection of the septum using a resectoscope. In this approach, the septum was electrocoagulated and morsulated. Laparoscopy was also performed at this time to exclude uterine perforation or thermal damage to the intestine. Nine of the 11 patients conceived postoperatively and carried to term.

Lindemann [49] has described hysteroscopic findings in 431 infertile patients. Forty-nine percent of these patients demonstrated an intracavitary irregularity. Presumably, hysterosalpingography had been used to select these patients for hysteroscopy. Forty percent (18 patients) of those who aborted habitually had intracavitary pathology; submucous myomas were found in 7, adhesions in 6, and septate uterus in 3 patients. The author [49] has described the extended sperm migration test, in which hysteroscopy and laparoscopy are performed simultaneously, approximately 3 hours after intercourse. An increased amount of transparent mucus was found extending from the endocervix to the cornual segment. It was theorized by Lindemann that sperm migration took place along this mucus, facilitating transport into the fallopian tube. Samples of mucus were taken from the endocervix, uterine corpus, and the pouch of Douglas for evaluation. Three examinations were performed; in only 40 percent of patients with a positive Sims' test were sperm found in the upper genital tract and pouch of Douglas. It was thought that decreased mobility of sperm in the upper genital tract suggested the presence of an immobilizing factor.

In conclusion, it appears that the recently introduced microhysteroscope offers an exciting opportunity for further study by the infertility specialist. The ability to magnify 50 to 100× may permit further evaluation of sperm activity inside the uterine cavity, as described by Lindemann. Careful evaluation of the endometrium should also provide insight into endocrine abnormalities, such as irregular shedding and inadequate luteal phase. Sites of implantation could also be monitored by this technique.

## Endoscopic Surgery Using the Laser
James F. Daniell

The use of the laser through an endoscope is not a new idea in medicine, having been previously applied in urology, orthopedics, ear, nose, and throat, and gastroenterology. Its use in gynecology, however, is recent and still limited to a few medical centers. Lasers have been used with both hysteroscopes and laparoscopes; however, this section will be devoted to the use of the argon or carbon dioxide laser during operative laparoscopy in the infertile patient.

### Hysteroscopic Use of Lasers
Goldrath [32] has reported the use of the neodymium-YAG laser for photovaporization of the endometrium to produce permanent amenorrhea. This was accomplished by firing the hysteroscopically directed laser through fiberoptics, using dextran or saline as the distending medium. This procedure, although innovative and successful for treating menorrhagia, does not appear to be an improvement in the field of operative hysteroscopy in the treatment of such infertility problems as Asherman's syndrome, submucosal fibroids, or uterine septae. The physical properties of the neodymium-YAG laser are such that only tissue coagulation is possible, which limits the use of this modality during hysteroscopy.

The carbon dioxide laser cannot yet be effectively fired through fibers and, thus, can be used only with carbon dioxide hysteroscopy. A prototype of a hysteroscope adapted to allow intrauterine aiming and firing of the carbon dioxide laser is being developed, but at this writing has not been clinically tested. Theoretically, the carbon dioxide laser is ideal for hysteroscopic resection of a uterine septum, removal of a solitary submucosal myoma, or removal of intrauterine adhesions. However, the technical problems of safe aiming and firing of the carbon dioxide laser hysteroscopically must still be overcome.

### Laparoscopic Use of the Laser
Two types of lasers have been used during operative laparoscopy, the argon and the carbon dioxide. The argon laser, which can be fired through fibers, has been used by Keye [42] to photocoagulate implants of pelvic endometriosis at laparoscopy. This technique seems promising, because the tissue effect is dependent on the tissue color (purplish) for beam absorption and action. The fiberoptic probe can be passed intraabdominally under laparoscopic control and the tissue (endometrial serosal implant) touched directly with the end of the probe. The argon laser is then activated, and the lesion absorbs the laser energy with resultant tissue necrosis to variable depths without surface vaporization. The limitations of this system are lack of fine control of depth of tissue destruction, tissue damage that may not be evident at the time of the procedure, and inability to incise or vaporize tissue. We have no personal experience with the argon laser at Vanderbilt University but encourage cautious further investigation of this process to determine if there may be benefits to patients that are not attainable with alternate forms of operative laparoscopy.

Investigation of the use of the carbon dioxide laser during operative laparoscopy began independently on three continents, with reports by Bruhat in France [6], Tadir in Israel [85], and Daniell in North America [14, 15]. Ideal operative laparoscopy should allow precise destruction of endometriotic implants and hemostatic lysis of adhesions or incision of a hydrosalpinx without injury to adjacent tissues. Risk of subsequent adhesion formation should be minimal. Because these conditions were not satisfactorily met with existing high frequency electrical systems used during operative laparoscopy, we investigated further the application of laser vaporization through the laparoscope. Investigators at Vanderbilt University have used two systems for delivery of carbon dioxide laser energy through the operating laparoscope. The first involves passage of the beam through the operating channel of the 12 mm laparoscope (Figs. 2-22, 2-23); the second, passage of the laser beam through a second-puncture instrument [15]. At present, because of design problems involving the use of the laser through the operating channel, which limits visibility and focusing of the beam, we favor delivery of the carbon dioxide laser beam through a second-puncture instrument. However, further modifications of the operating laparoscope may result in a workable single-puncture system in the near future.*

*Editor's Note: At this writing Eder Instrument Company and Sharplan Instrument Company market a carbon dioxide laser laparoscope set. This set includes a coupler that will articulate the laser arm to either the channel of an operating telescope or a second puncture laser guide. The set marketed by Eder Instrument Company can be adapted for use with most carbon dioxide laser generators. The Sharplan set can only be used with the Sharplan carbon dioxide generator.

**Figure 2-22.** 12 mm operating telescope adpated for use with the carbon dioxide laser. The trochar and trochar sleeve are also shown. The small handle (joy stick) can be used to manipulate the carbon dioxide laser beam through the telescope.

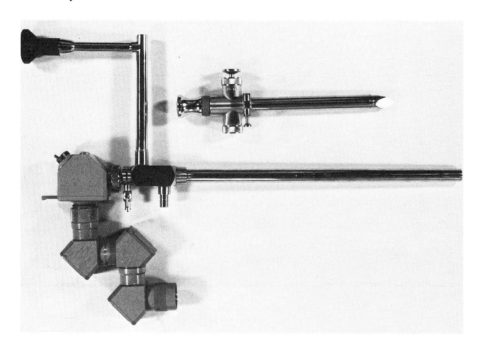

**Figure 2-23.** Early design of the articulation between the operating telescope and carbon dioxide laser.

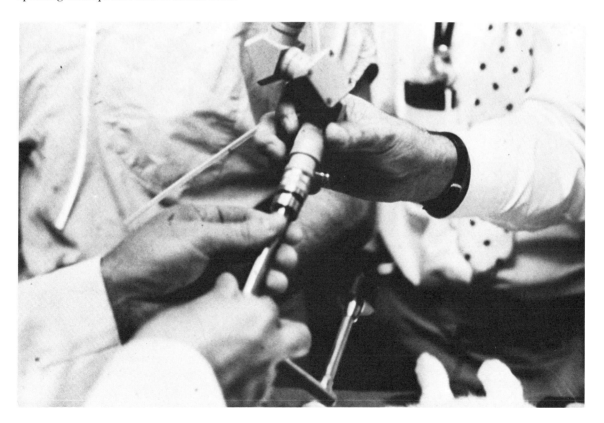

**Figure 2-24.** Instruments used to direct the carbon dioxide laser through a second puncture guide. Included from top to bottom are the coupler, which connects the Sharplan carbon dioxide laser to the laser guide, the second puncture trochar, the second puncture trochar sleeve, and at the bottom, the second puncture carbon dioxide laser guide.

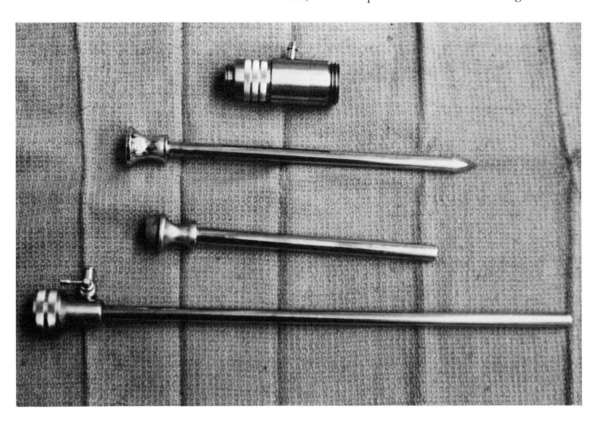

*Initial Experience with a Second-Puncture System for Laser Use at Laparoscopy*

A special 8.5-mm (external diameter) trochar and sheath were designed, as well as a 28 cm (7 mm diameter) hollow probe that attaches to a 300 mm zinc arcenide focusing lens and articulates to the arm of a Sharplan 733 laser unit (Fig. 2-24).* The lens focuses the beam to a spot size of 0.5 mm at a distance of 2 cm from the end of the instrument. A 1 mm channel mounted inside the aiming probe leads to a control valve just distal to the focusing lens and allows egress of smoke. This system permits the use of a standard laparoscope with the carbon dioxide laser beam being aimed, focused, and fired through the special laser probe placed through a second-puncture site. The probe was initially introduced in the midline just at the pubic hairline. However, after the first few cases, the site was moved to midway between the laparoscope and the pubic hairline to improve the angle at which the laser beam was directed into the pelvis. With this system a third-puncture trochar could be used to pass a 5 mm grasping forceps to expose and position pelvic structures. Using this system, visibility of the orange optical aiming beam was excellent, and the intraperitoneal smoke from vaporization of the tissue could be continuously removed by suction and did not interfere with visualization of the pelvis. Test aiming and firing in New Zealand rabbits demonstrated that this carbon dioxide laser system, with appropriate focusing and wattage settings, could be used for both vaporizing and incising tissue.

Fifteen patients with mild or moderate endometriosis without significant adhesions had operative laparoscopy with use of the carbon dioxide laser for vaporization of the implants of endometriosis. A setting of 5 to 10 watts was used to vaporize endometriotic implants on the ovaries, the pelvic side walls, and the uterosacral ligaments. No attempt was made to vaporize lesions near the bladder, the bowel, or the ureter. All procedures were performed with informed consent under general endotracheal anesthesia in the proliferative phase of the cycle, using a triple-puncture technique. These patients received no medical therapy for their endometriosis either prior to or after laser laparoscopy.

---

*Physical principles and specific instruments involved in the use of the carbon dioxide laser are discussed at length in Chapter 6.

After gaining experience using the second-puncture laser probe for vaporization, the incisional use of the laser was examined intraperitoneally under laparoscopic control. Patients with a large hydrosalpinx who did not desire major surgery were offered an attempt at laparoscopic terminal salpingostomy. Five patients who gave informed consent for this procedure were considered good candidates at the time of laparoscopic screening of the pelvis. The criteria used for performing this procedure were the following: patient's desire for the procedure and acceptance of the conditions of treatment, lack of significant ovarian adhesions, ability of the distal hydrosalpinx to be distended by dye at laparoscopy, absence of adhesions around the distal end of the tube, and the ability to safely focus the laser beam at right angles to the end of the fallopian tube. At a setting of 25 watts, the laser beam was focused by positioning the end of the probe at 2 cm from the end of the fallopian tube. After identifying the area of thinnest scarring on the distal end of the tube, the laser was used to make a linear incision in the distal end of the tube. A 3 mm grasping forceps was used through the operating channel of the laparoscope, as well as a 5 mm grasping forceps through the third-puncture site to grasp the edges of the tube for traction. After making the initial incision at the end of the fallopian tube, a second incision was made at right angles, using the accessory instruments for traction. The laser beam was then defocused by pulling the probe back 3 to 4 cm from the end of the fallopian tube and reducing the power to 3 watts. The incised tube was everted using the low-power setting to cause shrinkage and contraction of the tubal ampullary peritoneum. This caused a "flowering effect" of the distal tube and everted the incised edges of the hydrosalpinx. This procedure was performed in all five patients, three with bilateral hydrosalpinges and two with hydrosalpinx in their only fallopian tube. These patients were observed in the hospital for 24 hours, given prophylactic antibiotics, and had 200 ml of 32% dextran 70 instilled into the peritoneal cavity at the end of the laparoscopy. Hydrotubation was performed with 40 ml of sterile saline on the morning following laparoscopy, prior to discharge from the hospital. Following the first menstrual period, the patients returned for outpatient hysterosalpingograms with antibiotic coverage.

*Results*

In all 15 patients undergoing laser vaporization of endometriosis, the procedure was carried out with no complications. After follow-up intervals ranging from 6 to 9 months, five of these patients have conceived and the other 10 are without symptoms of endometriosis. None of the patients have been treated with any medical therapy and none have had a second-look laparoscopy. There were no operative complications in the five patients with hydrosalpinges treated with laparoscopic terminal salpingostomy. All five had patent tubes demonstrated by hysterosalpingography performed during the 6-month postoperative evaluation. Two patients have thus far conceived, one with an intrauterine gestation that is progressing normally, and one with an ectopic pregnancy that was operated on 3 months after the laparoscopic procedure. The ectopic implantation was in the ampullary portion of the oviduct. At the time of surgery the other fallopian tube was patent. No significant adhesions were seen, nor was there reagglutination of the distal tube on either side.

*Discussion of the Carbon Dioxide Laser*

The carbon dioxide laser has now been employed in a variety of gynecologic operations. However, its use intraperitoneally at open surgery or through laparoscopy is still considered incipient therapeutics. The characteristics of the laser beam are particularly applicable to laparoscopic surgery. The beam is very collimated and coherent and, with proper lenses, can be focused to a very fine point. By controlling the beam density and the length of continuous exposure, the depth of laser vaporization can be limited to less than 1 mm. Similarly, with proper focusing and power density settings, a bloodless incision can be made with a carbon dioxide laser under laparoscopic control. This laser system can deliver precise destruction of tissue without risk of electrical injury or significant thermal damage. The use of the carbon dioxide laser through the laparoscope may prove to be an ideal technique for vaporizing implants of endometriosis, because tissue reaction has been shown to be minimal with this technique [4].

The introduction of the carbon dioxide laser beam through the second-puncture probe avoids the initial technical problems encountered when the laser was directed through the operating channel of the laparoscope. In addition, the triple-puncture technique described earlier resulted in adequate tissue exposure, position, and traction, although it did require a surgical assistant experienced in operative laparoscopy. Because the laser beam travels in a straight line from the distal end of the second-puncture probe, the operator must always have good visibility of the impact site before firing. The ability to use this system without complications in this early group of carefully selected patients was encouraging. The fact that distally obstructed fallopian tubes could be safely opened using the carbon dioxide laser with a laparoscope suggests that this type of tubal surgery on the distal end of the fallopian tube may be efficacious. Controlled studies evaluating this form of laparoscopic surgery will be necessary before any firm conclusions can be drawn. Nevertheless, if this type of surgery is shown to be of value it would reduce the cost, inconvenience, and discomfort to patients and decrease the number of laparotomies necessary during infertility treatment.

## References

1. Baggish, M. S., and Barbot, J. Contact hysteroscopy for easier diagnosis. *Contemp. OB/GYN* 16:93, 1980.
2. Balin, H., Wan, L. S., and Israel, S. L. Recent advances in pelvic endoscopy. *Obstet. Gynecol.* 27:30, 1966.
3. Behrman, S. J., and Kistner, R. W. (eds.). *Progress in Infertility* (2nd ed.). Boston: Little, Brown, 1975.
4. Ben-Bassatt, M., and Kaplan, I. An Ultrastructural Study of the Cut Edges of Skin and Mucous Membrane Specimens Excised by Carbon Dioxide Laser. In I. Kaplan (ed.), *Laser Surgery.* Jerusalem: Jerusalem Academic Press, 1976.
5. Bronson, R. A., and Wallach, E. E. Lysis of periadnexal adhesions for correction of infertility. *Fertil. Steril.* 28:613, 1977.
6. Bruhat, M., Mage, G., and Manhes, M. Use of the $CO_2$ laser via laparoscopy. In I. Kaplan (ed.), *Laser Surgery III.* Tel Aviv: International Society for Laser Surgery, 1979.
7. Bumm, E. Experimente und Erfahrungen mit der Hysteroskopie. *Verhandl. d. Gesellsch. f. Geburtsh. u. Gynäk. zu Leipz.* 6:524, 1895.
8. Cohen, M. R. Culdoscopy vs. peritoneoscopy. *Am. J. Obstet. Gynecol.* 31:310, 1968.
9. Cohen, M. R. Photography. In J. M. Phillips (ed.), *Laparoscopy.* Baltimore: Williams & Wilkins, 1977.
10. Cohen, M. R. Laparoscopic diagnosis and pseudomenopause treatment of endometriosis with danazol. *Clin. Obstet. Gynecol.* 23:901, 1980.
11. Coltart, T. M. Laparoscopy in the diagnosis of tubal patency. *J. Obstet. Gynecol.* 77:69, 1970.
12. Corson, S. L. Use of the laparoscope in the infertile patient. *Fertil. Steril.* 32:359, 1979.
13. Corson, S. L., and Bolognese, R. J. Laparoscopy: An overview and results of large series. *J. Reprod. Med.* 9:148, 1972.
14. Daniell, J., and Brown, D. Carbon dioxide laser laparoscope: Initial experience in experimental animals and humans. *Obstet. Gynecol.* 59:761, 1982.
15. Daniell, J., and Pittaway, D. Use of the $CO_2$ laser in laparoscopic surgery: Initial experience with the second puncture technique. *Infertility* 5:15, 1982.
16. David, C. Endoscopie de l'uterus apres l'avortement et dans les suites de couches normales et pathologiques. *Bull. Soc. Obstet. Paris* 10:288, 1907.
17. DeCherney, A. H. Müllerian fusion defects. Presented at the First World Congress of Hysteroscopy, Jan. 1982, Miami, Florida.
18. Diamond, E. Lysis of postoperative pelvic adhesions in infertility. *Fertil. Steril.* 31:287, 1979.
19. Drake, T. C., and Grunert, G. M. The unsuspected pelvic factor in the infertility investigation. *Fertil. Steril.* 34:27, 1980.
19a. Drake, T., Treadway, D., Buchanan, G., Takaki, N., and Daane, T. Unexplained infertility. *Obstet. Gynecol.* 50:644, 1977.

20. Duignan, N. M., Jordan, J. A., and Coughlan, B. M. One thousand consecutive cases of diagnostic laparoscopy. *J. Obstet. Gynecol. of Br. Comm.* 79:1016, 1972.

21. Edgerton, W. D., and Kleppinger, R. Laparoscopy in a Community Hospital. In J. M. Phillips (Ed.), *Laparoscopy.* Baltimore: Williams & Wilkins, 1977.

22. Edström, K., and Fernström, I. The diagnostic possibilities of a modified hysteroscopic technique. *Acta Obstet. Gynecol. Scand.* 49:327, 1970.

23. Edwards, R. G. Cauterization of Stages I & II Endometriosis and the Resulting Pregnancy Rate. In J. M. Phillips (ed.), *Endoscopy in Gynecology.* Downey, Calif.: American Association of Gynecologic Laparoscopists, 1978.

24. El-Minawi, M., Abdel-Hadi, M., Ibrahim, A. A., and Wahby, O. Comparative evaluation of laparoscopy and hysterosalpingography in infertile patients. *Obstet. Gynecol.* 51:29, 1978.

25. Fear, R. E. Laparoscopy: A valuable aid in gynecologic diagnosis. *Am. J. Obstet. Gynecol.* 31:297, 1968.

26. Frangenheim, H. Vergleichende unter-suchungen zwischen dem wert der Hysterosalpingographic und der coelioskopic bei der Sterilitats-diagnostik. *Arch. Gynaekol.* 204:167, 1967.

27. Frangenheim, H. *Laparoscopy and Culdoscopy in Gynecology.* Stuttgart: G. Thieme, 1972.

28. Gabos, P. A comparison of hysterosalpingography and endoscopy in evaluation of tubal function in infertile women. *Fertil. Steril.* 27:238, 1976.

29. Gallinat, A., Lucken, R. P., and Lindemann, H. J. Hysteroscopy as a diagnostic and therapeutic tool in sterility (abstract). Presented to First World Congress of Hysteroscopy, Jan. 1982, Miami, Fla.

30. Gauss, C. J. Hysteroskopie. *Arch. Gynaekol.* 133:18, 1928.

31. Goldenberg, R. L., and Magendantz, H. G. Laparoscopy and the infertility evaluation. *Obstet. Gynecol.* 47:410, 1976.

32. Goldrath, M., Fuller, T., and Segal, S. Laser photovaporization of endometrium for the treatment of menorrhagia. *Am. J. Obstet. Gynecol.* 140:14, 1981.

33. Gomel, V. Laparoscopic tubal surgery in infertility. *Obstet. Gynecol.* 46:47, 1975.

34. Gomel, V. Laparoscopy prior to reconstructive tubal surgery for infertility. *J. Reprod. Med.* 18:251, 1977.

35. Gomel, V. Salpingostomy by laparoscopy. *J. Reprod. Med.* 18:265, 1977.

36. Gomel, V. Microsurgery in gynecology. In S. J. Silber (ed.), *Microsurgery.* Baltimore: Williams & Wilkins, 1979.

37. Hamou, J. Microhysteroscopy—A new procedure and its original applications in gynecology. *J. Reprod. Med.* 26:375, 1981.

38. Hutchins, C. J. Laparoscopy and hysterosalpingography in the assessment of tubal patency. *Obstet. Gynecol.* 49:325, 1977.

39. Israel, R., and March, C. M. Diagnostic laparoscopy: A prognostic aid in the surgical management of infertility. *Am. J. Obstet. Gynecol.* 125:969, 1976.

40. Jewelewicz, R. Newer methods of diagnosing and treating Asherman's syndrome. *Contemp. OB/GYN* 14:117, 1979.

41. Keirse, M. J., and Vandervellen, R. A comparison of hysterosalpingography and laparoscopy in the investigation of infertility. *Obstet. Gynecol.* 41:685, 1973.

42. Keye, W. The argon laser used laparoscopically for photocoagulation of endometriosis. Presented to the 2nd Congress of the Gynecologic International Laser Society, May 1982, Montreal, Canada.

43. Kistner, R. W. Endometriosis and infertility. *Clin. Obstet. Gynecol.* 22:101, 1979.

44. Kistner, R. W., and Patton, G. W. *Atlas of Infertility Surgery.* Boston: Little, Brown, 1975.

45. Kleppinger, R. K. Ovarian cyst penetration via laparoscopy. *J. Reprod. Med.* 21:16, 1978.

46. Knott, D. F. Photography, Cinematography, and Television in Microsurgery. In J. M. Phillips (ed.), *Microsurgery in Gynecology.* St. Louis: Christian Board of Publishers, 1977.

47. Kreitmann, O., and Hodgen, G. D. Low tubal ovum transfer: An alternative to in vitro fertilization. *Fertil. Steril.* 34:375, 1980.

48. Levine, R. U., and Neuwirth, R. S. Evaluation of a method of hysteroscopy with the use of thirty percent dextran. *Am. J. Obstet. Gynecol.* 113:696, 1972.

49. Lindemann, H. J. Eine neue Untersuchungsmethode für die hysteroskopic. *Endoscopy* 4:194, 1971.

50. Liston, W. A., Bradford, W. P., Downie, J. and Kerr, M. G. Laparoscopy in a general gynecologic unit. *Am. J. Obstet. Gynecol.* 113:672, 1972.

51. Maathius, J. B., Horbach, J. G., and Hall, E. V. A comparison of the results of hysterosalpingography and laparoscopy in the diagnosis of fallopian tube dysfunction. *Fertil. Steril.* 23:428, 1972.

52. March, C. M., and Isr'ael, R. Gestational outcome following hysteroscopic lysis of adhesions. *Fertil. Steril.* 36:455, 1981.

53. March, C. M., Israel, R., and March, A. O. Hysteroscopic management of intrauterine adhesions. *Am. J. Obstet. Gynecol.* 130:653, 1978.

54. Mercer, J. P., et al. Spring clip tubal sterilization. *Obstet. Gynecol.* 44:449, 1974.

55. Moghissi, R. S. Correlation between hysterosalpingography and pelvic endoscopy for the evaluation of tubal factor. *Fertil. Steril.* 26:1178, 1975.

56. Neuwirth, R. S., and Amin, H. K. Excision of submucous fibroids with hysteroscopic control. *Am. J. Obstet. Gynecol.* 126:95, 1976.

57. Palmer, R., Laparoscopies opératoires dans le traitement de la stérilité féminine. *Acta Endoscopia* 1:19, 1971.

58. Pantaleoni, D. On endoscopic examination of the cavity of the womb. *Med. Press. Circ.* London 18:25, 1869.

59. Parent, B., et al. Metrorrhagies postmenopausiques diagnostique pur l'hysteroscopic de contact. *Acta Endoscopia* 8:18, 1978.

60. Patton, G. W. Report of results of 637 laparoscopies. Unpublished data, 1975–1982.

61. Peterson, E. P., and Behrman, S. J. Laparoscopy of the infertile patient. *Obstet. Gynecol.* 36:363, 1970.

62. Prescott, R. Optical principles of endoscopy. *J. Med. Primatol.* 5:136, 1976.

63. Quint, R. H. Endoscopic instrumentation. *Clin. Obstet. Gynecol.* 12:463, 1969.

64. Rioux, J. E., and Cloutier, D. Bipolar cautery for sterilization by laparoscopy. *J. Reprod. Med.* 13:6, 1974.

65. Rubin, I. C. Uterine endoscopy, endometrioscope with the aid of uterine insufflation. *Am. J. Obstet. Gynecol.* 10:313, 1925.

66. Ruddock, J. C. Peritoneoscopy. *Surg. Gynecol. Obstet.* 651:623, 1937.

67. Saidi, M. H., and Zainie, C. M. *Female Sterilization—A Handbook for Women.* New York: Garland STPM Press, 1980.

68. Schroeder, C., Uber den Ausbau und die Leistungen der Hysteroskopie. *Arch. Gynaekol.* 156:407, 1934.

69. Semm, K. *Atlas of Gynecologic Laparoscopy and Hysteroscopy.* Philadelphia: Saunders, 1975.

70. Semm, K. Endocoagulation: A new field of endoscopic surgery. *J. Reprod. Med.* 16:195, 1976.

71. Semm, K. Change in the classic gynecologic surgery: Review of 3,300 pelviscopies in 1971–1976. *Int. J. Fertil.* 24(1):13, 1979.

72. Semm, K. Treatment of female infertility due to tubal obstruction by operative laparoscopy. *Fertil. Steril.* 32:384, 1979.

73. Semm, K., and Mettler, L. Technical progress in pelvic surgery via operative laparoscopy. *Am. J. Obstet. Gynecol.* 138:121, 1980.

74. Silander, T. Hysteroscopy through a transparent rubber balloon in patients with uterine bleeding. *Acta Obstet. Gynecol. Scand.* 42:300, 1963.

75. Sjovall, A. Size measuring at laparoscopy. *Acta Obstet. Gynecol. Scand.* 42:279, 1963.

76. Soderström, R. M. Operative Sterilization, an Overview. In J. M. Phillips (ed.), *Laparoscopy.* Baltimore: Williams & Wilkins, 1977.

77. Soulas, A., Dubois De Montreynaud, J. M., Edwards, R. J., and Gladu, A. J. Bronchoscopy and television. *Dis. Chest* 31:580, 1957.

78. Steptoe, P. C. Gynaecological endoscopy—laparoscopy and culdoscopy. *J. Obstet. Gynecol. Br. Comm.* 72:535, 1965.

79. Steptoe, P. C. *Laparoscopy in Gynecology.* London: Livingstone, 1967.

80. Steptoe, P. C. Gynecologic laparoscopy. *J. Reprod. Med.* 10:211, 1973.

81. Steptoe, P. C., and Edwards, R. G. Laparoscopic recovery of preovulatory human oocytes after priming of ovaries with gonadotrophins. *Lancet* 1:683, 1970.

82. Sugimoto, Osamu. *Diagnostic and Therapeutic Hysteroscopy.* Tokyo-New York: Iguku-Chvin, 1977.

83. Swolin, K. Laparoscopy as an operative tool in female sterility. *J. Reprod. Med.* 19:167, 1977.

84. Swolin, K., and Rosencrantz, M. Laparoscopy vs. hysterosalpingography in sterility investigation: A comparative study. *Fertil. Steril.* 23:270, 1972.

85. Tadir, Y., Ovadia, J., Zuckerman, A., and Kaplan, I. Laparoscopic application of the $CO_2$ laser. Presented at the 4th Congress of International Society for Laser Surgery, 1981, Tokyo, Japan.

86. Taylor, P. J., and Leader, A. Combined laparoscopy and hysteroscopy in the investigation of infertility (abstract). Presented to the First World Congress of Hysteroscopy, Jan. 1982, Miami, Florida.

87. Valle, R. F. Hysteroscopy. *Obstet. Gynecol. Ann.* 7:245, 1978.

88. Valle, R. F., and Sciarra, J. J. Hysteroscopic treatment of intrauterine adhesions (abstract). Presented to the First World Congress of Hysteroscopy, Jan. 1982, Miami, Florida.

89. Wheeless, C. R. A rapid, inexpensive and effective method of surgical sterilization by laparoscopy. *J. Reprod. Med.* 3:65, 1969.

90. Wheeless, C. R. Laparoscopic sterilization, review of 3600 cases. *Obstet. Gynecol.* 42:751, 1973.

91. Yoon, I. B., and King, T. M. A preliminary and intermediate report on a new laparoscopic tubal ring procedure. *J. Reprod. Med.* 15:54, 1975.

92. Yuzpe, A. A. Operative laparoscopy. *J. Reprod. Med.* 13:27, 1974.

93. Yuzpe, A. A. Television in laparoscopy. In J. M. Phillips (ed.), *Laparoscopy.* Baltimore: Williams & Wilkins, 1977.

The importance of the postcoital test was emphasized in Chapter 1. The endocervical canal is lined by racemose glands composed of mucus-containing columnar cells. These cells produce a secretion that contains a variety of sugars and amino acids, and although the effects of these substances on sperm metabolism and migration are not completely known, spermatozoa maintain motility longer in favorable cervical mucus than in seminal fluid.

Traditionally, the endocervical glands have been described as racemose in type, that is, made up of numerous branching ducts terminating in acini. Fluhmann [11], however, has shown that these glands consist merely of deep clefts in the stroma, from which multiple blind tunnels branch forth in all directions. Cross-sections of these tunnels appear to be acini. It may be that the tunnels are the early tubular "glands" that have been carried downward with the formation of clefts and whose ostia, henceforth, open into the clefts.

Two types of cells are found in the endocervix, a mucus-secreting cell and a ciliated cell, which is located in patches in the cervical canal and in gland orifices. Although the concept of clefts and tunnels described above renders the term *gland* a misnomer, common usage most likely will dictate continued reference to endocervical glands. The cleft arrangement increases the surface area of endocervical mucosa and permits increased mucus production.

The stroma of the cervix is composed of connective tissue with unstriated muscle fibers and elastic tissue. The elastic tissue is found chiefly around the walls of the larger blood vessels. Danforth [5] has emphasized that the cervix is composed predominantly of fibrous connective tissue. The so-called musculature consists of isolated, attenuated strands of smooth muscle which are embedded in a heavy collagenous matrix. These strands of cervical muscle are continuous with the muscle of the corpus, but despite this continuity, they are entirely dissimilar to the powerful, closely packed, collagen-sparse corporeal musculature.

Hormonal, anatomic, and infectious aspects of the cervical factor are important. Stated simply, estrogen stimulates the secretory activity of the endocervical glands, and progesterone inhibits this activity. The estrogen effect may be assayed by microscopic examination of the mucus, which demonstrates the fern pattern, and by gross inspection, which reveals the formation of spinnbarkeit. Furthermore, estrogen produces specific anatomic changes in the isthmic canal. Two days before ovulation this area assumes a funnel shape owing to relaxation of the sphincteric constriction, and it becomes shorter and wider. After ovulation the canal becomes longer and narrower. If estrogen deficiency is detected, exogenous estrogen may be administered, but care must be taken to keep the dose low enough so that ovulation is not inhibited. Ethinyl estradiol (Estinyl), 0.02 mg, may be given daily for several months under these circumstances. Some patients, however, will note delay of ovulation and prolongation of cycles even at this low dose. This may be important if artificial insemination is being performed. In such patients the estrogen should be given from day 5 through day 12 of the cycle.

Anatomic variations in the position of the cervix do not seem to be as important as was previously suggested by various observers. Spermatozoa enter the anteriorly directed cervix that is associated with a third-degree retroversion of the uterus as readily as they enter the cervix that is directed into the mythical seminal pool. However, the cervix that is prolapsed beyond the introitus is poorly positioned to accept the seminal fluid. Correction of the prolapse by pessaries, cervical cups, or surgery is frequently followed by pregnancy. Although the size and shape of the cervix may not be related to infertility, the hypoplastic cervix may be a predisposing factor because of scant mucus. Similarly, a small, tight endocervical canal and a tight internal os may be improved by careful but not overzealous dilatation. It has been suggested that the passage of sounds or dilators through the cervix is attended by a large measure of success in overcoming infertility. Such success cannot be assigned to the process of dilatation alone, however, because it was also recommended that this procedure be followed by coitus with the woman in the knee-chest position. Thus, hypothalamic and other stimuli might have had more effect than the cervical dilatation. If one chooses to follow this advice, care should be taken not to traumatize the endocervix by the use of large dilators and, perhaps, predispose the patient to subsequent midtrimester abortion because of cervical incompetence.

Specific cervical lesions and infections demand careful and individual attention. If biopsy reveals invasive carcinoma, the indicated treatment immediately ends reproductive potential. If carcinoma in situ is found, conservative therapy may allow further childbearing if the patient agrees to frequent follow-up examinations. Large endocervical polyps should be excised and the bases lightly cauterized. Although cervical erosions and eversions are commonly found in infertile patients, their etiologic significance has been overemphasized. Nevertheless, erosions and eversions should be corrected through cryosurgery, but care should be taken not to destroy the endocervical mucosa. Gentle passage of a uterine sound should be performed after healing is com-

plete, to prevent stenosis. Severely lacerated and distorted cervices occasionally may be improved by meticulous plastic surgery, comprising excision of the scar and restoration of as much as possible of the normal anatomy of the portio vaginalis cervicis.

Acute cervicitis should be treated with antibiotics specifically indicated by cultures and by sensitivity study of the responsible organism. *T. mycoplasma* should be suspected, and appropriate cultures performed in patients who are habitual aborters. Patients and husbands with positive cultures should be treated with tetracycline. At a later date, chronic foci of infection in the cervix should be obliterated by cauterization or by the use of topically or systemically administered antibiotics, or both. Recent evidence suggests that enzymatic debridement with fibrinogen-deoxyribonuclease preparations may be less traumatic to the cervix than cautery. In certain instances the anatomic or physiologic insufficiency of the cervix may be overcome by artificial insemination with the husband's semen. The use of polyethylene cups that are trimmed to fit the contours of the grossly abnormal cervix has simplified this technique.

Recent studies have shown that cervical secretions may contain ABO antibodies, thus suggesting an etiologic concept of infertility based on agglutination of the sperm by these secretions in incompatible ABO matings [6, 7, 17]. Therefore, blood types should be checked in all patients who have infertility of apparently unknown cause. Research in the field of immunology will undoubtedly clarify many unsettled questions in the field of infertility, but direct clinical application is not possible at this time.

Various diagnostic tests have been designed to test the cervical factor in infertility. These are (1) evaluation of cervical mucus for arborization and spinnbarkeit, (2) the postcoital test, (3) an in vitro test of mucus penetration by spermatozoa, (4) determination of pH of cervical mucus, (5) tests of cervical glucose, (6) test of cervical mucus chloride, (7) assays of changes in cervical mucus proteins, and (8) cultures of the cervix.

For a complete review of the cervical factor in infertility the reader is referred to Davajan [6, 7].

### The Incompetent Cervix

The first operation for repair of incompetence of the internal os was performed by Douay in France in 1938 [8], although the first case report is credited to Palmer and Lacomme. Since the report of the latter authors in 1948 [24], a variety of operations for surgical correction of this condition, in either the gravid or nongravid state, have been described. Among them are those suggested by Baden and Baden, Barter and associates, Lash, McDonald, and Shirodkar [1, 2, 18, 20, 26].

The incompetent internal os of the cervix is due to an abnormally enlarged canal at the corporocervical junction; the degree of this enlargement varies. When the enlargement is moderate or severe, repeated abortions occur, particularly during the second trimester, regardless of whether the patient is in a constant supine position or has been subjected to medical therapy.

The causes of incompetence of the internal cervical os often are related to rapid and traumatic dilatation secondary to (1) overzealous dilatation of the cervix for diagnostic curettage or abortion, (2) wide conization of the cervix, (3) precipitate delivery due to tumultuous uterine contractions (spontaneous or drug induced) or to an obstetrical operation involving forceps or version and extraction, or (4) poor uterine wound healing due to improper myometrial coaptation or infection after a cesarean section. However, since cervical incompetence has been reported in primiparous women [18] who have had no previous cervical manipulation, it is felt that a congenital factor is responsible in some patients. One might also conclude that a latent weakness in the sphincter mechanism of the internal os is aggravated in certain individuals; this is termed *functional incompetence* by Mann [19]. This form was undiagnosable in most patients until its onset and accounted for 10 percent of patients in this series. Obviously, because the procedures mentioned here occur more often than does the incompetent cervix, many cervical injuries heal primarily without leaving a scar or defect in the circumference of the corporocervical area.

One of the major causes of cervical incompetence is wide conization of the cervix. In the past there has been a tendency to resort immediately to diagnostic conization if cytologic studies indicated the possibility of dysplasia or carcinoma in situ. Fortunately, diagnostic conization is no longer the keystone of pretreatment evaluation in most clinics in the United States. The wide application of culposcopy and selected cervical biopsy has largely replaced diagnostic cone biopsy.

For more than forty years, the diagnostic regimen for patients with abnormal cytologic findings at the Boston Hospital for Women (now part of the Brigham and Women's Hospital) consisted of multiple biopsies combined with endocervical curettage. The most serious error encountered in the evaluation of a cervix is that which leads to inadequate treatment of invasive cancer. The fear of overlooking invasive cancer when biopsies alone are employed is given as the primary reason for conization. It should be emphasized, however, that unsuspected invasive cancer has been found in 0.8 to 4.0 percent of hysterectomy specimens in which the preoperative conization disclosed only carcinoma in situ. At the Boston Hospital for Women (now part of the Brigham and Women's Hospital) the diagnostic accuracy in 513 patients who were evaluated by multiple biopsies and endocervical curettage was 94.7 percent, and no patient was undertreated.

If the patient agrees to prolonged follow-up and is anxious to have children, and if the carcinoma in situ is

limited to the squamocolumnar junction in an everted cervix and the canal is normal, a therapeutic conization is recommended. If dysplasia is the only lesion found, cryosurgery is performed. Of 34 patients so treated, 12 have had a total of 21 children and 7 miscarriages. If electrocauterization is performed, care should be taken to avoid the endocervical canal. Dilatation of the cervix should be performed subsequent to healing. This permits better drainage and minimizes the possibility of subsequent stenosis. Local antibiotics should be used after electrocauterization and cryosurgery. If conization is performed, the endocervical canal should not be excised, and care should be taken not to carry the incision too deeply into the stroma. Increased use of the carbon dioxide laser for treatment of cervical dysplasia should reduce the use of cone biopsy and cryosurgery.

*Diagnosis*

The diagnosis of the incompetent cervical os is based on a history of repeated abortions, especially during the second trimester of pregnancy. These repeated or habitual abortions are characterized by a painless presentation of the bulging membranes at the external os of the cervix, and this is usually followed by rupture of the membranes and relatively painless expulsion of the fetus (Fig. 3-1). Occasionally, slight spotting or an increase in cervical secretions may precede the rupture. Upon examination with a speculum, there is the unusual sight of the bulging membranes and the occasional moving extremity. In the nonpregnant state, however, physical examination reveals no abnormality. Only

**Figure 3-1.** Incompetent cervical os seen during the thirty-second week of gestation. The cervix is widely patulous and the membranes are clearly visible. (From C. L. Easterday and D. E. Reid, The incompetent cervix in repetitive abortion and premature labor. *N. Engl. J. Med.* 260:687, 1959. Reprinted with permission.)

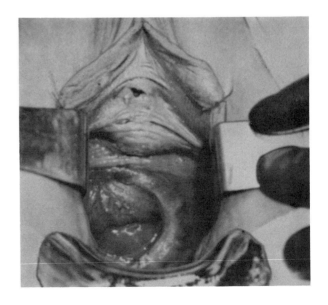

by exploration of the cervical canal with a uterine dressing forceps or Hegar dilator is the lack of resistance at the internal os discovered.

If a No. 9 Hegar dilator can be passed through the cervix without resistance, the internal os is theoretically incompetent. However, this sign may be present in many multiparous women in whom habitual abortion does not occur.

Hysterography has been utilized for the detection of the incompetent cervical os, and it has been stated that an isthmic width of 8 mm or more is a definite sign of incompetence. This corresponds to a No. 8 Hegar dilator. By hysterography, the width of the internal os may be noted to change during various phases of the menstrual cycle, and therefore the test is ideally performed during the secretory phase, when the natural width of the internal os is smallest.

Another observation made in patients having cervical incompetence is that at the time of dilatation and curettage, the distinct snapping closure of the internal os that is characteristic as the dilator is withdrawn does not occur.

Although all of the previously mentioned techniques are helpful, the only certain way to diagnose cervical incompetence is to suspect it from the history and then, by weekly vaginal examinations, take notice of the gradual opening of the internal os.

The history is all-important. In a typical case of cervical incompetence, 2 or more painless abortions have occurred between the sixteenth and twenty-eighth weeks. There may be a mucoid discharge followed by rupture of the membranes and expulsion of the fetus or the entire ovisac without appreciable discomfort and without bleeding. A history of the membranes rupturing first is believed by some to be a diagnostic sign, but this is not invariably true. Whenever the history is not typical, all other causes of abortion should be eliminated by thorough investigation.

### Cervical Incompetence Associated with Diethylstilbestrol Exposure in Utero

There are a number of case reports of "incompetent cervix" successfully treated with cervical cerclage among women exposed to diethylstilbestrol (DES) in utero. The documented anomalies of the uterus found in such patients make the possibility of cervical defects likely. In 1978, Singer and Hochman [27] reported incompetent cervix in a female thought to have been exposed to DES in utero. Goldstein [12] followed nine DES-exposed pregnant females and noted that 5 developed cervical incompetency during the second trimester of pregnancy. Only 1 of these patients had experienced a previous second trimester loss, and she was treated with a perma-

nent cerclage (Mersilene band) and subsequently delivered by cesarean section. Three of the remaining 4 patients had experienced early spontaneous abortion, and 1 patient had not been pregnant previously. All 4 were followed at weekly intervals and, when painless effacement of the cervix was noted, were treated with a modified Shirodkar cerclage, and all 4 carried to term. Goldstein stated that 3 of these 5 patients had vaginal adenosis in the nonpregnant state and "all patients had markedly abnormal appearing cervices which were hypoplastic, flush with the vaginal apex, and measured less than 1 cm in length" [12].

Recently, Herbst [14] reported a study of pregnancy experience in DES-exposed daughters and confirmed a higher rate of premature birth in this group. Among women in the exposed group, term pregnancy occurred in 40 and premature stillborn births in 25. Also among this exposed group, 5 women had cervical cerclage after experiencing prior premature stillbirth or miscarriage, and all 5 subsequently delivered live infants.

The cause of cervical incompetence in these DES-exposed patients is unknown; however, it has been suggested that the fibromuscular junction might be misplaced from the internal os to a lower site in the cervical canal, and therefore, it might interfere with the sphincter mechanism of the internal os [27]. Kaufman et al. [15] demonstrated a T-shaped anomaly of the uterus in DES-exposed women by hysterography; however, the endocervical canal was not specifically examined in that study. Nunley and Kitchin [22] recently reported a single case in which a 28-year-old nulligravida female known to have been exposed to DES in utero became pregnant. This patient demonstrated a T-shaped uterine cavity on previous hysterogram. Progressive cervical effacement began at 14 to 16 weeks, and a McDonald cerclage was placed. She delivered at 38 weeks after going into spontaneous labor. Cesarean section was performed because of failure to dilate. At present, a specific uterine anomaly has not been associated with cervical incompetence. However, all patients exposed in utero to DES should be followed carefully during early pregnancy, and the possibility of this defect considered.

### Cervical Incompetence Associated with an Anomalous Uterus

Dr. William Keetle [16] appears to have been the first to call attention to the association between cervical incompetence and congenital uterine defects. Dr. Keetle related the courses of five patients with uterine anomaly who were treated successfully with a permanent Shirodkar cerclage procedure at the University of Iowa. Four of these patients had a bicornuate uterus and one a unicornuate uterus. The first patient found to have a bicornuate uterus had undergone a unification procedure only to subsequently suffer three spontaneous abortions and one premature delivery. A Shirodkar cerclage was then placed while the patient was not pregnant; she later gave birth to a term infant. The other four patients all had a similar cerclage prior to pregnancy. Three of these patients then had term deliveries, and the fourth failed to conceive because of divorce. Dr. Keetle concluded, "It is our present belief that certain patients with congenital defects of the uterus also have defects of the internal os" [16].

Ten years later, Craig [4] reported the use of a Shirodkar cervical cerclage combined with a Tompkins metroplasty to improve postoperative pregnancy results. This surgeon performed a Tompkins metroplasty on 23 patients, 14 of whom underwent combined metroplasty-cerclage procedure. Of interest, 1 additional patient with a unicornuate uterus was also successfully treated with a cerclage procedure. Postoperative pregnancy results were not reported for individual groups; however, preoperatively, only 15 of 115 pregnancies resulted in live infants, compared to 55 of 57 pregnancies following surgical intervention. Craig concluded that "any case of incompetent cervix should have an investigation of the fundus of the uterus performed before a Shirodkar suture is employed as definitive treatment" [4].

Two reports from Israel appear to support a primary role for cervical cerclage in the prevention of pregnancy wastage due to a uterine anomaly. In 1974 Gros et al. [13] reported their experience with 61 patients who had uterine anomaly. In this group, 57 patients had bicornuate uteri, 2 had unicornuate uteri, and 2, didelphic uteri. A treatment plan was reported in which 30 patients were not treated, and 26 patients, including 2 with unicornuate uteri and 24 with bicornuate uteri, were treated with cervical cerclage. Five additional patients had a surgical unification procedure. In the entire group prior to treatment, 161 pregnancies had resulted in 95 spontaneous abortions, 17 missed abortions, and only 28 term deliveries. Postoperatively, 26 patients in the cerclage treatment group produced 20 viable pregnancies and three spontaneous abortions. Twenty of 26 patients produced living infants. In 1977, Blum [3] reported the results of primary therapy with a McDonald cerclage procedure in 43 patients with uterine anomaly and poor obstetrical history. This group included bicornuate uterus in 23 patients, arcuate uterus in 13, uterus didelphys in 5 and unicornuate uterus in 2. Preoperatively, only 19 of 106 pregnancies resulted in a living infant, compared to 48 of 55 pregnancies following treatment with a McDonald cerclage.

Although cervical cerclage has not been considered a primary form of treatment in the United States for patients with bicornuate or septate uterus, it certainly may be a useful adjunct in those patients who have undergone a unification procedure. The therapeutic valve of cerclage in patients with a uterine anomaly is discussed in Chapter 4.

*Therapeutic Principles*

Following the original articles on cervical cerclage by Palmer and Shirodkar, numerous articles have been written and opinions expressed both for and against the procedure [1, 2, 9, 10, 25, 28]. Furthermore, modifications of the operation have been suggested that vary the sutures or their method of placement. However, the principle of producing an area of resistance to increasing intrauterine pressure is the same.

We prefer a slight modification of the Shirodkar procedure but agree that the most important part of the procedure is the placement of the suture or sutures as far as possible above the internal cervical os. By placement at this point, constant protrusion of the membranes, which may stimulate uterine contractions, is prevented. Those surgeons who place the suture below the internal os claim a large measure of success, and no doubt it simplifies the operation and minimizes hemorrhage [20]. However, we have not been impressed by excessive bleeding with our technique. Some workers have recommended a procedure (McDonald) in which a purse-string suture of braided silk is put around the cervix [20]. Others have described a method in which a suture actually closes the external os [20]. However, the original method of Shirodkar is so simple and free from hemorrhage that we have continued to use it.

One of the major controversial points is whether the operation should be done with the patient in the pregnant or the nonpregnant state. We agree with Shirodkar that the operation is best performed during pregnancy. The nonpregnant cervix is not pliable and, therefore, it is impossible to judge the tightness of the closure. However, there are certain instances in which the procedure is indicated during the nonpregnant state, and, therefore we have included the Lash operation in this chapter.

Surgery is usually scheduled about the fourteenth to sixteenth week of gestation, because the cervix at this time is soft, and closure is accomplished quite easily. The vaginal walls are not as friable or excessively vascular as during the later weeks of pregnancy. However, cerclage can be performed as late as the twenty-seventh week.

CERVICAL CERCLAGE

*Temporary.* The procedure may be done under light general, low spinal, or epidural anesthetic. The bladder should be emptied by catheterization. The cervix is exposed with a Sims' speculum, and a culture is taken from the external os. The field is prepared with tincture of benzalkonium chloride (Zephiran) and a pelvic examination is performed. The size and shape of the uterus and the position of the cervix are noted. A self-retaining retractor is placed over the posterior vaginal wall and perineal body.

A solution of epinephrine (1:1000 in saline) is injected into the anterior vaginal mucosa at the level of the internal cervical os. This is repeated posteriorly at the level of the insertion of the uterosacral ligaments.

The anterior vaginal mucosa is then stretched with a thumb forceps, and a transverse incision is made. Figure 3-2 shows this incision and describes the remainder of the operative procedure.

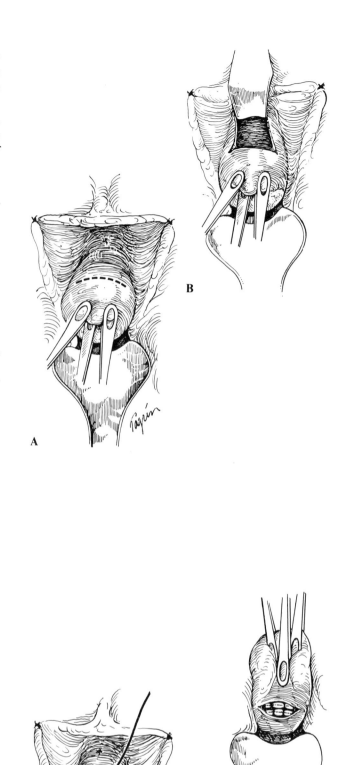

**Figure 3-2.** Temporary cervical cerclage. **A.** A transverse incision is made in anterior vaginal mucosa. The incision is extended laterally on either side for a distance of about 1.5 cm. **B.** After a few fibers of the vesicouterine ligament have been divided, the lowermost portion of the bladder may be easily advanced, and a small speculum is inserted under the bladder. **C.** The mucosa of the posterior vaginal wall is similarly incised, care being taken not to enter the posterior cul-de-sac. Therefore, the incision should be made about 1 cm from the insertion of the uterosacral ligaments on the cervix. The incision is similarly extended laterally. **D.** An Allis clamp is placed across the anterior and posterior edges of the lateral vaginal mucosa, folding it together and facilitating passage of the needle. The suture material is a tubule of 0 surgical steel encased in 26-gauge polyethylene tubing measuring 0.2 inches by 0.067 inches (inside diameter, 0.047 inches). The large needle is swedged on both ends of the tubule (Ethicon No. D-3865). A 5 mm Mersilene tape, produced by Ethicon, is also used. The needle is passed from the anterior incision submucosally around the lateral aspect of the cervix at 9 o'clock. **E.** The needle is brought out through the posterior incision. **F.** The needle is then directed around the 3 o'clock position and emerges anteriorly at the same level as the proximal end. This suture is not tied at this time, but is held for traction. **G.** Because the placement of the temporary suture is usually found to be below the desired level, a second suture is placed in exactly the same fashion at a slightly higher level. The second suture is usually adjacent to the internal cervical os. Traction on the cervix is then made toward the operator with DeLee's clamps. The operator inserts the index finger of his or her left hand into the patulous cervix and determines the level of the internal os. The assistant then ties the suture at that level as the operator's finger is gradually withdrawn. The previously placed suture is then tied in similar fashion. **H.** The excess suture material is then removed with a wirecutter, and a small bead of lead shot is clamped over the short ends of the wire. **I.** The wire sutures are then fixed into position both anteriorly and posteriorly with two interrupted sutures of 2-0 Mersilene (Ethicon). **J.** The anterior and posterior mucosal incisions are then closed with interrupted sutures of 3-0 chromic catgut. Neither vaginal packing nor an indwelling catheter is used.

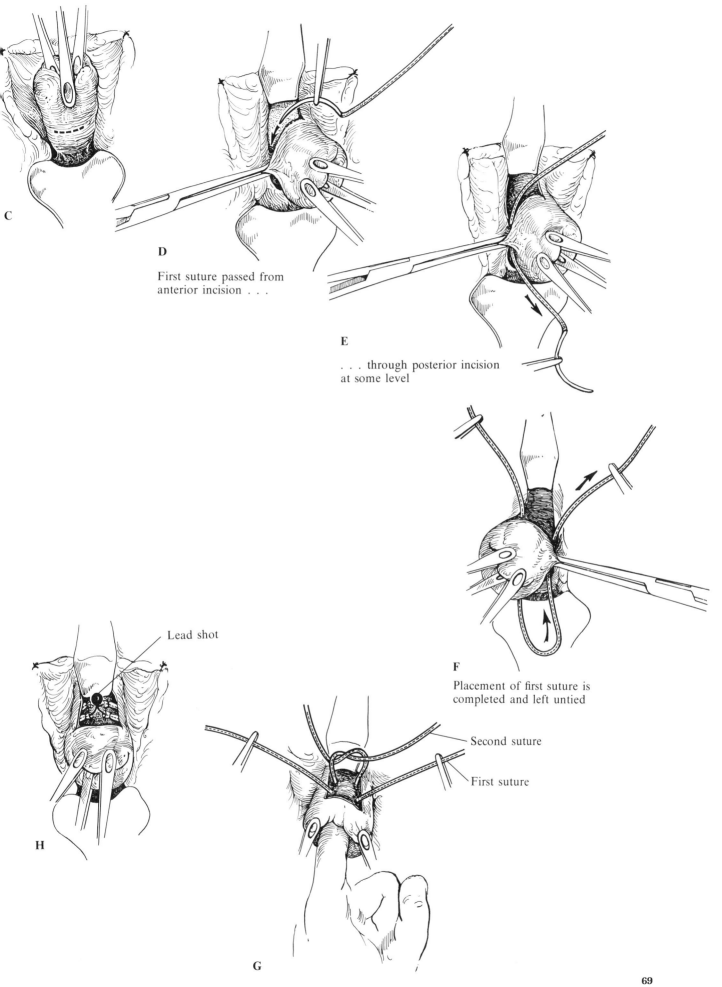

**C**

**D**

First suture passed from
anterior incision . . .

**E**

. . . through posterior incision
at some level

**F**

Placement of first suture is
completed and left untied

Second suture

First suture

Lead shot

**H**

**G**

69

*Permanent (Mersilene Band Technique).* The vaginal preparation and mucosal incisions are performed as in the temporary cerclage procedure. The technique of permanent cerclage is shown in Figure 3-3.

The patient is kept in bed for the first 24 hours postoperatively, and ambulation is initiated on the second postoperative day. Postoperative pain is minimal, but analgesic drugs may be used as necessary for uterine cramping. The effectiveness of progesterone or synthetic progestins is difficult to evaluate and is infrequently used by us.

The patient is usually discharged on the third postoperative day and is cautioned against having douches, intercourse, and tub baths for the first 2 weeks after surgery. She is examined in the office 2 weeks after surgery, at which time the position and integrity of the cerclage are evaluated.

**Figure 3-3.** Permanent cervical cerclage. **A.** A special curved clamp with perforated tip is inserted through the posterior incision and curved around the 3 o'clock position of the cervix, emerging through the anterior incision. One edge of the Mersilene band (woven strip 5 mm wide [Ethicon No. RS-20]) is grasped with the clamp and brought submucosally around the cervix and out through the posterior incision. (The Mersilene band is also supplied with swedged-on needles, eliminating the use of the grasping clamp.) **B.** A curved clamp is placed through the anterior incision and curved around the 9 o'clock position of the cervix, emerging through the posterior incision. The end of the Mersilene suture is grasped and brought around the curvature of the cervix and out through the anterior incision. **C.** The Mersilene may be folded through a small aperture in the band and drawn to the proper degree of occlusion. This should be accomplished with a finger in the cervix to determine the exact aperture desired. **D.** The Mersilene band is fixed both anteriorly and posteriorly with interrupted sutures of 2-0 Mersilene to prevent the band from slipping off. **E.** The mucosa is closed both anteriorly and posteriorly with interrupted sutures of 3-0 chromic catgut.

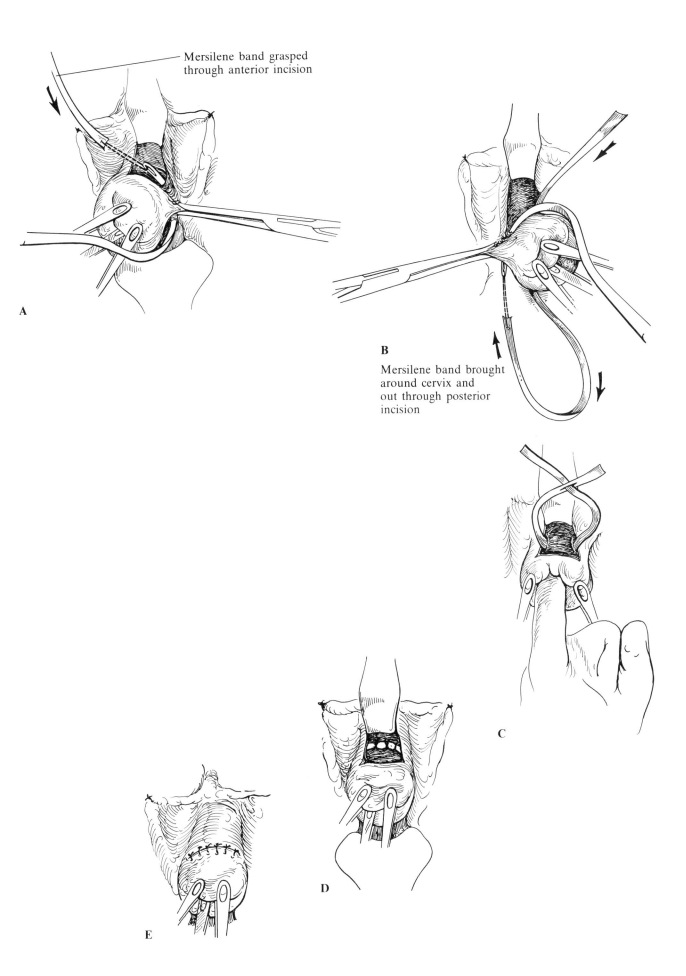

Mersilene band grasped through anterior incision

**A**

**B**

Mersilene band brought around cervix and out through posterior incision

**C**

**D**

**E**

*Method of Lash.* Lash [18] has long been of the opinion that when a scar is present in the enlarged isthmic ring of the uterus in a nonpregnant patient, it should be removed and the normal status of the supportive ring restored along surgical principles. Lash disagrees with the position of delaying surgery until the patient is pregnant. He has stated that treatment of the incompetent cervical os aims to restore the normal caliber of the isthmus either by closure of the defect or by excision of the scar tissue in the area of the defect. This defect may range from 1.5 to 2.0 cm in width and from 2.5 to 3.5 cm in length. With a Hegar dilator placed in the canal, palpation of the corporocervical junction discloses a defect in the ring that is usually found anteriorly but occasionally is situated obliquely or laterally. Occasionally this condition is associated with a longer cervical laceration through the external os. Sometimes a hypoplastic or retrodisplaced uterus is found associated with this large opening into the uterine cavity. Figure 3-4A shows a typical defect producing cervical incompetence. Figure 3-4B through I shows Lash's technique of repairing such a defect.

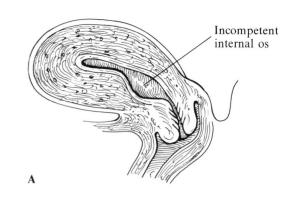

Incompetent internal os

A

**Figure 3-4.** Lash procedure for repair of the incompetent internal os of the cervix. **A.** Representative defect in cervical incompetence. The site of the defect may be anterior, lateral, or oblique. **B.** A semicircular incision is made in the vaginal mucosa over the defect. **C.** The mucosal flap is dissected free and held under a retractor. An elliptical incision is made around the defect. **D.** The wedge-shaped portion of endocervix removed should be adequate to cover the entire defect. It approximates 3 to 4 cm in length, 2 to 3 cm in width, and 0.5 cm in depth. A No. 4 Hegar dilator is inserted through the external os into the uterine cavity. **E.** The first layer of 0 chromic catgut sutures is placed directly over the dilator. There should be no tension on the suture line. **F.** A second layer of 0 chromic catgut sutures is placed above the first. If the tissues appear poorly vascularized, Mersilene or stainless steel suture material may be used. **G.** The second-layer sutures are tied. **H.** The cardinal ligaments are imbricated over the upper portion of the suture line for added support at the level of the internal os. **I.** The mucosal flap is closed over the repair with interrupted sutures of 0 chromic catgut.

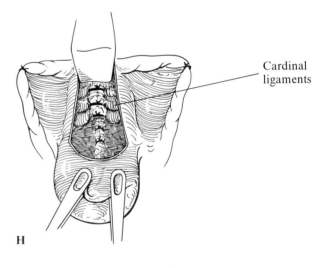

Cardinal ligaments

H

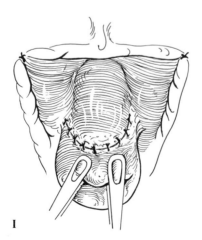

I

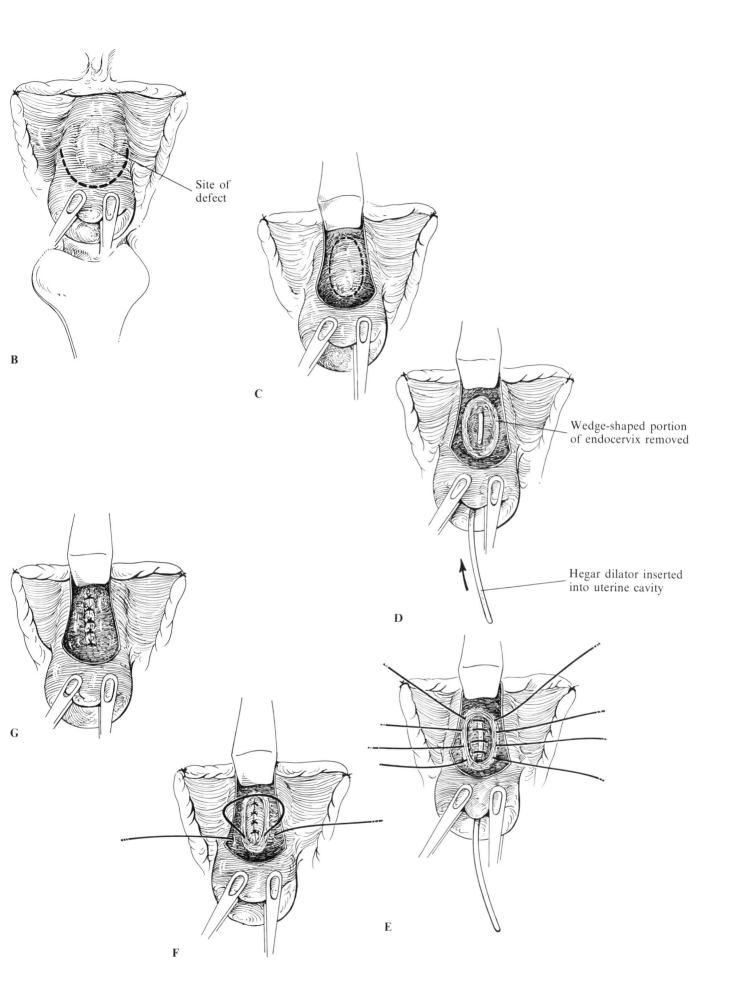

**B**

Site of
defect

**C**

**D**

Wedge-shaped portion
of endocervix removed

Hegar dilator inserted
into uterine cavity

**G**

**F**

**E**

When the Lash procedure is performed on patients who have had previous unsuccessful cerclages during pregnancy or reconstructive cervical surgery, one may see that the bladder was drawn down into the cervical defect and is intimately attached to it. In order to avoid entrance into the bladder, a Kelly clamp should be introduced through the urethra after the mucosal flap has been reflected. This will delineate the lowermost portion of the bladder. Indigo carmine solution may be instilled into the bladder to detect minute perforations during the dissection. Reflection of the bladder from the cervix in such patients demands meticulous dissection.

Following surgery the patients are ambulatory during the first 24 hours and are discharged the next day. Patients are advised not to have intercourse for at least 1 month and to avoid pregnancy for at least 6 months.

*Balloon Technique.* Yosowitz and associates [29] more recently introduced an inflatable silicone cuff for treatment of the incompetent cervix. This device is a plastic ring with two fluid-inflatable balloons attached to its inner and outer surfaces. The procedure is carried out in the physician's office, eliminating the need for surgery and anesthesia. Problems associated with placement of the silicone cuff have been minimal. Several women had vaginal discharge, apparently due to the foreign body, but they were treated successfully with appropriate antibiotic suppositories. There were no instances of vaginal discomfort or bleeding. None of the patients aborted. The data on the silicone cuff are preliminary, but there is a question as to whether it will be able to prevent cervical effacement and dilatation after the thirty-sixth week. The end result will be a viable but premature infant.

First the cuff is placed on the cervix. The cervix is then pulled through the center of the cuff with ring forceps, and the balloon adjacent to the cervix is inflated with 6 ml of saline solution. The filling tube is ligated with nonabsorbable suture as close to the vagina as possible. The outer balloon is also inflated with saline and ligated. The excess tubing is cut from both balloons distal to the ligating sutures.

After placement of the cuff, the patient should be permitted to resume normal activities but should refrain from coitus for a 2-week period. Ideally, the cuff should be placed in position during the middle trimester and observed weekly. When dilatation occurs at the end of normal gestation, the cuff usually slips off the cervix and is easily removed from the vaginal canal without deflating the balloons. If the balloons must be deflated for premature removal, the filling tubes may be cut distal to the cuff, thus permitting escape of the saline solution.

TRANSABDOMINAL ISTHMIC CERCLAGE

Most patients found to have cervical incompetence will be treated with a temporary vaginal cerclage procedure, as was described earlier. There appears, however, to be a small group of patients in whom this is not possible, either because the cervix is extremely short or because it has been deeply lacerated and scarred during a previous delivery or traumatic dilatation and curettage. Recently, Novy [21] has drawn attention to the benefit of transabdominal cervical cerclage in this group of patients.

Originally described by Benson and Durfee, the technique of transabdominal cerclage has since been described in detail by Novy [21]. This procedure is usually performed in the pregnant patient at 13 to 15 weeks' gestation, although it has been performed as late as 24 weeks. A Mersilene tape is threaded between the uterine vessels and placed around the cervix at the level of the isthmus. Most patients have been delivered by cesarean section, although it has been stated that removal is possible through a posterior colpotomy incision.

Novy has stated that at the University of Oregon School of Medicine, one transabdominal cerclage procedure was performed for each 5 vaginal procedures. Although the authors of this text have not employed transabdominal cerclage in the treatment of cervical incompetence, it would appear that a small group of patients may benefit from this procedure. In particular, the hypoplastic cervix found in the female exposed to DES in utero may occasionally require this type of cervical cerclage.

*Results*

Shirodkar [26] has reported a series of 305 cases in which the rate of fetal salvage was 10.1 percent prior to cervical cerclage. Subsequent to the surgical procedure, the fetal salvage rate was 81 percent. Lash [18] treated 117 patients between 1941 and 1963, but was able to report follow-up data on only 93 of these. Seventy-six percent of these patients became pregnant and 85 percent of these progressed to term. Seppala and Vara [25] reported results of 163 cerclages performed on 159 women. Most of the operations were done at about 14 weeks of gestation, and the pregnancies usually lasted 35 weeks. The success rate was 83.2 percent, as compared with 30.8 percent for the previous pregnancies of the same patients. Recently, O'Brien and Murphy [23] performed a McDonald cerclage procedure in 100 patients. An 88 percent success rate was achieved in this group. There were only 10 cesarean sections performed in this group, 7 of which were due to the patients' poor obstetrical histories. In the experience of one of us (G.W.P.) using a modified Shirodkar procedure described earlier in 20 patients, all of whom had lost at least 1 previous pregnancy, 18 achieved living infants following surgery.

The speculation that patients treated for cervical incompetence may subsequently have some impairment of fertility has had no real documentation. It has been postulated that there may be interference with the so-called insuck reflex and with spermatozoal migration [24]. However, because secondary infertility itself is not a rare phenomenon, it is difficult to incriminate the correction of the cervical incompetence per se as the cause of the subsequent infertility.

Lash, in evaluating this problem with respect to his operative procedure, pointed out that advancing age may play a role; 55 percent of his patients who had had surgery and failed in attempts to conceive were over 35 years of age and may have had other pathologic conditions of the uterus that were detrimental to fertility. He also observed that the time required for conception following surgery was not increased over the time required for individual patients' first conception, and that certain patients who had had 2 or 3 operations for cervical incompetence had no subsequent difficulty in conceiving.

Yosowitz and associates have reported [29] results of the balloon technique in 30 patients with cervical incompetence. The results were comparable to cerclages performed by the McDonald or Shirodkar techniques (roughly 80 to 85 percent). The average length of gestation was 36 weeks and the average birth weight was 5 lb 2 oz. This technique cannot be used when cervical dilatation and effacement have progressed to any significant degree. Because the balloon method is a simple office procedure, it should be used at 12 to 14 weeks of gestation, before changes in the cervix have occurred. The simplicity of the procedure should allow latitude regarding indications.

## References

1. Baden, W. F., and Baden, E. E. Cervical incompetence: Current therapy. *Am. J. Obstet. Gynecol.* 79:545, 1960.
2. Barter, R. M., Dusbabek, J. A., Tyndal, C. M., and Erkenbach, R. V. Further experiences with the Shirodkar operation. *Am. J. Obstet. Gynecol.* 85:792, 1963.
3. Blum, M. Prevention of spontaneous abortion by cervical suture of the malformed uterus. *Int. Surg.* 62:213, 1977.
4. Craig, C. J. T. Congenital abnormalities of the uterus and fetal wastage. *S. Afro. Med. J.* 47:2000, 1973.
5. Danforth, A. N. Fibrous nature of the human cervix in its relation to the isthmic segment in gravid and nongravid uteri. *Am. J. Obstet. Gynecol.* 53:541, 1947.
6. Davajan, V., and Kunitake, G. M. Fractional in vivo and in vitro examination of postcoital cervical mucus in the human. *Fertil. Steril.* 20:197, 1969.
7. Davajan, V. The Cervical Factor. In S. J. Behrman and R. W. Kistner (eds.), *Progress in Infertility* (2nd ed.). Boston: Little, Brown, 1975.
8. Douay, M. E. Discussion of paper by R. Palmer and M. Lacomme. *Gynecol. Obstet.* 47:905, 1948.
9. Durfee, R. B. Surgical treatment of the incompetent cervix during pregnancy. *Obstet. Gynecol.* 12:91, 1958.
10. Easterday, C. L., and Reid, D. E. The incompetent cervix in repetitive abortion and premature labor. *N. Engl. J. Med.* 260:687, 1959.
11. Fluhmann, C. F. *The Cervix Uteri and Its Diseases.* Philadelphia: Saunders, 1961.
12. Goldstein, D. P. Incompetent cervix in offspring exposed to diethylstilbestrol in utero. *Obstet. Gynecol.* 52[suppl.]:73, 1978.
13. Gros, A., David, A., and Serr, D. M. Management of congenital malformation of the uterus: Fetal salvage. *Acta Eur. Fertil.* 5:301, 1974.
14. Herbst, A. L., Hubby, M. M., Blough, R. R., and Freidoon, A. A comparison of pregnancy experience in DES-exposed and DES-unexposed daughters. *J. of Reprod. Med.* 24:62, 1980.
15. Kaufman, R. H., Binder, G. L., Gray, P. M., and Ervin, A. Upper genital tract changes associated with exposure in utero to diethylstilbestrol. *Am. J. Obstet. Gynecol.* 128:51, 1977.
16. Keetle, W. C., Comments in R. M. Barter et al., Further experiences with the Shirodkar operation. *Am. J. Obstet. Gynecol.* 85:802, 1963.
17. Kunitake, G. M., and Davajan, V. A new method of evaluating infertility due to cervical mucus-spermatozoa incompatibility. *Fertil. Steril.* 21:706, 1970.
18. Lash, A. F. Review of more than 20 years' experience with the incompetent internal os of the cervix. *Fertil. Steril.* 15:254, 1964.
19. Mann, E. C. Comments in R. M. Barter et al., Further experiences with the Shirodkar operation. *Am. J. Obstet. Gynecol.* 85:804, 1963.
20. McDonald, I. A. Suture of the cervix for inevitable miscarriage. *J. Obstet. Gynaecol. Br. Emp.* 64:346, 1957.
21. Novy, M. J. Managing reproductive failure by transabdominal isthmic cerclage. *Contemporary OB/GYN* 10:17, 1977.
22. Nunley, W. C., and Kitchin, J. D. Successful management of incompetent cervix in a primigravida exposed to diethylstilbestrol in utero. *Fertil. Steril.* 31:217, 1979.
23. O'Brien, D. P., and Murphy, J. F. The value of cervical cerclage in the treatment of cervical incompetence. *Ir. J. Med. Sci.* 147:197, 1978.
24. Palmer, R., and Lacomme, M. La béance de l'orifice interne, cause d'avortements à la petition? Une observation de déchirure cervical isthmique reparée chirugicalment, avec gestation à larme consécutive. *Gynecol. Obstet.* 47:905, 1948.
25. Seppala, M., and Vara, P. Cervical cerclage in treatment of incompetent cervix. *Acta Obstet. Gynecol. Scand.* 49:343, 1970.
26. Shirodkar, V. N. *Progress in Gynecology.* New York: Grune & Stratton, 1963. P. 260.
27. Singer, M. S., and Hochman, M. Incompetent cervix in a hormone-exposed offspring. *Obstet. Gynecol.* 51:625, 1978.
28. Stromme, W. B., Reed, S. C., Wagner, R. M., and Haywa, E. W. Surgical management of repeated late abortions. *Minn. Med.* 41:843, 1958.
29. Yosowitz, E. E., Haufrect, F., Kaufman, R. H., and Goyette, R. E. Silicone-plastic cuff for the treatment of the incompetent cervix in pregnancy. *Am. J. Obstet. Gynecol.* 113:233, 1972.

### The Double Uterus

The gynecologic surgeon usually encounters congenital anomalies of the female generative tract as an incidental finding unrelated to the chief complaint of the patient. Occasionally a patient may note dyspareunia caused by a vaginal septum, and, even less often, a uterine anomaly may be found as the major factor in the etiology of habitual abortion. This orientation is important because the isolated finding of a double uterus does not prove its role in infertility. This section describes the embryologic deviations that lead to abnormal uterine formation, the clinical evidence that relates certain uterine abnormalities to pregnancy wastage, and, finally, the surgical correction of these abnormalities. A new group of uterine defects found to occur in females exposed to diethylstilbestrol (DES) in utero will also be discussed.

The incidence of congenital abnormalities of the vagina and uterus in the general population is difficult to determine, because the vast majority of these anomalies are compatible with normal pregnancy. They are casually noted during routine obstetrical delivery or yearly examination but usually are not recorded. Jarcho [31] concluded that "lack of fusion of the müllerian ducts, either complete or incomplete, occurs once in 15,000 deliveries and once in 2000 gynecologic cases." Moore [47], however, stated that "the incidence of congenital abnormalities in the female genitalia is probably much higher . . . one in five or six hundred women present some definite congenital deviation from the normal." This higher incidence is supported by many studies, including that of Jones [36], who found the incidence of "women with genital anomalies" at the Providence Lying-in Hospital to be about 1 in 700. Semmens [60] found the incidence of uterine anomalies at two naval hospitals to be 1 in 625 births; only 33 of 59,170 outpatients had gynecologic complaints related to uterine anomalies, an incidence of 1 in 1800. Fenton and Singh [19] reported an incidence of 1 in 633 deliveries.

The number of patients who require medical attention because of genital anomalies, including habitual abortion, is not clear. During the years 1936 to 1975, 210 patients with double uterus were seen at the Johns Hopkins University Hospital [55]. One hundred twenty-nine of these patients (61 percent) received only routine care, although 29 of these patients demonstrated a poor obstetric history. Only 81 patients (39 percent) were actively treated for infertility, and 43 of these (20 percent) subsequently had corrective surgery. It should be noted that patients are referred to this hospital from all parts of the United States and foreign countries because of its interest in this problem.

Among 55 couples with histories of recurrent abortion evaluated by Byrd et al. [12], müllerian abnormalities were identified in 7 patients (11.7 percent). The uterine abnormality in each instance was a septate uterus. This group consisted of 44 couples with pure abortion histories and 11 couples with a mixed history of abortion and delivery of an abnormal child. Four of the patients with septate uteri did not undergo chromosome analysis, because they had not had an abnormal child, and it was assumed that such an analysis would have been normal. Therefore, the incidence of müllerian defects would appear to have been 7 of 48 patients. In contrast, chromosome defects were found in 3 of 44 couples without a living child, and in 7 of 11 couples who had experienced recurrent abortion and had delivered an abnormal child. Six of these individuals were found to be carriers of a balanced translocation.

*Embryology*

It is convenient to consider congenital anomalies of the female genital tract in relation to the stage of maturation at which deviation from normal development occurred. We have divided the process of müllerian duct formation into four embryologic stages to facilitate this correlation. These are (1) müllerian duct elongation, (2) fusion, (3) canalization, and (4) septum resorption.

The gonadal wolffian and müllerian ducts are mesodermal elements that arise from the urogenital ridge on the dorsal surface of the embryo lateral to the aorta. Because the development of the wolffian (male) ducts, müllerian (female) ducts, and urinary system of the female are closely intertwined, and congenital abnormalities of the uterus are often associated with anomalies of the renal collecting system, the embryology of both systems should be considered.

In the human embryo the urinary tract develops in three stages. The earliest and simplest organ, actually functionless, is termed the *pronephros* and consists of a pair of longitudinal pronephric ducts that extend along the dorsal surface of the embryo and empty into the cloaca (future bladder). These longitudinal ducts are retained throughout embryologic development and are a key structure, because they are incorporated into the mesonephric urinary system and are then called mesonephric ducts. In the male, these ducts in the indifferent stage are termed *wolffian ducts*; they are later incorporated into the genital system as the vas deferens. In the female these early ducts provide a guide for müllerian duct development. The remaining portions of the first urinary system are the pronephric tubules, which occur at each mesoblastic segment of the embryo as conduits which extend laterally, one end opening into the coelomic cavity and the other end into the collecting (pronephric) duct.

In the second stage the pronephros is replaced by a second, more complex collecting system termed the *mesonephros*. It functions only temporarily in the embryo. The essential elements of this second stage are more complicated tubules that interface with blood vessels as a glomerulus. They drain into the pronephric ducts which, as was noted above, are now called mesonephric ducts.

The third stage consists of the development of the adult kidney and its collecting system; it is termed the *metanephros*. In the present discussion it is convenient to refer back to the mesonephric (wolffian) ducts and recall the paired tubular structures coursing on the dorsal surface of the embryo and emptying into the cloaca. At about the fourth week of development (5 mm) in the human embryo the mesonephric (wolffian) duct makes a sharp bend before entering the cloaca. At this level (twenty-eighth somite, or future first sacral vertebra) a bud, or outgrowth, of tissue appears. This bud, termed the *ureteric bud*, grows at two points to form a tubelike structure that later separates from its early attachment to the mesonephric (wolffian) duct. It subsequently becomes the ureter and renal collecting system. The proximal portion of the ureteric bud differentiates into the future ureter and extends to the anterior portion of the cloaca. The distal blind end of this tube dilates and becomes the renal pelvis. This portion pushes into a mass of condensed tissue, a part of which separates and surrounds the future renal pelvis like a cap. This caplike tissue and future renal pelvis from the ureteric bud then differentiate into an adult kidney. Double ureters accompanied by double renal pelves, therefore, arise as double ureteric buds, and a branched ureter is caused by a forking of the proximal segment of the bud.

About the fifth or sixth week of embryologic development (5 to 12 mm) the genital tract begins to differentiate and enters the *indifferent stage* (Fig. 4-1). The gonad first appears as a thickening in part of the urogenital ridge that subsequently enlongates. These indifferent gonads subsequently differentiate into ovary and testis, depending on their genetic coding. The primordial germ cells are thought to originate in a separate area of the embryo, the yolk-sac entoderm, and later migrate into this mass of gonadal tissue. It is important to recall that because ovarian development is separate from that of the müllerian ducts, abnormalities of the uterus and tubes are usually associated with normal ovarian development.

**Figure 4-1.** Plan of the urogenital system at an early stage when it is still sexually undifferentiated. (Modified from Hertwig and presented in Bradley M. Patten, *Human Embryology* (3rd ed.). New York: McGraw-Hill, 1968. P. 476. Reprinted with permission.)

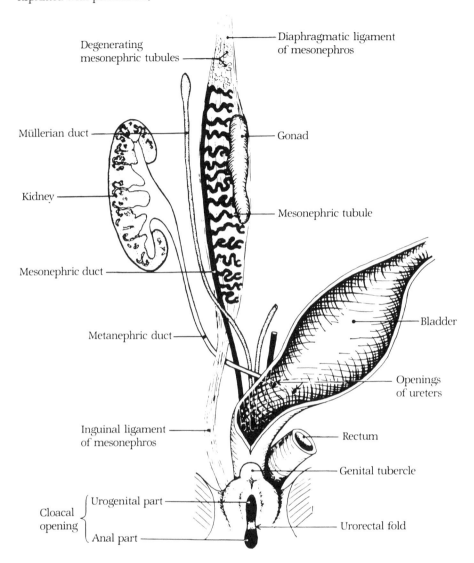

At this early stage (5 to 6 weeks) the müllerian ducts are first evident as an involution of the lateral portion of the urogenital ridge. A tubelike structure is formed bilaterally; in this structure the cranial end remains open to the abdominal (coelomic) cavity and later becomes the fimbriated end of the oviduct, whereas caudally the solid blind end advances by progressive growth. These ducts course laterally to the mesonephric ducts, but then swing toward the midline of the embryo and come to lie side by side. At 9 weeks the müllerian ducts end blindly in Müller's tubercle on the urogenital sinus. The cloaca is a saclike area in the distal embryo into which the ureters course anteriorly (site of future bladder), and the wolffian ducts and müllerian ducts enter posteriorly (site of future vagina).

The bilateral fused müllerian ducts later form the upper vagina, cervix, and uterus, and the nonfused ends become the oviducts (Fig. 4-2). Thus far we have described a process of müllerian duct descent and fusion. Absence of the duct unilaterally results in a hemiuterus (uterus unicornis), and lack of fusion results in a double hemiuterus (uterus didelphys, with double vagina, cervix, and uterus).

**Figure 4-2.** Plan of developing female reproductive system. The position of the ovary and uterine tube after their descent into the pelvis is indicated (*dashed lines*). (Modified from Hertwig and presented in Bradley M. Patten, *Human Embryology* (3rd ed.). New York: McGraw-Hill, 1968. P. 477. Reprinted with permission.)

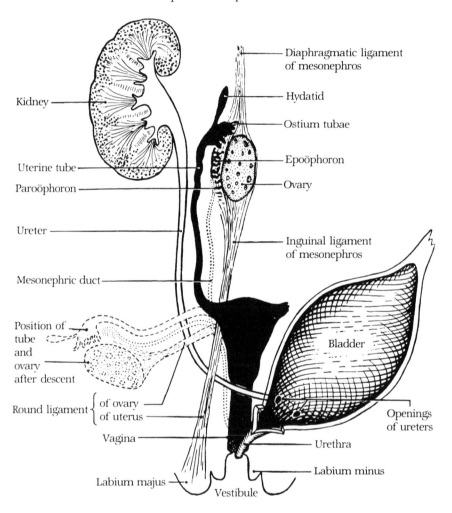

Embryos of the second month (8 weeks), therefore, have a double set of reproductive ducts, wolffian (mesonephric) and müllerian. By inference from experiments in other mammals, apparently in humans the presence of male hormone results in future wolffian duct development. Lack of this hormone and, perhaps, the presence of estrogen, causes müllerian duct development. Remnants of the wolffian ducts occur in the female pelvis and vagina as Gartner's duct cysts.

In the process of müllerian system elongation, each duct develops two curves that, after fusion, result in three anatomic regions: (1) the cranial, longitudinal portion, which becomes the oviduct, (2) the middle, transverse portion, which becomes the uterine corpus, and (3) the caudal, longitudinal portion, which differentiates into the cervix and upper vagina. Shortly after fusion, the solid cordlike structures canalize and lie adjacent to each other as hollow tubes. Subsequent differentiation results in development of myometrial and epithelial elements and resorption of the medial, fused

area, termed the *septum*. Vaginal development also occurs during this stage by canalization and resorption of the midline septum, but this process is not completed until week 20 to 22. A schematic summary of the stages of müllerian duct development is presented in Figure 4-3.

An outline of these stages of embryologic development of the urogenital system in the female is as follows:

  I. Pronephros: first stage of kidney
     Pronephric duct - becomes mesonephric duct in later stage
 II. Mesonephros: second stage of kidney
     Mesonephric ducts - previously called pronephric ducts; these paired tubular structures are also called wolffian ducts; form vas deferens in adult male; act as guide for müllerian ducts in female
III. Metanephros: adult kidney
     Metanephric ducts are the ureters; formed as outbudding from mesonephric (wolffian) ducts
 IV. Müllerian ducts
     Separable tubular structures that descend in path of mesonephric ducts and fuse to form upper vagina, uterus, and oviducts

**Figure 4-3.** Developing female reproductive system. Gradual fusion and canalization of the müllerian ducts in human embryo are shown. (Modified from Hertwig and presented in Bradley M. Patten, *Human Embryology* (3rd ed.). New York: McGraw-Hill, 1968. P. 478. Reprinted with permission.)

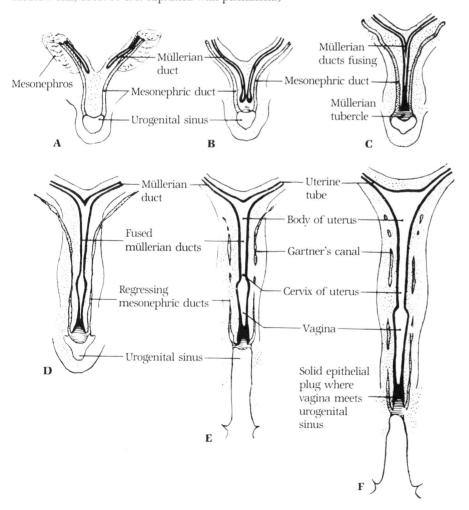

EMBRYOLOGIC CLASSIFICATION

The concept of dividing uterine anomalies into groups based on faulty embryologic development is not new. In 1922, Kaufman (37) divided anomalies of the uterus into four groups, including malformation due to faulty juxtaposition of Müller's ducts (fusion), faulty absorption of septa, aplasia (i.e., failure to descend), and hypoplasia. In the first edition of this atlas, the authors proposed a classification based on embryologic development. Failure of development or abnormality at four stages of development was noted as follows:

1. Those due to failure of müllerian duct descent
2. Those due to failure of distal ducts to canalize
3. Those due to abnormal fusion
4. Those due to failure of resorption of the midline uterine septa

If descent of one müllerian duct fails to occur or ceases before reaching the urogenital sinus, only the opposite duct completes its development. The result is a unicornuate, or single-horned, uterus. A single cervix, fallopian tube, and round ligament are present, and vaginal development is normal. Studies by Gruenwald [25] relate this failure of müllerian duct descent or elongation to abnormal development of the wolffian duct, because the absence of the wolffian duct in experimental animals results in cessation of müllerian duct descent. Whether a rudimentary horn is an anomaly of this type is not clear; it could also be an abnormality of fusion or inadequate differentiation of uterine wall elements.

A second type of anomaly relates to the failure of the distal ducts to canalize and form lumina. This rare abnormality has been elucidated by Bowles, MacNaughton-Jones, and, recently, Crosby and Hill [8, 15, 41]. Examples of this defect include a rudimentary horn without an endometrial cavity and, perhaps, hypoplasia of the upper vagina and cervix.

A third type of uterine anomaly is that associated with abnormal fusion of the müllerian ducts, an event usually completed by the sixteenth week of embryologic development. This failure may result in numerous anatomic variations. For example, there may be a double set of reproductive organs, in which both müllerian ducts develop normally but do not fuse. This results in a double vagina, double cervix, and double uterus (didelphic). Less severe forms of this abnormality include a single vagina with double cervix and uterus (duplex), single vagina and single cervix with a double uterus (bicornuate) and a uterus with slight fundal indentation (arcuate).

Descent of the müllerian ducts may occur normally and be followed by normal fusion and canalization. However, during differentiation of the myometrial and stromal elements of the uterine wall, the midline septum may fail either totally or partially to be resorbed. Puddicombe [53] stated that disappearance of the septum may start in any part of the fused ducts and proceed in either direction. The resulting septate or subseptate uterus is the anomaly most often associated with problems of pregnancy wastage [11, 33, 34, 35, 36, 55].

Jones, in 1957 [36], emphasized the role of the three developmental processes of fusion, canalization, and unilateral development in the etiology of uterine anomalies. He proposed a classification based on functional uterine capability and unrelated to embryologic factors.

Crosby and Hill, in 1962 [15], divided the embryologic development of the female generative tract into four stages. The earliest stage (3 to 8 weeks) included the "production of the müllerian cleft and ended with the formation of the tubal ostium." Anomalies of unilateral müllerian duct development occurred at this stage. Stage 2, the intermediate stage (8 to 12 weeks), included müllerian duct fusion and canalization. Maldevelopment during this stage resulted in uteri without lumens (faulty canalization), the didelphic uterus (double uterus, cervix, and vagina), and the bicornuate uterus. Stage 3 (12 to 16 weeks) included completed fusion and canalization, with myometrial differentiation and septum resorption. The septate and subseptate anomalies were placed in stage 3. Stage 4 involved development of the vagina and included all anomalies of this structure.

The major criticism of the scheme proposed by Crosby and Hill is that their emphasis is on a temporal division of developmental stages; overlap in the processes of fusion and septum resorption occurs between stages 2 and 3. These authors were primarily concerned with the uterine anomaly caused by absent canalization, and they reported in their paper 3 patients with this defect. Furthermore, stage 4, vaginal development, is a departure from the temporal order and, in fact, bridges the first three developmental stages.

FUNCTIONAL CLASSIFICATION

The preceding discussion of the embryologic development of the female generative tract elucidated the correlation between defects in this process and observed uterine anomalies. There are, however, other classifications of uterine anomalies, both anatomic and functional. Jarcho, in 1946, published a classic article [31] in which he established an anatomic grouping of uterine anomalies that is still used in most gynecologic textbooks. Seven variations were described by Jarcho. The rudimentary uterine horn was felt to be a variation of the partial bicornuate uterus. We have grouped these seven uterine forms plus the rudimentary horn into 5 categories, as noted in Figure (4-4A-E) Jarcho failed to mention the defect associated with absent canalization, that of a uterine mass without a lumen. The more recent defects associated with DES exposure in utero were also not included by Jarcho.

Other gynecologists, including H. W. Jones, Strassman, W. S. Jones, and Semmens [35, 36, 60, 66], have attempted to define functional or clinical classes of abnormal uteri. H. W. Jones divided his patients into two groups on the basis of the ability to palpate "with certainty, the raphe separating the two halves." A hysterogram was necessary to identify two endometrial cavities. All patients were then "considered to have either a bicornuate or a septate uterus, either partial or complete." Strassman, in 1961 [66], stated, "so-called double uteri that require entirely different surgical management are asymmetric double formations and symmetric ones." The asymmetric group includes the unicornuate uterus and those uteri with a rudimentary horn. The symmetric group is divided into the externally unified uterus (septate and subseptate) and the externally divided uterus (bicornuate and didelphic).

Semmens [59] proposed a functional classification of uterine anomalies based on the potential capacity of the uterine cavity and its musculature:

Group 1: Functional uteri of single müllerian origin
  A. Didelphic uterus
  B. Unicornuate uterus
  C. Bicornuate uterus with one horn rudimentary
Group 2: Functional uteri of dual müllerian origin
  A. Bicornuate uterus
  B. Septate uterus
  C. Arcuate uterus

Hysterosalpingography and a careful bimanual examination are necessary when using this classification, and direct visualization is necessary to establish the presence of a rudimentary uterine horn. The intent of this grouping was to separate uteri derived from single and double müllerian origin. According to Semmens, group 1 patients, most of whom have didelphic uteri, had a 33 percent rate of fetal wastage (abortion and premature labor). In a literature review about group 1 patients, Semmens noted that the fetal wastage was 23.3 percent for didelphic uterus, 21 percent for unicornuate uterus, and 34.3 percent for bicornuate uterus with a rudimentary horn. Of 572 pregnancies that occurred in the normal hemiuterus, 111 resulted in abortion and 27 in the delivery of stillborn infants, for a fetal wastage of only 24.1 percent. In contrast, 25 group 2 patients seen by Semmens demonstrated a fetal wastage of 49.3 percent, and in the 202 cases from the literature of the same group, the overall fetal wastage was 37.1 percent. The rate of late abortion in group 2 was twice that in group 1 (34.7 percent compared with 17.3 percent). It thus appears that the hemiuterus functions slightly less well than a normal uterus, but better than the double

uterus with a bicornuate or septate defect. The significant point is that certain individuals with these anomalies appear to have repetitive pregnancy loss either as late abortion or premature delivery.

W. S. Jones [36] recognized four types of uterine abnormality: single (normal and arcuate), septate, bicornuate, and double uterus. He attempted to arrange these defects in terms of "gestational capacity" in the order given above. This classification and its rationale will be discussed later in this chapter.

PRESENT CLINICAL CLASSIFICATION
In the first edition of this atlas, uterine anomalies were classified as defective müllerian duct elongation, canalization, fusion and septum resorption, as was discussed earlier. In an effort to standardize the nomenclature of uterine anomalies and to permit the comparison of surgical results from different medical centers, a classification scheme proposed by Buttram and Gibbons [11] (1979) that appears to combine this earlier embryologic approach with the groups listed by Kaufman [37] and Jarcho [31], has been modified and is summarized in Table 4-1 and Figure 4-4. The major additions in this new classification are a category for müllerian agenesis and hypoplasia (i.e., absence of the cervix or a portion of the uterine body) and four subdivisions of the unicornuate uterus. Also included in this scheme is a class of uterine anomaly not recognized in 1975, that associated with maternal DES ingestion. The authors have modified the classification by Buttram and Gibbons [11]

**Table 4-1.** Classification of müllerian anomalies

---

Segmental müllerian agenesis/hypoplasia
  Vaginal
  Cervical
  Fundal
  Tubal
  Combined anomalies
Unicornuate
  With rudimentary horn
    With endometrial cavity
      Communicating
      Noncommunicating
    Without endometrial cavity
  Without rudimentary horn
Didelphys
Bicornuate
  Complete (division down to internal os)
  Partial
  Arcuate
Septate
  Complete (septum to internal os)
    With single cervix
    With double cervix
  Incomplete
DES-related
  T-shaped uterus
  T-shaped with dilated horns
  T-shaped with dilated lower uterine segment

---

by adding a third form of septate uterine anomaly to the two proposed earlier, because the presence of a double cervix requires a unique surgical approach.

It is axiomatic that the diagnosis of a uterine anomaly should be made by the combined diagnostic studies of hysterosalpingography and laparoscopy. Nowhere is the concept that these two studies are complementary more applicable than in the study of uterine contour.

*Class I: Segmental Müllerian Agenesis/Hypoplasia.* This group of anomalies includes absence of a segment of a fallopian tube or cervix, or part of the uterine body or upper vagina (Fig. 4-4A). Few patients in this group will present an anomaly amenable to surgical repair. Segmental tubal agenesis can theoretically be corrected, although that is rarely indicated. Segmental uterine agenesis is not reparable; however, cervical agenesis has been successfully repaired [49]. The wisdom of attempting conservative surgical repair of cervical agenesis has recently been questioned by Niver et al. [49], who reported a significant morbidity and mortality at the Columbia Presbyterian Medical Center. The three patients included in this report had both vaginal agenesis and absence of the cervix. One death resulted from postoperative sepsis in a patient whose initial surgical procedure was conservative. All 3 patients eventually underwent hysterectomy. Eleven cases of congenital cervical atresia were found in a literature review through 1973 by Zarou et al. [74], who published a paper reporting the only known pregnancy following cervical repair for this disorder. Since 1973, 8 cases have been reported by Greary and Weed [23] (2 of them with absent vagina), 1 case by Williams [72], and 2 cases by Faber and Marchant [18] (1 of them with absent vagina). At the time of initial surgery, hysterectomy was performed on only 4 of the patients referred to above. Eleven of the 22 patients in this series eventually underwent hysterectomy, however. Of the 10 patients who did not undergo hysterectomy, 8 had restoration of menses; 1 pregnancy occurred and was carried to term. One patient was lost to follow-up. All told, 22 adolescent females underwent a total of 45 surgical procedures and 2 died of sepsis.

*Class II: Unicornuate Uterus.* This classification identifies the four forms in which a unicornuate uterus may occur (Fig. 4-4B). Defective unilateral müllerian duct descent combined with defective canalization or fusion would appear to be the responsible embryologic defect. A rudimentary horn may be present either as a solid mass, termed *uterus solidaris* by one author [4] or may contain an endometrial cavity. This cavity may communicate with the primary uterine cavity or be noncommunicating. Surgical intervention is necessary only when a rudimentary horn with an endometrial cavity is found. Both communicating and noncommunicating remnants with a functional cavity should be removed. More often the surgeon will encounter a solid mass to which is attached a fallopian tube and ovary that appear to be normal. This structure should be left intact.

---

**Figure 4-4.** Clinical abnormalities of the uterus. The classification proposed by Buttram and Gibbons has been modified to include three forms of septate uteri. **A.** Class I. Five forms of müllerian agenesis or hypoplasia. **B.** Class II. Four forms of the unicornuate uterus, including variations of rudimentary horns. **C.** Class III. Uterus didelphys. **D.** Class IV. Two forms of bicornuate uteri and the arcuate uterus. **E.** Class V. Three forms of septate uteri. **F.** Class VI. Three forms of DES-related anomalies: (1) T-shaped uterus; (2) T-shaped cavity with widening of the interstitial and isthmic parts of the oviducts; (3) T-shaped cavity with widening of the lower two-thirds of uterine cavity and constriction at level of upper uterine cavity. (Modified from V. C. Buttram and W. E. Gibbons, Müllerian Anomalies: A proposed classification. *Fertil. Steril.* 32:40, 1979. Reprinted with permission.)

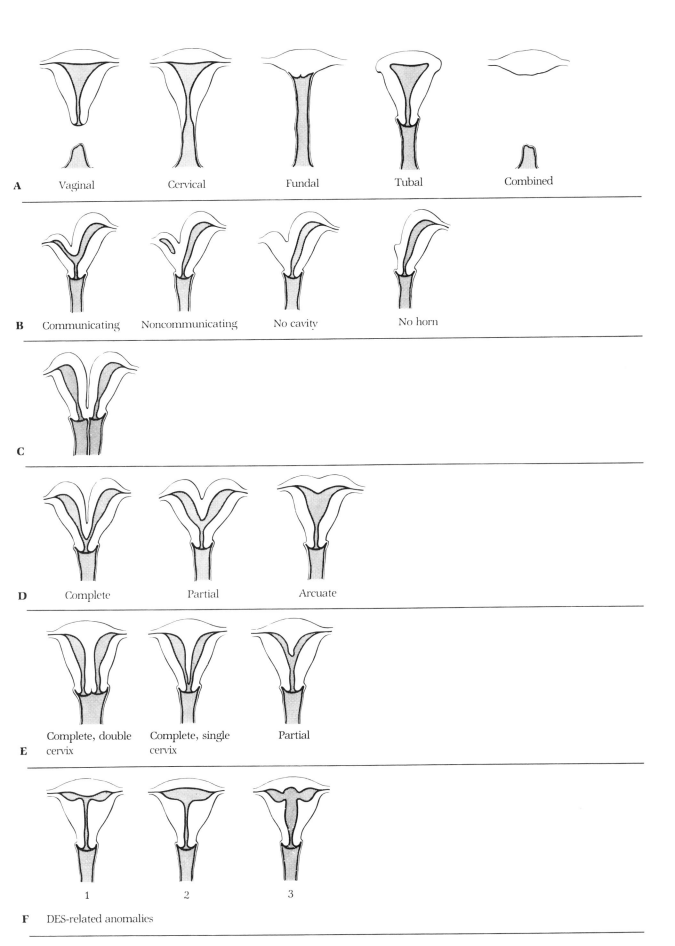

A    Vaginal       Cervical       Fundal       Tubal       Combined

B    Communicating    Noncommunicating    No cavity      No horn

C

D    Complete       Partial       Arcuate

E    Complete, double cervix    Complete, single cervix    Partial

F    DES-related anomalies

1      2      3

Cervical incompetence and attendant cerclage should be considered in the patient with a unicornuate uterus who has experienced midtrimester pregnancy loss. A review of this subject is presented later. Figure 4-5 demonstrates a typical unicornuate uterus, in this instance associated with a hydrosalpinx.

**Figure 4-5.** This hysterographic study revealed a unicornuate uterus (class II, no horn) deviated to the right. Distal fimbrial occlusion was confirmed at laparoscopy. The left ovary was seen high along the left pelvic brim.

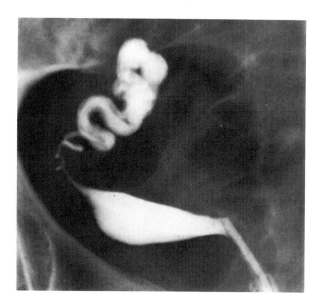

*Class III: Uterus Didelphys.* This anomaly (Fig. 4-4C) represents a failure of müllerian duct fusion that, in a mild degree, produces the bicornuate uterus (Class IV). It is practical to separate these two types of uterine anomaly because the prognosis for pregnancy differs in the two groups. Surgical unification of uterus didelphys is rarely necessary, although it has been successfully performed [69]. Figure 4-6 is a photograph of a hysterogram performed by this author (G.W.P.) on a patient with this anomaly following midtrimester loss; the patient then underwent cervical cerclage of the involved cervix and, subsequently, delivered two term infants.

**Figure 4-6.** Hysterogram of a uterus didelphys (class III). This patient demonstrated cervical incompetence and required cervical cerclage to achieve a viable child.

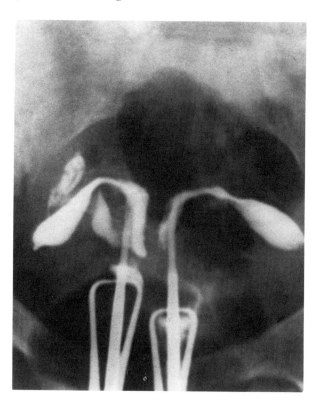

*Class IV: Bicornuate Uterus.* This form of uterine anomaly (Fig. 4-4D), as was noted above, represents a defect in müllerian duct fusion that may extend to the internal os (complete) or only to a midpoint along the uterine body, producing a partial defect (Fig. 4-7). Involvement of the cervix resulting in a double cervix would create a uterus didelphys. A bicornuate uterus is infrequently associated with pregnancy wastage and occurred rarely among the surgical unification procedures [55, 33, 11] performed at Johns Hopkins University Hospital or at Baylor College of Medicine. Metroplasties performed on subseptate uteri in 12 patients and bicornuate uteri in 6 patients, reported by Musich and Behrman [48], were the exceptions. The bicornuate uterus was the anomaly encountered by Dr. Strassman and should be repaired by the technique he described [66].

**Figure 4-7.** Bicornuate uterus (class IV, Partial). A single cervix was present, and filling of both uterine horns during hysterography was possible through a single cervical cannula. At laparoscopy, separate uterine bodies were seen extending laterally, to which were attached a normal oviduct and ovary. This investigation was performed because of the presence of bilateral adnexal masses.

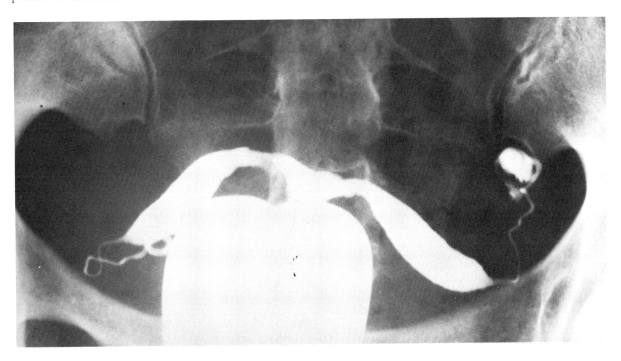

*Class V: Septate Uterus.* The septate uterus (Fig. 4-4E) represents an embryologic defect in septum resorption that may be partial or complete. The complete septum is defined as that extending to the internal os, and it will usually involve a single cervix (Fig. 4-8). Rarely, a complete septum (Fig. 4-9) will include a double cervix; this category is included by the authors in Buttram's classification. This anomaly may be distinguished from uterus didelphys (class III) by pelvic examination but must be confirmed by laparoscopic visualization of the pelvis.

**Figure 4-8. A.** This preoperative hysterogram demonstrates separate uterine cavities associated with a single cervix (class V, Partial). As defined at surgery **(B),** this pattern is that of a complete septate uterine anomaly associated with a single cervix. This author (G.W.P.) has recently encountered a complete septum associated with a double cervix, and has included that in the classification of müllerian defects (see Fig. 4-4E). **B.** This intraoperative photograph of the uterus outlined by hysterography **(A)** demonstrates the uterine contour of a typical septate uterine anomaly. Note the mild midfundal indentation. A Tompkins metroplasty was performed successfully on this patient.

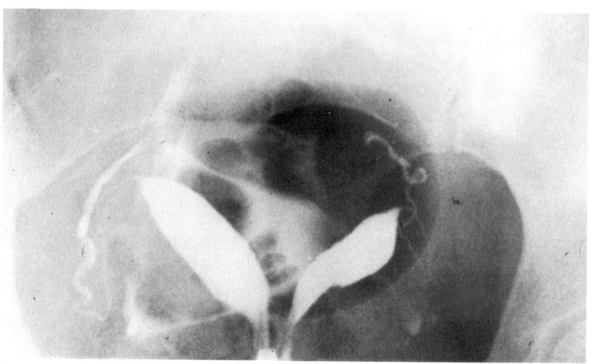

**A**

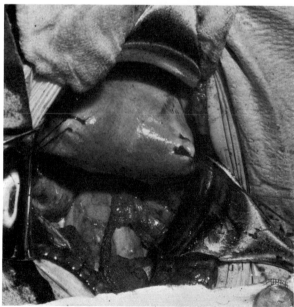

**B**

**Figure 4-9.** This hysterographic study outlines 2 uterine cavities and 2 cervical openings (class V, Complete double cervix). A vaginal septum had been removed years earlier. This patient had experienced 3 first-trimester losses. A septate uterus similar to that shown in Figure 4-8B was found, and a Tompkins metroplasty was performed with conservation of the double cervix.

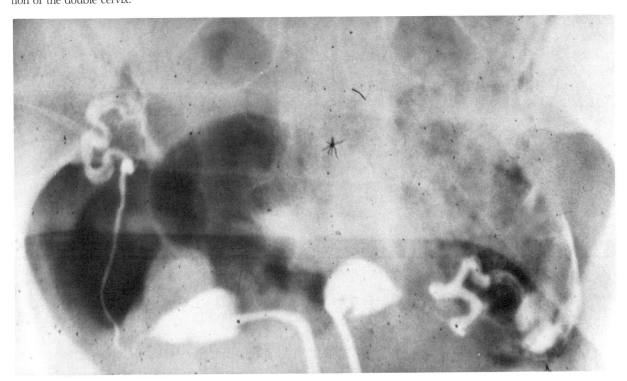

Most patients who experience pregnancy wastage due to a uterine factor will be found to have a septate uterine anomaly. This is dramatically shown by the surgical experience of Buttram and Gibbons [11], who found that 46 of 47 metroplasties performed were on septate uteri. A similar experience was noted at Johns Hopkins Hospital [35]. In contrast, Musich and Behrman [48] noted the ratio of septate to bicornuate anomalies to be 12 : 6 in patients undergoing metroplasty procedures. Rock and Jones [55] reviewed their patients who underwent uterine metroplasty and were unable to relate the extent of a septum to the degree of pregnancy loss. The surgical unification of a septate uterus is a highly satisfactory procedure as is described later. However, when one uterine cavity is markedly smaller than the other, an unusual circumstance (see Fig. 4-8A), it may be preferable, as suggested by John Rock [54], to simply remove the oviduct and ovary on that side. A typical pre- and postoperative hysterosalpingogram of a partial septate anomaly (class V, Partial) repaired by a Tompkins metroplasty procedure is shown in Figures 4-10 A and B.

**Figure 4-10. A.** This preoperative hysterogram demonstrates the characteristic appearance of a partial subseptate uterine anomaly (class V, Partial). This patient had undergone 2 spontaneous abortions and 1 midtrimester loss prior to evaluation. **B.** A Tompkins metroplasty was performed on the uterus **(A).** This postoperative hysterogram revealed a uterine contour that was almost normal. Unfortunately, the uterus was slightly flexed at this time. This patient subsequently delivered 2 term infants.

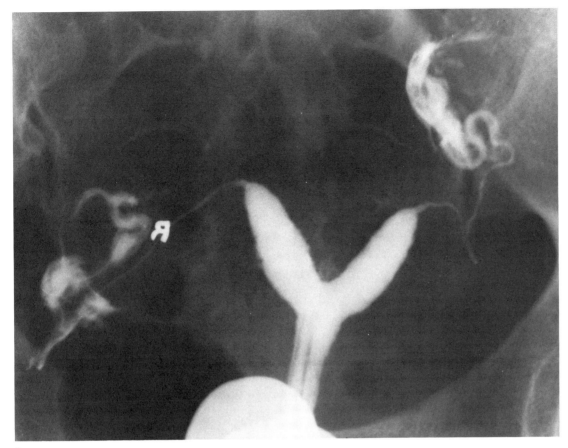

**A**

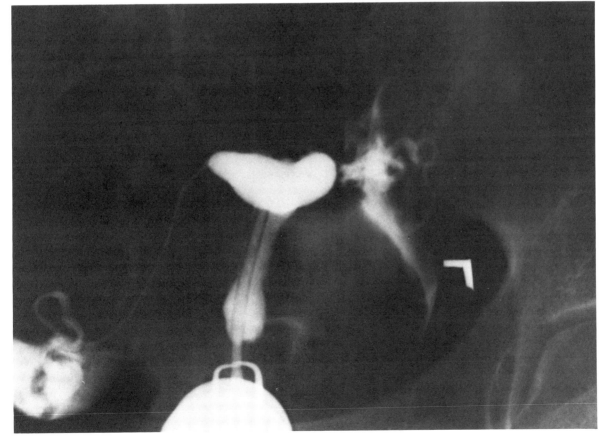

**B**

**Table 4-2.** Hysterographic observations
in patients exposed to DES

| No. of patients | Uterine anomaly |
| --- | --- |
| 21 | T-shaped appearance<br>Widening of the interstitial and isthmic portions of oviducts<br>In some cases, constriction bands that cause narrowing of the hornlike extension of the uterus<br>Lower two-thirds of the uterine cavity appeared to be considerably narrowed<br>Raggy uterine border, in some cases |
| 7 | Uterus T-shaped with widening of lower two-thirds<br>In several patients, constriction bands noted in the dilated lateral portions of the T<br>In some cases, a constriction of the junction of upper one-third and lower two-thirds of uterine cavity noted |
| 5 | Uterus small in size without gross changes noted above |
| 4 | Intrauterine defects noted—"filling defects" |
| 3 | Intrauterine synechiae; 1 unicornuate uterus, 1 lower uterine constriction |

Source: R. H. Kaufman, G. L. Binder, P. M. Gray, and E. Adam, Upper genital tract changes associated with exposure in utero to diethylstilbestrol. *Am. J. Obstet. Gynecol.* 128:51, 1977.

*Class VI: DES-related Uterine Anomalies.* In 1977, 6 years after the Herbst [28] report of an association between adenocarcinoma of the vagina and in utero DES exposure, Kaufman and coworkers [38] reported that in utero DES exposure also caused a unique T-shaped uterine anomaly (Fig. 4-4F). The earlier emphasis in this chapter on embryologic relationships and congenital uterine anomalies also has relevance to DES-related uterine defects. Kaufman et al. [38] stated ". . . it is well known that the uterus and oviduct arise from the same müllerian duct system as the cervix and upper vagina. It is logical to suspect that if intrauterine exposure to DES results in gross anatomic changes in the cervix and upper vagina, changes would be induced in the upper genital tract as well" (p. 56). The remarkable fact is that it took 6 years to establish this relationship.

Kaufman and coworkers at Baylor Medical School performed hysterosalpingography on 60 young women felt to have been exposed to DES in utero. Documentation of DES exposure was established in 46 patients and in 14 additional young women ". . . the patients' mothers were sure they had received stilbestrol" (p. 51). Gross anatomic changes in the vagina and cervix were present in 49 of the 60 women. In 28 of these 46 women with documented exposure, DES had been started prior to the thirteenth week of pregnancy. An abnormal hysterosalpingogram was found in 40 of the 60 patients. These x-ray findings are outlined in Table 4-2.

The Baylor group [38] found that 36 of 40 patients (90 percent) who had abnormal hysterosalpingograms also demonstrated an abnormality of the cervix (Fig. 4-11). In contrast, abnormal cervices were found in only 4 of 20 patients who had normal hysterosalpingograms. Adenosis occurred in 28 of 40 patients with abnormal uterine cavities, compared to 10 of the 20 patients whose uterine contour was normal. Of 38 patients in this series with adenosis, 74 percent had abnormal hysterosalpingograms.

From an embryologic point of view it is interesting to review the 28 patients exposed to DES in utero prior to the thirteenth week of pregnancy. Twenty of these patients had abnormalities of the cervix. Eight patients in this group had normal x-ray studies; however, 2 of these patients had abnormal cervices and 4 had adenoses.

The initial observations of Kaufman et al. have been confirmed by others [26, 52, 61], although little change in the original anatomic description of the T-shaped uterus has been made. Three variants of the T-shaped uterus are shown in Figure 4-4F.

**Figure 4-11.** This hysterogram demonstrates a T-shaped uterine anomaly that combines dilatation of the interstitial oviductal segments and widening of the lower uterine cavity with constriction at the junction of the upper one-third (class VI, 3). This young female, who was known to have been exposed to DES in utero, has had 2 spontaneous abortions and has not had a living child.

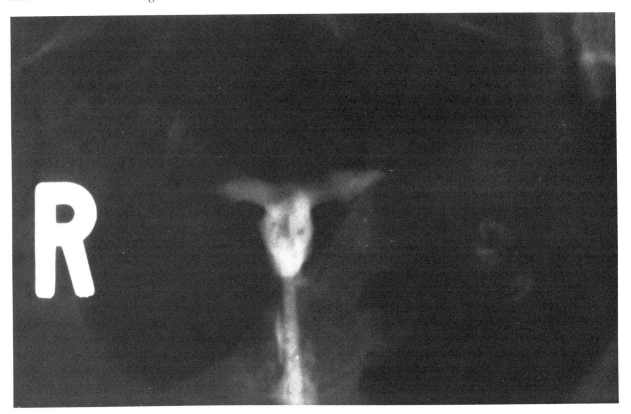

*Indications for Surgery*

In 1884, Ruge [58] reported that after Schroeder performed vaginal removal of a uterine septum in a patient with two previous abortions, the patient carried to term. It is Paul Strassman, however, who deserves credit for initiating the surgical approach to unification of the double uterus, a procedure he termed *metroplasty*. In 1907, Strassman (as quoted by his son Erwin Strassman [65]) reported the case history of a patient who had had 8 prior pregnancies, all of which ended in abortion or premature delivery. Strassman performed a unification of her bicornuate uterus vaginally through an anterior colpotomy incision, using the technique that now bears his name. Postoperatively this patient had 6 term deliveries. All of the infants were delivered vaginally and all survived. Erwin Strassman [65] commented that his father performed 8 of his 18 operations vaginally. Most of these patients had bicornuate uteri, because hysterosalpingography was not available, and the preoperative diagnosis of septate uterus was almost impossible.

In 1952, a literature review by Erwin Strassman [65] revealed 84 cases in which surgical unification of a double uterus (metroplasty) had been performed for the following indications (some patients had more than one indication):

1. Menometrorrhagia (22 cases, 26 percent)
2. Dysmenorrhea (33 cases, 39 percent)
3. Dyspareunia (9 cases, 11 percent)
4. Primary infertility (13 cases, 15 percent)
5. Habitual abortion or premature delivery (39 cases, 46 percent)

MENOMETRORRHAGIA

Bainbridge [2] stated that menstruation in a patient with a double uterus may take place every 2 weeks, first from one side, then from the other. Puddicombe [53] reported from the Free Hospital for Women (now part of the Brigham and Women's Hospital) 11 patients with bicornuate uteri, 5 of whom complained of menorrhagia.

Although dysfunctional uterine bleeding may occur in patients with uterine anomalies, the cause of this abnormality is usually considered to be hormonal rather than anatomic. Luteal phase insufficiency has been demonstrated in patients with a double uterus, and anovulatory cycles may also occur [35]. However, cases have been reported in which abnormal bleeding patterns have ceased following a unification procedure [59]. Steinberg [63] postulated that the abnormal bleeding was due to irregular endometrial shedding in the two uterine horns.

It has been suggested that pregnancy wastage associated with a septate uterus may be due to abnormal placentation in the area of the septum [59]. Vascular insufficiency and inadequate endometrial development are thought to be the major factors producing this situation. The same structural deficiencies in a midline uterine septum might also produce dysfunctional uterine bleeding because of irregular shedding and inadequate hemostasis. However, the evidence regarding this conclusion is not clear. Semmens [59] noted that 36 percent of his 25 patients with septate or bicornuate uteri subsequently developed moderate to severe menorrhagia refractory to treatment, necessitating hysterectomy.

In spite of the theoretical possibility that a uterine septum may contribute to irregular or profuse vaginal bleeding, we consider this symptom to be a rare indication for uterine unification.

DYSMENORRHEA

When associated with severe cervical stenosis or hematometra in a rudimentary uterine horn, painful menstrual periods justify surgical correction of this anomaly. Although surgery was performed during the late nineteenth and early twentieth centuries for dysmenorrhea associated with a rudimentary uterine horn, it is interesting to consider the first surgical repair of this anomaly, reported by Jones and Jones in 1953 [34]. They reported finding a rudimentary uterine horn in a 14-year-old girl operated on for severe dysmenorrhea. The septum was excised and the two halves united. H. W. Jones subsequently [33] described a surgical technique for repair of the septate uterus that will be described later.

Dysmenorrhea may exist without obstruction to blood flow from the uterus. For example, in the series reported by Semmens [59], 60 percent of group 1 patients (uteri of single müllerian origin) complained of dysmenorrhea, but only 15 percent required medication. However, 20 percent of group 2 patients (septate and bicornuate uteri) were incapacitated by pain and required medication. Most patients who have primary, incapacitating dysmenorrhea do not have congenital uterine anomalies as the cause of their pain, but improvement does occur frequently after cervical dilatation.

An example of the complexity of evaluating dysmenorrhea in patients with a double uterus is reflected in a case reported by Semmens [59] in which "one patient who had 5 consecutive spontaneous abortions and disabling dysmenorrhea was treated by presacral neurectomy, and a diagnosis of bicornuate uterus was made. Although no corrective surgery of the uterine anomaly was attempted, this patient was relieved of her dysmenorrhea and carried her sixth and eighth pregnancies to term." Semmens wondered whether a "neurogenic factor" might have been responsible for the repetitive uterine wastage.

We have not performed uterine unification for relief of dysmenorrhea, except when it is associated with obstruction, as in the case of a rudimentary uterine horn.

Pain during sexual intercourse occurring in patients with a double uterus is usually caused by a vaginal septum. Steinberg noted that a septate vagina might also be a cause of sterility in patients with a didelphic uterus if intercourse were to take place consistently on the nonovulating side [63]. One of us (R.W.K.) had a patient who claimed to have control of conception by directing the penis into the right or left vaginal compartment. The right side connected with an atrophic cervix and a noncanalized uterus. The left vaginal compartment was in continuity with a functional uterus.

Excision of a vaginal septum is always indicated. Parenthetically, this type of vaginal septum frequently does not totally separate a double vagina and may be recognized only as a source of vaginal dystocia during labor.

### PRIMARY STERILITY

The inability to conceive is not usually considered an indication for metroplasty, although Strassmar and others have reported favorable results in patients with this condition following surgical unification (66). As was previously noted, 15 percent of the 84 cases reviewed in 1952 by Strassman were operated on because of primary sterility. Genell [21], in 1952, reported a series of 88 metroplasties in Swedish hospitals, 9 of which were done for primary sterility. In a later report (1959) Genell and Sjovall [21] reported 13 patients with uterine anomalies and primary infertility of 1 to 12 years' duration 5 of whom achieved pregnancy following metroplasty. Zourlas (1975) [75] reported 2 patients with primary infertility and a uterine anomaly who conceived following metroplasty. Recently, Tulandi, Arronet, and McInnnes (1980) [71] described 2 patients with long-standing primary infertility who were found to have bicornuate uteri; they conceived 12 months and 17 months following metroplasty. These authors theorized that ". . . since the customary fundal implantation is not anatomically feasible in the abnormal uterus, septal implantation or lateral wall implantation occurs. With the altered myometrial organization and blood supply and, perhaps, even alteration of the endometrium in this area, early undiagnosed abortion due to an inadequate implantation may be the result, with the patient presenting with 'primary' infertility."

We do not feel that a double uterus is responsible for an inability to conceive and rarely recommend surgical correction for primary sterility. This opinion was expressed by Rock [54] in commenting on the report by Jones and associates, when he said "like previous commentators, the present essayists find no proof that the so-called double uterus prevents pregnancy but . . . it may be an effective factor in prevention of normal growth and parturition."

Rock has commented further that "infertility is a sad affliction but being unproductive in spite of conception is worse" [54]. Te Linde [67] stated that "probably the most important indication for surgery of the double uterus is for the cure of habitual abortion." One must not assume, however, that the mere presence of a bicornuate or septate uterus dictates repetitive pregnancy wastage and, therefore, indicates surgery. The following discussion will attempt to elucidate the frequency of fetal wastage associated with various uterine anomalies and identify the patient with an anomalous uterus who may be expected to achieve improved functional capability following surgical unification.

The pitfalls encountered in evaluating obstetric performance in patients with anomalous uteri are many. The following discussion is based on retrospective studies published by W. S. Jones and by Semmens [36, 59]. Jones theorized that "gestational capability," or uterine function, was best in the normal single uterus and was least affected by the septate uterus. The bicornuate uterus was "the next step removed from the normal," and, theoretically, in a bicornuate uterus "the obstetric performance will be in inverse proportion to the degree of muscular distortion produced by the forking." The "hemiuterus is the ultimate stage of abnormality . . . whether it is a didelphys uterus or a unicornuate uterus" (Fig. 4-12).

**Figure 4-12.** Hysterographic study revealed a left unicornuate uterus, a noncommunicating rudimentary horn, and a normal fallopian tube (class II, Noncommunicating). Evidence of cervical incompetence seen in this photograph was confirmed clinically. Habitual abortion in this patient was successfully treated by cervical cerclage.

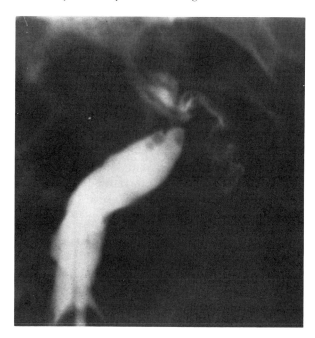

This functional classification was supported by the obstetrical histories of 103 women with uterine anomalies at the Providence Lying-in Hospital. It is significant that W. S. Jones reported only 11 women with a septate uterus. The fetal wastage in this group was only 22.2 percent—the best performance for any of the patients with uterine anomaly. (This favorable performance might have been due to a small patient sample, because H. W. Jones has found this anomaly to be the most frequent indication for metroplasty.) Sixty-four patients with bicornuate uteri had a 33.8 percent abortion rate and total fetal wastage of 40.2 percent. The hemiuterus in 16 patients resulted in an early abortion rate of 32.4 percent and total fetal wastage of 46.0 percent. In the total group of patients with uterine anomalies, spontaneous abortion occurred in 27.2 percent and premature delivery in 13.2 percent; the total fetal wastage was 33.9 percent. Forty percent of viable infants in a hemiuterus were in breech position; cesarean section was performed in 68 percent, because of cervical dystocia.

Semmens [59] evaluated the obstetrical performance of 556 patients with congenital uterine anomalies. He added 56 of his own cases to 500 obtained from a review of the literature. As was noted previously, these patients were classified as group 1 (uteri of single müllerian origin) and group 2 (uteri of dual müllerian origin). The hemiuterus in this series was thought to be "functionally superior to the anomalies of group 2 in terms of viable infants delivered." It is significant that didelphys uteri accounted for 225 cases of group 1 defects, as compared with only 15 cases of unicornuate uteri. Fetal wastage was 32 percent in group 1, compared with 42 percent in group 2. It may be that the unicornuate uterus functions less well than a single horn of the didelphic uterus; the high fetal wastage in the series by W. S. Jones occurred in a group of 16 patients 25 percent of whom had unicornuate uteri. Unfortunately, Semmens did not separate group 2 patients into those with septate uteri and those with bicornuate uteri, so a comparison of these anomalies is not possible. Breech presentation occurred in 30 percent of patients in group 1 and 20 percent in group 2. In comparison to the 68 percent rate for cesarean section reported by Jones, this procedure was performed in only 20 percent of patients. Semmens did not note, however, that the 49.3 percent fetal wastage in group 2 of his series was unusually high because of 4 patients who, together, had 17 abortions. This observation lends support to the belief of H. W. Jones that certain patients with septate uteri have repetitive obstetrical difficulty.

A direct clinical approach to selection of patients for surgical unification was evaluated in the series of patients with double uteri reported by Rock and Jones [55]. Two groups were studied. Group A consisted of 129 patients admitted to Johns Hopkins University Hospital between 1936 and 1975 and who received routine obstetrical care. One hundred of these patients gave an essentially normal reproductive history, and 71 percent of their pregnancies resulted in the birth of a living infant. However, 29 percent of these patients had previously demonstrated poor reproductive performance, and only 39 percent of the pregnancies in this group resulted in the birth of a living child. Designation of septate and bicornuate uteri was not made in this group. This update supported the previous conclusion from this medical center that "there seem to be patients with a double uterus who are characterized by repetitive reproductive problems rather than individual problem pregnancies in all patients with a double uterus" [35].

Group B consisted of 81 patients who were studied because of reproductive difficulty and who were found to have double uteri. All were treated initially by hormonal therapy, usually progesterone replacement for correction of possible luteal phase insufficiency. In the earlier report of this series during the years 1936 to 1964, 31 of 53 patients had at least 1 living child subsequent to hormonal therapy. Prior to hormone therapy, the 31 patients had had 72 pregnancies; of these, 8 went to term and 7 resulted in premature births. In contrast, after progesterone therapy there were 58 pregnancies; of these, 44 were carried to term, and 8 resulted in premature births. It should be noted that all of the patients who did not have a living child by medical management became candidates for surgery [62], and only 22 of the 53 patients in this group subsequently underwent a metroplasty procedure. During the years 1964 to 1975, 28 patients were noted to be in group B and 21 of 28 underwent a metroplasty, which apparently indicated a decreased interest in hormonal replacement therapy at the Johns Hopkins University Hospital [55]. Rock and Jones reported a total of 43 patients in group B who underwent surgical unification, and all but 2 had a septate uterus. Prior to surgical intervention, 4 patients (8 percent) had living children after a total of 140 pregnancies. Ninety-four percent of the pregnancies ended in abortion and 6 percent were premature. There were no term infants in this preoperative series that resulted in 4 living children, for a 3 percent fetal salvage rate. Among 28 patients in group B followed during the interval from 1964 to 1975, 36 percent had one spontaneous abortion; 32 percent, two abortions; and 32 percent, three or more abortions. This was in contrast to the earlier group of 22 patients operated on between the years 1936 and 1964, 16 of whom had a history of three or more consecutive miscarriages and, thus, could be classified as habitual aborters.

The etiology of congenital uterine anomalies is not clear. Hereditary factors associated with these congenital anomalies have been reviewed [62] and the possibility suggested that they may be the manifestation of a single mutant gene. Uterine anomalies have also been described in sisters, raising the possibility of recessive forms of inheritance. Simpson concluded, however, that "most uterine anomalies probably result from deleterious environmental factors." The nature of these factors is not clear, however.

ASSOCIATED RENAL ANOMALIES

The earlier discussion of the embryologic development of the female genital tract emphasized the close relationship between müllerian duct development and the metanephros, or adult kidney. Signs of abnormal müllerian duct development would be expected to accompany serious renal anomalies, and this is supported by numerous clinical observations. Jones [35] reported absence of the uterus and vagina associated with anomalies of the urinary tract in a large number of patients. He noted a rate of 48 percent in 17 patients studied by Thompson and coworkers [68] and of 12 percent of major anomalies reported by Phelan and coworkers [51]. Obviously, an intravenous urogram should be taken in all patients with congenital absence of the vagina, a vaginal septum, a double cervix, or a uterine anomaly. Conversely, patients who have a congenital abnormality detected by urography should have hysterosalpingography performed if subsequent pregnancies are planned. Collins reported genital anomalies in 90 percent of 231 patients with unilateral renal anomalies [13].

Woolf and Allen [73] found that all 15 cases of unilateral müllerian duct development in their series were associated with unilateral renal defects. Semmens [59] noted that 37.5 percent of his patients and 50.8 percent of patients in the literature with uteri of single müllerian duct origin (unicornuate and didelphys) had renal agenesis. Forty-three percent of patients with septate or bicornuate uteri had renal agenesis.

Urologic evaluation is recommended for all patients undergoing surgical unification of a double uterus. Whether this study is of more than academic interest is questionable, because the surgical approaches do not usually involve the kidney, ureter, or bladder. However, maximum concern for the urologic system should be exercised in all patients undergoing metroplasty, and urinary infection should be prevented or controlled.

UNIFICATION OF THE SEPTATE UTERUS

Most patients who demonstrate habitual abortion or repetitive midtrimester loss and whose infertility evaluation indicates that this process is caused by a double uterus will be seen to have a septate or subseptate uterus at the time of surgical exploration. There are two surgical procedures for removing the uterine septum in patients with this anomaly, and both techniques will be described. A third surgical approach described by Strassman [65] to unify a bicornuate uterus or uterus didelphys will also be described here. The lines of surgical incision used in these three procedures are shown in Figure 4-13.

**Figure 4-13.** The lines of surgical incision required by the three procedures of uterine unification are shown. **A.** The uterine cavity and fundal shape of a typical subseptate uterus. The line of incision used during Tompkins metroplasty is carried through the midseptal area into the endometrial cavity. **B.** The wedge incision used by Jones for repair of a similar subseptate anomaly. **C.** The line of incision used by Strassman to repair a bicornuate uterus runs from fundus to fundus and is a transverse line, in contrast to the line of incision used by Jones and Tompkins during repair of a septate uterus.

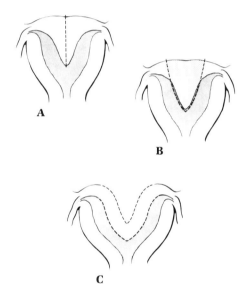

Prior to laparotomy a pelvic examination is performed, and if a vaginal septum is present it is excised and the vagina is reconstructed using interrupted sutures of 2-0 chromic catgut or 4-0 Dexon. The cervix is dilated and the uterine cavity stained with indigo carmine dye. If two cervices are present, each endometrial cavity is carefully stained. This dark blue color aids in identifying the endometrial cavity and also permits the surgeon to avoid this layer during closure of the uterus. Alternative methods are packing of the endometrial cavity with gauze, or introduction of a uterine sound into each horn.

The Tompkins procedure for unification of the septate uterus is shown in Figure 4-14.

The Jones procedure for unification of a subseptate uterus differs from that used by Tompkins in that the uterine septum is actually removed by a wedge-shaped incision (Fig. 4-15). Figure 4-15A illustrates the same subseptate uterus that was noted in the discussion of the Tompkins procedure and describes the Jones method of unification.

**Figure 4-14.** Unification of a septate uterus (Tompkins procedure). **A.** A septate uterus characterized by the presence of 2 distinct uterine cavities (see Fig. 4-13) and a small dimple or indentation in the midfundal area. Retraction sutures of 2-0 polyglycolic acid are placed near the junction of the round ligaments. Bulldog clamps are placed over the ovarian vessels and a No. 12 rubber tourniquet is placed around the uterine vessels. The line of incision is injected with dilute vasopressin (Pitressin, 1 ampule in 100 cc NaCl). These procedures will assure almost complete hemostasis during the operation. **B.** The midfundal incision (**A,** dotted line) is described by Tompkins [69]. The apex of the incision is placed in the midline of the fundus (the site is frequently identified by a small dimple or groove running vertically over the dome of the fundus). The incision is carried to the junction of the 2 uterine cavities. If a complete septum is present, the incision is carried to the level of the internal cervical ring or the junction of the lower uterine segment and the cervix. **C.** After the fundal incision has been carried to the point of entering the uterine cavity, the knife blade should be turned 90 degrees and an incision made in the central portion of each uterine horn until the blue-stained endometrial lining is clearly exposed. If gauze or a metal probe have been used, they should be removed vaginally at this time, if possible. **D.** At times excess septal tissue will appear to prevent a smooth closure. This author (G.W.P.) has found it convenient to trim the edges of each cavity as shown in this drawing. **E.** A linear incision is made in the midportion of the myometrium to facilitate a three-layer closure. The dark blue endometrium is visible. **F.** The first layer of myometrial suture employs 2-0 synthetic absorbable suture material. A running suture is begun on each side and carried to the midfundal site where the two are joined. **G.** A second layer of myometrial closure also utilizes 2-0 Dexon or Vicral and, again, a running suture is used and is joined at the midfundus. **H.** The uterine serosa is approximated with a subcuticular running suture of 4-0 Dexon or Vicral. This presents a smooth linear incision that is thought less likely to be a site of subsequent adhesion formation.

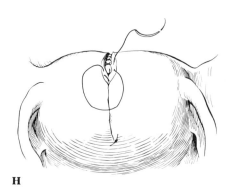

**H**

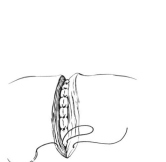

**G**

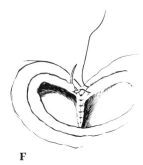

**F**

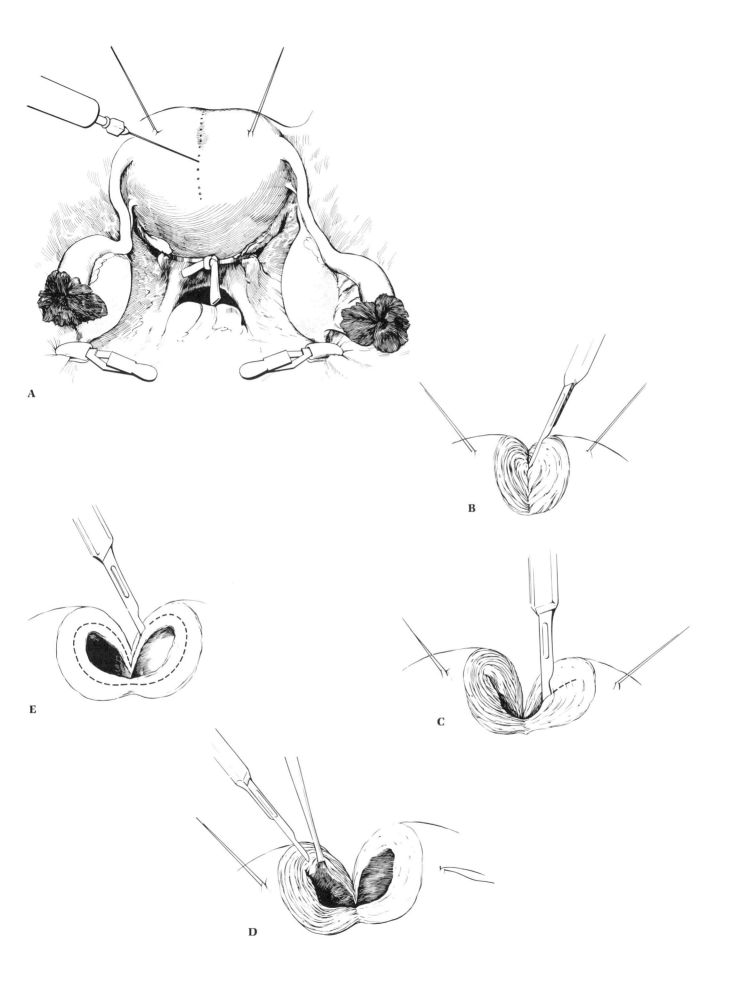

A

B

C

D

E

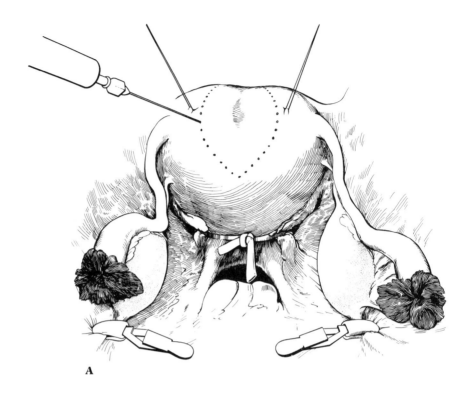

**A**

**Figure 4-15.** Unification of a subseptate uterus (Jones procedure). **A.** Subseptate uterus showing the line of incision necessary to excise the central septum (*dotted line*). The incision should begin 1 to 2 cm from each cornu, and the surgeon must keep in mind that the final uterine fundus will be the sum of these two distances. The site of incision is marked with vital dye and injected with dilute vasopressin (Pitressin). The tourniquet technique described earlier is also used. **B.** The line of wedge excision is carried to the junction of the two uterine cavities if a partial septum is present. If a complete septum is being excised, the excision extends to the lower uterine segment. Additional myometrium is excised to enter the endometrial cavities. **C.** Because the myometrial wall is quite thick an incision should be made in the long axis of the uterine horn. This permits a more precise two-layer closure. **D.** A three-layer closure is used as described in the Tompkins procedure. First, a layer of running 2-0 synthetic absorbable suture (Dexon or Vicral) progresses evenly on the anterior and posterior uterine wall to achieve a symmetrical closure. The endometrium is excluded from this suture. **E.** The second myometrial layer is closed in a similar manner with a similar suture. **F.** The uterine serosa is approximated with a running subcuticular suture of 4-0 Dexon or Vicral. A smooth closure with minimal bleeding is achieved.

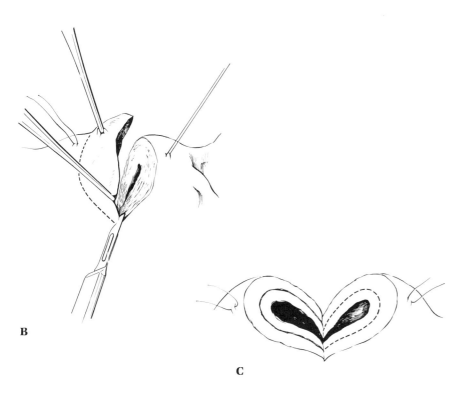

**B**

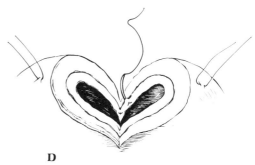

**C**

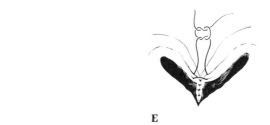

**D**

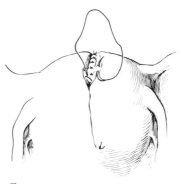

**E**

**F**

Although habitual abortion and repetitive midtrimester loss are not usually associated with a bicornuate uterus of minor degree, a cause-and-effect relationship does exist in certain patients when the abnormality is severe. It is our opinion that a Strassman metroplasty (Fig. 4-16) is the procedure of choice for reconstruction of this uterine anomaly. And the caveat here is "Don't cut out—cut in" [47].

**Figure 4-16.** Unification of the bicornuate uterus (Strassman's metroplasty). **A.** A typical bicornuate uterus, characterized by 2 endometrial cavities and a single endocervical canal and lower uterine segment. Traction sutures of 2-0 Dexon are placed near the round ligaments' junction with the uterine fundus. The line of incision is that advocated by Strassman (*dotted line*). Preliminary staining of the endometrial cavity with methylene blue dye, or insertion of gauze packing or a uterine sound into each horn prior to laparotomy assists in identifying the endometrial cavities at the time of incision, thereby reducing blood loss. Blood loss is further minimized by placing rubber shod bulldog clamps over the infundibulopelvic ligaments and a tourniquet around the uterine vessels. Vasopressin (Pitressin) should be injected along the proposed site of incision. **B.** Both endometrial cavities have been entered. The vesicorectal ligament is ligated and cut in the midportion. The incision of the common lower uterine segment is completed. **C.** The uterine closure used in the Strassman procedure is identical to that described for the Tompkins and Jones procedures. A linear incision has been made in the myometrium to facilitate three-layer closure of the uterus. The first layer uses a running 2-0 synthetic absorbable suture that excludes the mucosal layer. **D.** The second myometrial layer is also closed with 2-0 Dexon or Vicral. Two running sutures begin in the lateral cornual area and carry to the central portion where they are tied. **E.** The serosal layer is approximated with 4-0 Dexon in a running subcuticular suture. The use of an omental graft to cover this suture line has been found necessary when this closure is used.

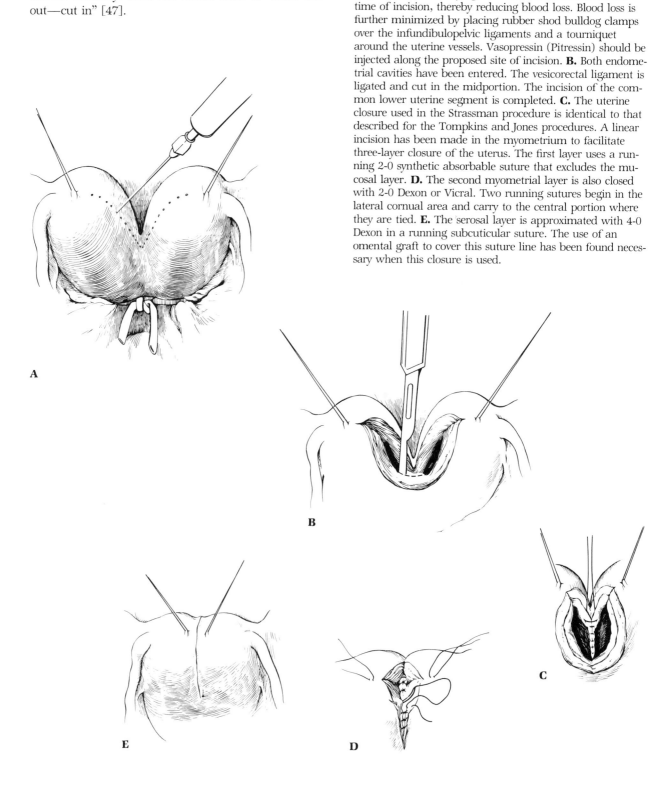

A

B

C

D

E

In January 1982 DeCherney (16a) presented the somewhat startling evidence that a uterine septum could be safely removed by an operative hysteroscopic technique. This surgeon utilized a resectoscope and electrocautery to remove a uterine septum in 11 patients found to have pregnancy wastage due to a septate uterus. Nine of the 11 patients subsequently achieved a successful pregnancy. The technique employed concurrent laparoscopy to insure that the intestine was not in contact with the uterus during electrocoagulation of the septum. Daly et al. [15a] appears recently to have confirmed the usefulness of this approach. These authors performed hysteroscopic septum removal in 25 patients without apparent complications. Minimal bleeding occurred at the time of septum incision, and blood transfusion was not performed in any of these patients. Laparoscopy was again performed concurrently as a safety measure. Adequate follow-up of these patients has not been possible, however, a preliminary report indicates that 10 of 11 patients with preoperative repetitive pregnancy wastage have had a successful pregnancy following this surgery.

The operative hysteroscopic approach to septum resection is of great interest because of apparent low morbidity and convenience to the patient. Certainly the vaginal approach would be preferable to an intraabdominal metroplasty if it proves to be of equal benefit. Most of these patients underwent vaginal delivery rather than the cesarean section commonly performed following metroplasty. Further study of this operative approach will be followed with interest.

Surgical removal of the uterine septum is not the only treatment for the patient with a septate or bicornuate uterus who has experienced repetitive pregnancy wastage. Cervical cerclage has been shown to improve pregnancy success rates in these patients whether or not it is combined with a metroplasty. Keetle's [39] early success with this technique in such patients led him to state the belief that "certain patients with congenital defects of the uterus also have defects of the internal os." Later, the combination of cervical cerclage and metroplasty in 14 patients by Craig (14) resulted in an improved pregnancy success rate.

The role of cervical cerclage as the primary therapy in patients with a symptomatic septate or bicornuate uterine anomaly has been studied by two Israeli investigators. Gross (24) treated 24 patients with a bicornuate anomaly by cervical cerclage and achieved a living child in 77 percent of these women. In 1977 Blum (6) reported that treatment of 13 patients who had a bicornuate uterus by cervical cerclage was successful in 88 percent. This compared to a preoperative pregnancy success rate of only 17 percent in these patients.

Although the use of cerclage as primary therapy for a patient with a septate uterine anomaly remains controversial, it is clear that the surgeon should at least consider such a course. The simplicity of this procedure in patients with a fixed septum not amenable to hysteroscopic resection makes it a potential therapy for individuals who do not quite meet the criteria for metroplasty but in whom a uterine septum appears to be an etiologic factor.

The benefit of cerclage in patients whose pregnancy wastage is thought to be related to a unicornuate uterus or uterus didelphys is clear. The authors have successfully treated such patients with a temporary Shirodkar cerclage removed approximately one week before the expected date of delivery and strongly recommend this therapeutic approach. The role of cervical cerclage as a form of treatment in patients with habitual abortion has been discussed at length in Chapter 3. Surgery of the cervix, including Shirodkar and McDonald cerclage procedures, have been outlined in detail in that section.

*Results of Surgical Procedures Involving the Uterus*

Paul Strassman performed the metroplasty that bears his name on only 18 patients with bicornuate uteri, and 8 of these were approached vaginally through an anterior colpotomy incision. His son, Erwin Strassman, operated on 22 patients with double uteri between 1954 and 1960 for reproductive failure. Preoperatively, these 22 patients had 44 pregnancies, 43 of which had ended in spontaneous abortion, and only one had resulted in a living child. Postoperatively 23 pregnancies were recorded, and 18 (78 percent) were carried to term and resulted in living children. The number of *patients* who achieved a living child was not reported. Eight of these operations were performed for primary sterility, and, postoperatively, in this group 9 pregnancies occurred and 7 patients achieved a living child.

As was discussed earlier, the series of patients with uterine anomalies followed at Johns Hopkins University Hospital [55] compared a group of patients with a normal obstetric history (group A) with patients in a treatment group (group B) who had achieved a living child in only 3 percent of 140 pregnancies. Group A patients were divided into those with normal obstetric histories and included 100 patients in whom 284 pregnancies had resulted in living children 70 percent of the time. Term pregnancy occurred in 67 percent, premature infants in 10 percent, and spontaneous abortion in 23 percent. There were 29 additional patients in group A with poor obstetrical histories who received no special medical care.

In comparison were 43 patients classified as group B-2 who underwent surgical metroplasty. Apparently 42 of 43 patients had septate uterine anomalies and all 42 underwent the Jones wedge-resection procedure. Preoperatively, 8 percent of the 43 patients had achieved living children, and this increased to 77 percent postoperatively. Among 140 preoperative pregnancies none were carried to term, and 3 percent of these pregnancies produced living children. Postoperatively, 58 pregnancies were carried to term in 42 patients (73 percent), and the 94 percent preoperative spontaneous abortion rate was lowered to 20 percent following surgical repair. Overall, 70 percent of pregnancies produced living children, a marked increase from the 3 percent preoperative level.

Tompkins [69, 70] using the metroplasty procedure described earlier, reported 14 cases, 9 of which were observed longer than 15 months, and all conceived postoperatively. This group had 12 pregnancies resulting in 10 term births, 2 premature deliveries, and 1 spontaneous abortion. Eight of the 9 patients had a living child postoperatively. All deliveries were by cesarean section at 39 weeks of gestation. Five patients have been followed less than 15 months postoperatively, and at this time none have conceived. No surgical complications occurred in this group of 14 patients.

Buttram [11] recently reported the obstetric outcome of 67 patients found to have poor obstetric histories associated with septate uterine anomalies. Fifty-three of these patients had partial uterine septa, and in 14 complete septa were found. Seven of the patients with complete septa underwent surgical unification, and 6 were followed for 12 months postoperatively. Five of these 6 patients conceived and all 5 pregnancies resulted in term infants. Among those patients with incomplete septa, 39 had uterine metroplasties; however, only 28 patients had been followed for 12 months at the time of the report. Twenty of the 39 patients conceived postop-

eratively, and 13/20 patients delivered term infants. Two of the 7 remaining patients had premature infants that lived, 1 had a spontaneous abortion, 1 an ectopic pregnancy, and 3 were lost to follow-up during the pregnancy.

*Approach to the Double Uterus*

In conclusion, a patient who has experienced 2 or 3 consecutive spontaneous abortions or who has had a midtrimester or premature fetal loss may be found at the time of hysterosalpingography to have a double uterus, either septate or bicornuate. Every effort should be made, however, by the usual diagnostic regimen to exclude other causes of pregnancy wastage, including luteal phase insufficiency, genetic abnormalities, mycoplasma infection, and cervical incompetence. The authors agree with Craig [14] that if the first pregnancy ended in either a premature loss or midtrimester abortion, then a second pregnancy will usually follow the same course. Yet, if the first pregnancy went to term and a congenital anomaly was found with a second pregnancy midtrimester loss, metroplasty should be delayed until after the third or fourth pregnancy loss. At least two successive first trimester abortions should occur before corrective surgery is recommended. Septate uteri have been most commonly associated with a high rate of pregnancy wastage [55]; however, others have noted similar histories in patients with bicornuate uteri [35]. We prefer the Strassman metroplasty for repair of a bicornuate uterus and have recently used with success the Tompkins technique for unification of a septate form. The available data indicate that properly selected patients who undergo unification can anticipate a 75 percent chance of having a living child. The role of cervical cerclage and hysteroscopic resection in treatment of the bicornuate or subseptate uterus has been discussed earlier.

The degree to which didelphic and unicornuate uteri are associated with increased pregnancy wastage is unresolved. Miller [46] noted in 1962 that in a patient with a didelphic uterus "the chance for a normal spontaneous birth at term is only 41.7 percent" and "28.3 percent of pregnancies . . . abort during the early period of gestation." Steinberg [63] reported from the literature 34 patients who underwent metroplasty for didelphic uteri. However, only 8 of these patients had a history of repetitive pregnancy loss; the others were operated on primarily for relief of dysmenorrhea. Postoperatively, 3 of the 8 patients were lost to follow-up, but 4 of the other 5 had a living child. Buttram and Gibbons [11] reported the occurrence of uterus didelphys in 4/100 patients with uterine anomalies and found that fetal survival occurred in 2 of 5 pregnancies. No surgical attempts were made to repair this anomaly. In contrast, Musich and Behrman [48] noted this uterine anomaly in 11 of 41 patients. Fetal survival occurred in 20/35 (57 percent) conceptions in this group. Both recent reports confirm the relatively favorable obstetric outlook associated with this type of uterine anomaly.

Occasionally, patients with didelphic uteri will be thought to benefit from uterine unification. However, as was noted earlier, the role of cervical incompetence should be considered and cervical cerclage performed if midtrimester pregnancy loss has occurred. The same criteria used to evaluate the patients with a bicornuate uterus should be applied here. The surgical metroplasty technique employed is one that leaves the double cervix in situ and unifies the corpus of the uterus in a manner similar to that described by Strassman for a bicornuate uterus.

The incidence of pregnancy wastage in a patient with a unicornuate uterus is difficult to determine because of the rarity of this anomaly. Semmens [59] in 1962 noted one personal case of unicornuate uterus and 14 case reports from the literature. These 14 patients had 19 pregnancies with a 21 percent fetal wastage rate, which is similar to the rate of 23.7 percent in patients with didelphic uteri. The fetal wastage rate was 37.1 percent in patients with bicornuate and septate uteri and 19 percent in a control group of patients with arcuate uteri. Four patients with a unicornuate uterus followed by W. S. Jones [36] had 10 pregnancies. These patients were combined with 12 who had complete müllerian doubling, and these 16 patients with hemiuteri were found to have an abortion rate of 37.4 percent; only 60 percent of pregnancies were carried to term. Gross fetal wastage was 46.0 percent. Buttram [11] reported the pregnancy outcome in 19 patients with unicornuate uteri in 1979. In this group, 14 pregnancies occurred in 10 individuals and 12/14 of the pregnancies ended in abortion. Two term infants resulted among the 6 patients who were placed in class II (Fig. 4-4B) that had an anomaly in which a communicating rudimentary horn is attached to the unicornuate uterus. Remarkably, only 1 of 6 patients with pure unicornuate uteri conceived. Five of 6 patients had undergone surgical excision of the communicating rudimentary horn and, among this group, 3 patients had endometriosis and 1 had pelvic adhesions. This low incidence of conception has not been this author's (G.W.P.) experience in dealing with unicornuate uteri. In 5 patients with unicornuate uteri, 4 have conceived and have eventually had a living infant. The fifth patient underwent salpingostomy and has not yet conceived. Cervical cerclage has been used successfully in 2 of these patients. Craig (1973) [14] and Michalas (1976) [45] have discussed the association of a unicornuate uterus and incompetent cervix, and in each instance used a Shirodkar-type cerclage successfully during treatment.

*Approach to DES-related Uterine Anomaly*

In the series of 60 patients reported by Kaufman in 1977 [38] only 12 had prior pregnancies and 5 of these had been voluntarily terminated. Of the remaining 7 pregnancies, 1 was ectopic, 2 ended in spontaneous abortion, 3 were premature deliveries, and 1 resulted in a term delivery. Of the 2 patients who had spontaneous abortions, 1 had an abnormal hysterosalpingogram, and 2 of the premature deliveries occurred in abnormal uteri. The only term pregnancy occurred in a patient with a normal uterus.

Berger and Goldstein [5] described the obstetric history of 69 women who demonstrated DES-related cervical-vaginal abnormalities. Pregnancy occurred in 46 of these patients (67 percent), and 32 of the patients who were followed had 62 pregnancies that resulted in only 26 living children. Among the 36 pregnancy losses were 19 first trimester abortions, 11 second trimester losses, 3 premature infants who died, and 3 ectopic tubal pregnancies. Five other premature infants survived, as did 21 term infants, although 2 of these patients were treated with cervical cerclage. In an earlier report, Goldstein [22] described the successful use of cervical cerclage in 5 patients found to have cervical incompetence who had been treated with DES in utero. The uterine contour of the patients followed by Berger and Goldstein was not reported. This study and others were discussed in a publication by Pillsbury in 1980 [52]. Table 4-3 summarizes the results of pregnancy in DES-exposed women.

**Table 4-3.** Results of pregnancies in DES-exposed women

| | No. of pregnancies | No. of women | Term delivery | Preterm delivery | 2Δ Spontaneous abortions | 1Δ Spontaneous abortion | Therapeutic abortions | Tubal pregnancy |
|---|---|---|---|---|---|---|---|---|
| Bibbo and associates | 41 | 41[a] | 30 | | | 11 | | |
| Kaufman and Adam | 14 | 14 | 2 | 3 | | 2 | 5 | 2 |
| Sandberg | 47 | 39 | 17 | 3 | | 3 | 23 | 1 |
| Singer and Hochman | 2 | 1 | | | 2[b] | | | |
| Berger and Goldstein | 80 | 46 | 21[c] | 8[c] | 11 | 19 | 18 | 3 |
| Totals | 184 | 141 | 70 | 14 | 13 | 35 | 46 | 6 |

[a]Numbers reported here were implied but not specifically stated.
[b]Both midpregnancy losses said to have been due to cervical insufficiency.
[c]Cervical cerclage said to have been required in 8 of the 26 pregnancies with surviving infants.
Source: S. G. Pillsbury, Jr., Reproductive significance of changes in the endometrial cavity associated with exposure in utero to diethylstilbestrol, *Am. J. Obstet. Gynecol.* 137:178, 1980.

Recently, Herbst et al. [27] compared the obstetric history of 226 DES-exposed females with 206 unexposed women whose mothers participated in a double-blind evaluation 27 years prior to this follow-up. These women were members of the study reported by Dieckmann et al. [17]. Primary infertility was somewhat higher in the DES-exposed group. These authors also noted that premature live births occurred in 22 percent of DES-exposed patients, compared to 7 percent of the control group. Nonviable outcomes, including stillbirth, neonatal death, miscarriage, and ectopic pregnancy occurred in 31 percent of DES-exposed, and 8 percent of unexposed patients. No correlation was found between intrauterine DES dosage and pregnancy outcome. Five DES-exposed patients reported by Herbst were treated with cervical cerclage after experiencing prior premature stillbirth or miscarriage. All 5 patients subsequently had a living child, 4 at term and 1 premature birth.

It has become clear that DES-exposed females may demonstrate uterine as well as cervical and upper vaginal anomalies. The presence of a cervical abnormality increases the possibility of finding a T-shaped uterus by hysterosalpingography. No surgical or hormonal therapy has yet been demonstrated to reduce the incidence of spontaneous abortion in these patients. An x-ray pattern demonstrates the frustration of this situation in a patient who experienced 2 spontaneous abortions and has no living children (see Fig. 4-11).

Prior midtrimester loss has been successfully treated with cervical cerclage. It is our opinion that this form of therapy should be offered to these patients. Whether cerclage would reduce the incidence of first trimester loss, as has been shown in two series of congenital uterine anomalies, is unclear.

## The Myomatous Uterus

Although pregnancy often occurs in myomatous uteri, the presence of such tumors imposes a considerable degree of relative infertility, although we know little as to the mechanism involved. In the management of sterility problems in the younger group of women, after elimination of other factors in husband and wife, I do not hesitate to advise myomectomy if one or more tumors of any real size are present. Such a considerable proportion of these patients become pregnant after these operations . . . as to leave no doubt, in my mind at least, as to the causative role of the myoma in infertility.

EMIL NOVAK [50]

The history of myomectomy appears to date from 1840, when Amussat, of Paris, removed a pedunculated uterine fibroid. In 1843 Atlee, of Lancaster, Pennsylvania, also removed a uterine fibroid, and in 1898 Alexander, of Liverpool, England, removed 25 fibromyomata from a single uterus. Conservative tubal surgery was also being suggested at this time, and this undoubtedly provided impetus to a few surgeons who attempted to

conserve myomatous uteri for further childbearing. Sepsis and hemorrhage were formidable obstacles to this procedure, however, and a significant mortality was reported. This is emphasized in the series of 96 patients reported by Martin in 1890 [44], in which 18 patients died following surgery. Some improvement occurred by 1909, when Kelly and Cullen [40] reported myomectomy on 296 patients at Johns Hopkins Hospital, 16 of whom died postoperatively.

Although myomectomy was recommended by Bonney in 1925 [7], it was not until the post–World War II era that the operative morbidity associated with this procedure reached an acceptable level. Israel, Ingersoll, and others in the United States suggested myomectomy for improving fertility and supported their views with statistically significant data [29, 30]. In 1951, Novak made the statement quoted at the beginning of this section. Additional reports advocating myomectomy have been published by Stevenson and by Finn and Muller [20, 64].

### Relationship of Leiomyomas to Sterility and Pregnancy Wastage

During a discussion of the relationship of leiomyomata and sterility, Rubin stated (1954) [56], "That the presence of these uterine tumors acts as a deterrent to conception and successful culmination of pregnancy, there can be no doubt." This surgeon observed (57) that ". . . about 40 percent of married women with multiple uterine fibroids have a history of childlessness." In a series of 481 married women operated on for myomas at Mt. Sinai Hospital in New York City, 42 percent had never conceived and 18.3 percent had delivered only a single child prior to surgery. Barter and Parks [3] have established that 5 percent of infertility patients have a myomatous uterus that is at least partially responsible for their inability to conceive.

It is likely that inability of patients with myomatous uteri to achieve pregnancy may in large measure be related to the difficulty of implantation in the area of a submucous fibroid. However, an intramural fibroid adjacent to the intramural tubal segment may cause cornual occlusion, and a large posterior fibroid may interfere with tubal function and prevent oocyte pickup (Fig. 4-17). The association between uterine leiomyomata and pregnancy wastage has received less scientific attention, although both Rubin [56] and Davids [16] noted an increase in spontaneous abortion among patients with a myomatous uterus. Recently, Wallach [9] stated

Despite all of these theoretical influences, it is relatively unusual for myomas to interfere with establishment of a pregnancy. Uterine myomas are more likely to have an adverse influence on the outcome of pregnancy once established. Impaired implantation, recurrent spontaneous abortion, premature labor, and abnormal fetal presentations are more commonly associated with myomas than is infertility per se.

**Figure 4-17.** Location of uterine leiomyomata. **A.** A submucous leiomyoma. **B.** Subserous leiomyomata. **C.** Three intramural leiomyomata. (From R. W. Kistner, *Gynecology: Principles and Practice* (3rd ed.). Chicago: Year Book, 1979. Reprinted with permission.)

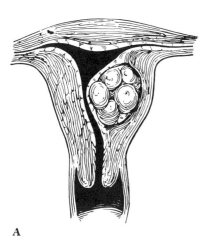

A

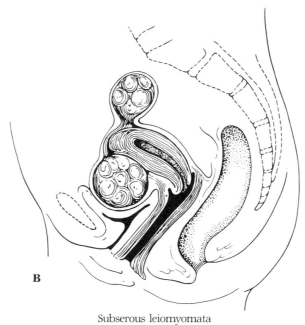

B

Subserous leiomyomata

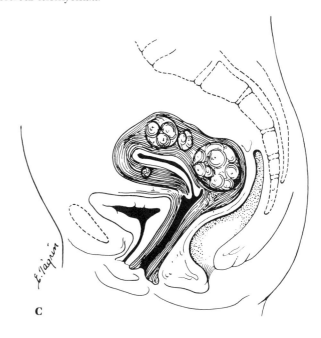

C

Despite the conviction that uterine myomas may be a significant cause of early pregnancy loss, little clinical data has been available to support this relationship. Davids [16] noted a history of spontaneous abortion in 41 percent of 432 married women with myomatous uteri, and observed that 69 of these patients had a history of 2 to 5 miscarriages. A recent retrospective study from Johns Hopkins Hospital [1] also supports this association. In this group of 46 patients who underwent myomectomy for infertility, 12 had secondary infertility. The group of 12 patients had achieved 21 preoperative pregnancies 16 of which ended in miscarriage, and 5 resulted in a living child. Following myomectomy in 6 patients, 8 pregnancies were carried to term.

In the past, most myomectomy procedures performed on infertile patients whose inability to conceive has been attributed to a myoma have been found to have a submucous or intraluminal fibroid. This association was due to the preoperative identification of endometrial distortion by hysterosalpingography, and, more recently, by hysteroscopy and the acceptance of this observation as an indication for myomectomy. Ingersoll [29] discussed the etiology of sterility in patients with myomatous uteri and noted that ". . . the mechanism by which a leiomyoma interferes with conception is dependent upon the location, size, and blood supply." In concert with this anatomic approach, there is recent evidence to support the notion of Rubin [56] and others that intramural and subserous myomas may also be a principle cause of sterility. In the study from Johns Hopkins Hospital referred to above, Babaknia, Rock, and Jones [1] found that among 44 patients with a preoperative hysterogram who underwent myomectomy for sterility, only 9 had uterine distortion apparent at this x-ray study. No other cause of sterility was found in the 33 patients who underwent myomectomy, and, postoperatively, pregnancy occurred in 16 patients. In contrast, 5 of 9 patients whose endometrial cavity was abnormal conceived following surgery. Somewhat difficult to explain was the observation in this series that only 6 of the 12 patients with secondary infertility had demonstrated an irregular uterine contour on a preoperative hysterogram. As expected following surgery, pregnancy occurred in 5 of these 6 patients, and 4 of these carried to term. Remarkably, however, 3 of the 6 patients whose preoperative hysterogram revealed a normal uterine contour conceived following myomectomy and 2 term pregnancies resulted. These authors did not offer an explanation for the pregnancy successes in this latter small group.

Uterine leiomyomas occur in the presence of other pelvic pathologic conditions that may interfere with fertility. Eighteen percent of patients undergoing hysterectomy or myomectomy for leiomyomata were found to demonstrate tuboovarian abnormalities [57], and Kelly and Cullen [40] found normal tubes in only 51.6 percent of 934 patients undergoing hysterectomy for myomatous enlargement. These data, however, add little to one's approach to the infertile patient, because the presence of tubal abnormalities is known preoperatively in the infertile patient and, in most cases, would be the primary indication for laparotomy. The combination of tubal pathologic changes and significant uterine distortion by a myoma is uncommon in our experience. Malone and Ingersoll [42, 43] found extensive endometriosis in 5 of 75 patients operated on for leiomyomas, and pelvic adhesions also occurred in 5 of these 75 patients. Thirty-five of the 75 patients had associated pelvic pathologic changes, most of which were minor.

In summary, the following list of six relationships between leiomyomata and sterility or pregnancy wastage proposed by Rubin [57] seems current. These have been paraphrased and are listed below.

1. The location of a myoma may impede oocyte pick-up or interfere with sperm transport.
2. Associated tubal and adnexal pathology may be falsely identified as a fibromyoma.
3. A submucous myoma may prevent implantation.
4. A submucous or intramural myoma may cause uterine contractions and produce abortion.
5. A premature delivery may be caused by torsion of a pedunculated fibroid.
6. A myoma in the lower uterine segment may lead to an obstructed labor.

## Preoperative Approach

A complete sterility evaluation should be performed on the infertile patient with a myomatous uterus. The presence of normal ovulation and normal cervical, tubal, and sperm factors should be determined. Hysterosalpingography will identify an intraluminal myoma as a lucent defect within the endometrial cavity that must be differentiated from an air bubble or polyp (Fig. 4-18). Further confirmation of this mass by direct endoscopic visualization is essential.

**Figure 4-18.** Intrauterine mass outlined during hysterography was later found by hysteroscopy to be an endometrial polyp.

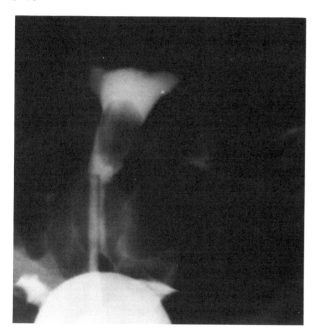

Hysteroscopic examination of the uterine cavity (see Chap. 2) is helpful in the diagnosis and management of a submucous or intraluminal fibroid. It permits direct observation of the intraluminal mass that may be an endometrial polyp and avoids opening the uterine cavity only to find that the mass was an artifact of the x-ray study. Figure 4-19 demonstrates the subtlety of hysterographic evaluation of an intraluminal fibroid.

Diagnostic laparoscopy is an essential test during evaluation of those patients thought to have myomatous uteri and in whom the hysterogram was normal. Not only does it permit careful evaluation of an abdominal mass, but it offers reevaluation of tubal function under direct vision.

Tubal patency should be verified at the time of hysterosalpingography and at laparoscopy, because a question of patency may arise during laparotomy. In most cases of questionable tubal patency, transfundal lavage is performed before and after myomectomy. Technical problems at the time of laparotomy may be associated with difficulty in placing the needle or catheter in a distorted uterine cavity; following myomectomy, small endometrial fragments or blood clots may transiently occlude the cornual opening and lead to an erroneous diagnosis of cornual occlusion. We have occasionally experienced such difficulty following removal of a large intraluminal fibroid.

**Figure 4-19.** Hysterographic study. **A.** Injection of water-soluble dye outlines an obvious intrauterine mass. **B.** Overfilling the uterus with dye almost obscures the mass and is responsible for false-negative results. **C.** A delayed x-ray film following aspiration of dye from the uterine cavity clearly outlines the mass later found to be an intraluminal leiomyoma. This patient conceived easily following myomectomy but required cervical cerclage because of cervical incompetence.

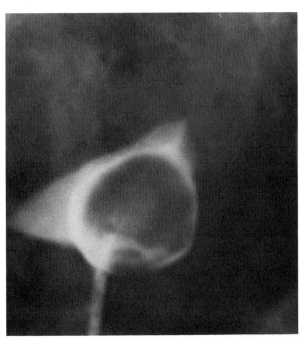

A

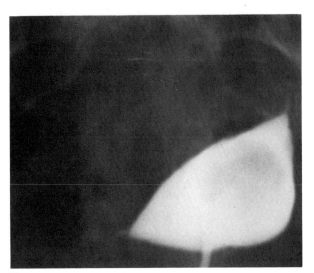

B

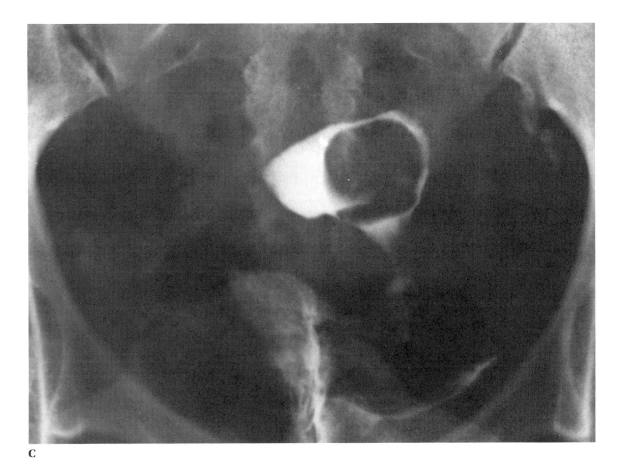

C

*Techniques of Myomectomy*

As with other operative procedures to improve fertility, the abdominal route is commonly used for myomectomy in the infertile patient. In most a transverse incision gives good exposure. The caveat here is "The fewer incisions in the uterus, the better" [30]. (See hysteroscopic resection of intraluminal myomas in Chap. 2.)

Hemostasis is a major factor during the abdominal procedure, and we recommend the tourniquet method popularized by Rubin [57] and described earlier in this chapter. A dry field is thus encountered on opening the uterus. This technique demands that careful apposition of reapproximated myometrium be accomplished to prevent bleeding following removal of the tourniquet. Hemostasis may also be achieved by using a Bonney clamp to occlude the uterine vessels and stabilize the uterus, or by injecting oxytocin or dilute epinephrine locally at the site of each uterine incision. These techniques of hemostasis are shown in Figure 4-20.

**Figure 4-20.** Technique of hemostasis. The following technique of hemostasis is described as it is used in a myomatous uterus, but it is also used by the author (Patton) during repair of a septate uterus. It has previously been referred to in the section on uterine metroplasty. **A.** A No. 12 rubber catheter is grasped by a mixter clamp passed through a small incision beneath the round and uteroovarian ligaments. Bulldog clamps have been placed on the ovarian vessels. **B.** A similar incision has been made in the opposite broad ligament through which a mixter clamp has been passed. The rubber catheter is pulled through this opening to encircle the lower uterine segment. **C.** The rubber tourniquet is tied tightly, thereby occluding the uterine vessels. **D.** Following application of the tourniquet and bulldog clamps, dilute Pitressin is injected along the line of incision shown as a dotted line both in myomectomy and metroplasty procedures.

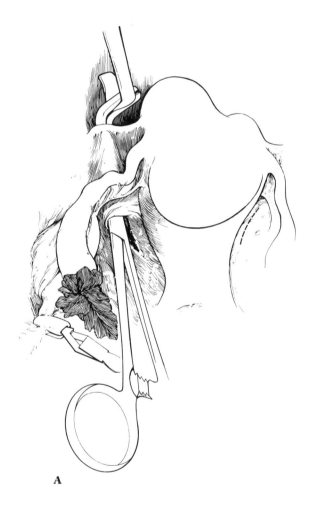

A

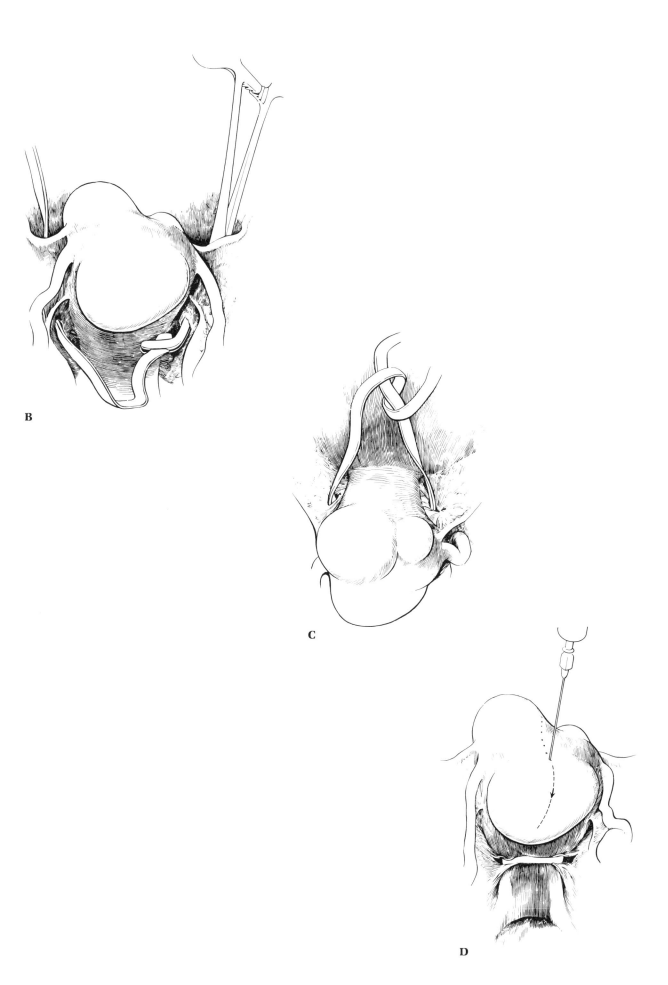

B

C

D

A midline incision is used whenever possible. Injection of dilute Pitressin and a rubber tourniquet are employed for hemostasis. Traction on the myoma is provided by grasping it with a small towel clip. The capsule is smooth and permits blunt dissection with either a knife blade or finger to pry it out of the surrounding myometrium. These points are demonstrated in Figure 4-21.

**Figure 4-21.** Surgical approach to an anterior fibroid. **A.** Following the application of the tourniquet and bulldog clamps, dilute Pitressin is injected along the line of incision. A midline incision is used whenever possible, utilizing the knife, as is shown in this drawing, or the electrode with cutting current, as is shown later. **B.** The myoma is grasped with a towel clamp to provide traction and pried from the surrounding myometrium by using a knife handle. **C.** Gentle dissection with an index finger also assists in separating the fibroid from surrounding myometrium. **D.** Improved hemostasis is achieved by ligating the vascular pedicle at the base of the myoma prior to removal. **E.** Additional myomata should be removed through a single midline incision whenever possible. Finger pressure on the myomata will often facilitate removal. Closure of the uterine wall is performed in layers using synthetic absorbable suture of 2-0 gauge. A subcuticular closure with 4-0 suture is used whenever possible.

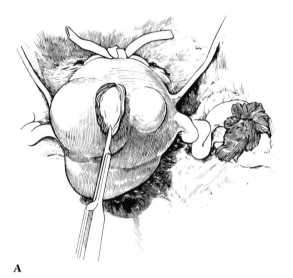

**A**

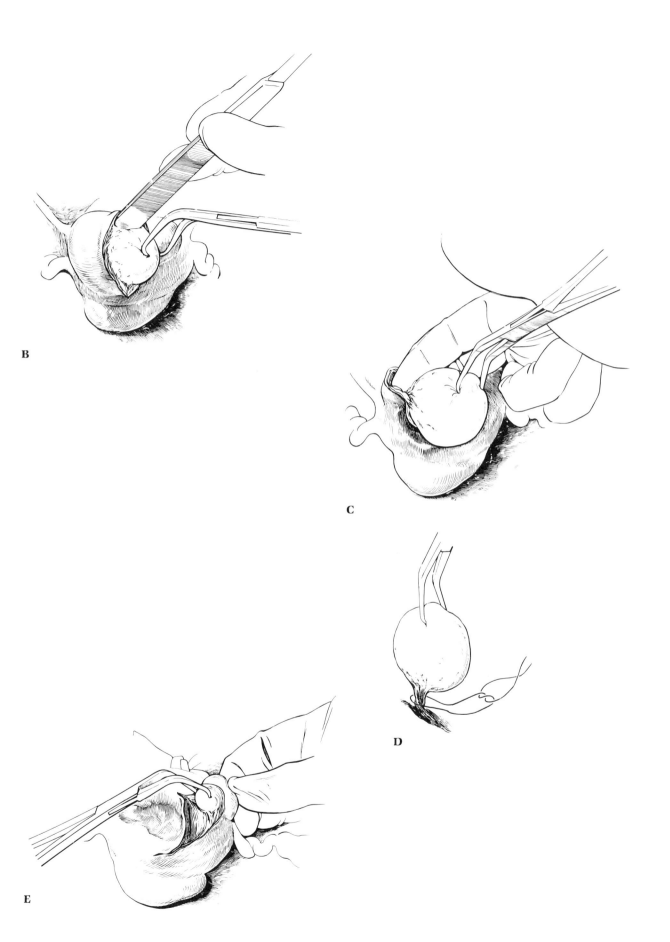

B

C

D

E

Removal of a posterior myoma is facilitated by first removing all anterior fibroids, thereby permitting improved posterior exposure. Again, a midline incision is used and hemostasis accomplished by the tourniquet technique shown earlier. Dilute Pitressin is also injected along the line of incision and a monopolar electrode used whenever convenient. This technique is shown in Figure 4-22.

**Figure 4-22.** Surgical approach to a posterior fibroid. **A.** A midline incision has been used to expose a large posterior fibroid. The fibroid is elevated with a towel clip and dissected with the electrosurgical needle, using a blended current. A small degree of coagulation produces excellent hemostasis during this procedure. Use of the fine tip permits dissection of the smooth capsule; however, it is still necessary to place a suture around the blood vessels in the pedicle. **B.** After the myoma has been removed, the endometrial cavity should be explored gently with a finger or blunt instrument to ascertain normal contour. Closure of the endometrial and myometrial layers is performed in three layers, as described earlier. A subcuticular serosal closure prevents subsequent adhesion formation.

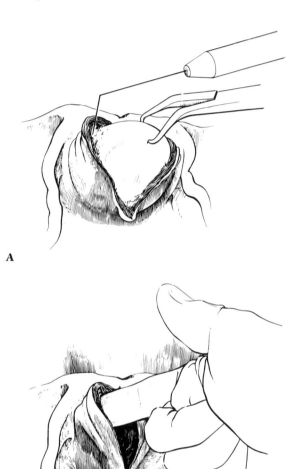

A

B

*Results of Myomectomy*

Pregnancy occurs postoperatively in about 50 percent of infertile patients carefully selected for myomectomy [20, 42, 64, 73]. The preoperative and postoperative hysterosalpingograms of a patient who successfully achieved a pregnancy following myomectomy by the author (G. W.P.) are shown in Figure 4-23A and B. Malone and Ingersoll [42] reported that 49 percent of 75 patients who were infertile for longer than 1 year, whose uteri were greater than twice normal size, and who underwent myomectomy conceived postoperatively, and 40 percent delivered term infants. Preoperatively, two-thirds of these patients had primary infertility, and only 17 percent had a living child. The average duration of infertility in this series was 3.9 years. Fifty-one percent of pregnancies occurred within the first postoperative year and 70 percent within the first two years.

Stevenson [64] reported results of myomectomy for the improvement of childbearing in 107 patients. This group included 69 infertile patients who underwent myomectomy in the nonpregnant state. In 17 patients, myomectomy was done to protect a concurrent pregnancy, and in 21 it was performed at the time of cesarean section.

In a group of patients who were comparable to those reported by Malone and Ingersoll, Stevenson followed 52 patients on whom myomectomy had been performed in the nonpregnant state to improve infertility. Patients with other causes of infertility were excluded. Fifty percent of this group had primary infertility, 25 percent had only spontaneous abortions, and 25 percent had term pregnancies. Among those with primary infertility, 58 percent conceived postoperatively and 50 percent had term pregnancies. In the entire group undergoing myomectomy, 63 percent conceived, and 54 percent carried to term.

**Figure 4-23. A.** This hysterogram demonstrates a large submucous fibroid in a patient with primary infertility. At the time of myomectomy, this was found to be a single large posterior fibroid. **B.** The postoperative hysterogram of this uterine abnormality **(A)** demonstrates a uterine cavity that appears to be almost normal.

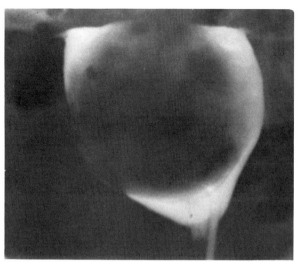

A

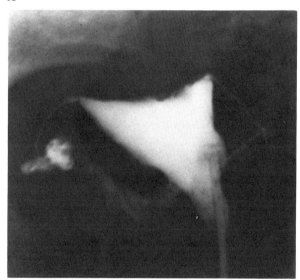

B

**Table 4-4.** Pregnancy rate in
infertile women following myomectomy

| Year | Reference | N | Infertile | Infertile patients who conceived |
|------|-----------|-----|-----------|-------------------|
| 1931 | Bonney | 210 | 77 | 30 (39%) |
| 1937 | Miller and Tyrone | 94 | 69 | 21 (30%) |
| 1937 | Counseller and Bedard | 523 | 196 | 68 (35%) |
| 1945 | Mussey et al. | 221 | 82 | 8 (10%) |
| 1950 | Finn and Muller | 432 | 46 | 17 (37%) |
| 1951 | Munnell and Martin | 370 | 23 | 13 (57%) |
| 1956 | Brown et al. | 335 | 21 | 11 (52%) |
| 1957 | Davids | 1335 | 310[a] | 140 (45%) |
| 1957 | Rubin | 167 | 73 | 21 (29%) |
| 1958 | McCormick | 66 | 20 | 6 (30%) |
| 1963 | Ingersoll | 139 | 56 | 28 (50%) |
| 1964 | Stevenson | 107 | 52 | 30 (58%) |
| 1967 | Brown et al. | 131 | 14 | 6 (43%) |
| 1968 | Malone and Ingersoll | 75 | 75 | 37 (49%) |
| 1970 | Loeffler and Noble | 180 | 23 | 9 (39%) |
| 1978 | Babaknia et al. | 46 | 46 | 22 (48%) |
| 1979 | Ranney and Frederick | 51 | 9 | 8 (89%) |
| 1980 | Buttram[b] | 59 | 10[c] | 5 (50%) |
| | Total | 4541 | 1202 | 480 (40%) |

[a] Assumed all married patients were infertile.
[b] Unpublished data.
[c] Patients with adequate follow-up greater than a year.
Source: V. C. Buttram and R. C. Reiter, Uterine leiomyomata: Etiology, symptomatology, and management. *Fertil. Steril.* 36:433, 1981. Reprinted with permission.

Babaknia, Rock, and Jones [1] reviewed patients who underwent myomectomy for sterility at Johns Hopkins University Hospital and found that, during the years 1950 to 1975, 48 percent of these 46 patients conceived postoperatively, and 42 percent had term pregnancies. Of 34 patients with primary infertility, pregnancy occurred postoperatively in 41 percent, and 38 percent had term infants. In contrast, 12 patients had secondary infertility, and 66 percent conceived postoperatively. It should be recalled that only 9 of these 46 patients had an abnormal hysterogram preoperatively, indicating that most patients had either intramural or subserous uterine leiomyomata responsible for sterility. A recent literature review is presented in Table 4-4.

Uterine myomata recur following myomectomy, and, occasionally, patients have undergone a second conservative procedure, although more often hysterectomy has been performed. Malone and Ingersoll found a recurrence rate of 30 percent, and reoperated on 18 percent of these patients. Israel and Mutch [30] recorded recurrence in 15 to 25 percent, Brown [10] in 31.3 percent, and Finn and Muller [20] in 23 percent. However, they did not report the frequency of a second operation whose indication was that of recurrent myomata only.

*Obstetric Management*
Postoperative conception control is advised for 3 months to ensure adequate healing before pregnancy. The authors recommend cesarean section if the endometrial cavity has been entered at the time of myomectomy. This is not a universal approach, however, and others have found vaginal delivery to be safe. Malone and Ingersoll (1975) [43] stated that "Cesarean section is advised only if extensive uterine surgery has been performed or if the endometrial cavity has been widely exposed" (P. 90). Of 30 patients with term pregnancies delivered by these authors, cesarean section was performed in only 9. Babaknia, Rock, and Jones (1978) [1] also recommended vaginal delivery "unless the uterine scars are known to have been weakened by postoperative infection" (P. 646). In their series of 19 term deliveries following myomectomy, cesarean section was performed in only 9 cases. No obstetric problems were encountered during vaginal delivery of the remaining 10 patients. The absence of a significant uterine incision during hysteroscopic resection permits these patients to undergo vaginal delivery without risk of uterine rupture.

# References

1. Babaknia, A., Rock, J. A., and Jones, H. W. Pregnancy success following abdominal myomectomy for infertility. *Fertil. Steril.* 30:644, 1978.
2. Bainbridge, W. S. Duplex uterus with multiple pregnancy. *Obstet. Gynecol.* 7:285, 1924.
3. Barter, R. W., and Parks, J. Myoma uteri associated with pregnancy. *Clin. Obstet. Gynecol.* 1:519, 1958.
4. Beernink, F. J., Beernink, H. E., and Chinn, A. Uterus unicornis with uterus solidaris. *Obstet. Gynecol.* 47:651, 1976.
5. Berger, M. J., and Goldstein, D. P. Reproductive outcome of diethylstilbestrol-exposed women (abstract). *Fertil. Steril.* 30:737, 1978.
6. Blum, M. Prevention of spontaneous abortion by cervical suture of the malformed uterus. *Int. Surg.* 62:213, 1977.
7. Bonney, V. Myomectomy as the treatment of election for uterine fibroids. *Lancet* 2:1060, 1925.
8. Bowles, H. E. Apparent congenital absence of the uterus and vagina. *Am. J. Obstet. Gynecol.* 38:723, 1939.
9. Bronson, R. A., and Wallach, E. Lysis of periadenexal adhesions for correction of infertility. *Fertil. Steril.* 28:617, 1977.
10. Brown, A. B., Chamberlain, R., and TeLinde, R. W. Myomectomy. *Am. J. Obstet. Gynecol.* 71:759, 1956.
11. Buttram, V. C., and Gibbons, W. E. Müllerian anomalies: A proposed classification (an analysis of 144 cases). *Fertil. Steril.* 32:40, 1979.
12. Byrd, J. R., Askew, D. W., and McDonough, P. G. Cytogenetic findings in 55 couples with recurrent fetal wastage. *Fertil. Steril.* 28:246, 1977.
13. Collins, G. E. Quoted by J. P. Semmens. *Obstet. Gynecol.* 19:328, 1962.
14. Craig, C. J. T., Congenital abnormalities of the uterus and fetal wastage. *S. Afro. Med. J.* 47:2000, 1973.
15. Crosby, W. M., and Hill, E. C. Embryology of the müllerian duct system. *Obstet. Gynecol.* 20:507, 1962.
15a. Daly, D. C., Walters, C. A., Soto-Albors, C. E., and Riddick, D. H. Hysteroscopic metroplasty: Surgical technique and obstetric outcome. *Fertil. Steril.* 39: No. 5, 1983.
16. Davids, A. M. Myomectomy. *Am. J. Obstet. Gynecol.* 63:592, 1952.
16a. DeCherney, A. H. Müllerian Fusion Defects. Presented at the First World Congress of Hysteroscopy, Jan. 1982, Miami, Fla.
17. Dieckmann, W. J., Davis, M. E., Rynkiewicz, I. M., and Puttinger, R. E. Does the administration of diethylstilbestrol during pregnancy have therapeutic value? *Am. J. Obstet. Gynecol.* 66:1062, 1953.
18. Faber, M., and Marchant, D. J. Congenital absence of the uterine cervix. *Am. J. Obstet. Gynecol.* 121:414, 1975.
19. Fenton, A. N., and Singh, B. P. Pregnancy associated with congenital abnormalities of the female reproductive tract. *Am. J. Obstet. Gynecol.* 63:744, 1952.
20. Finn, W. F. and Muller, P. F. Abdominal myomectomy. *Am. J. Obstet. Gynecol.* 60:109, 1950.
21. Genell, S., and Sjovall, A. The Strassman operation. *Acta Obstet. Gynecol. Scand.* 38:477, 1959.
22. Goldstein, D. P. Incompetent cervix in offspring exposed to diethylstilbestrol in utero. *Obstet. Gynecol.* 52:73ₛ, 1978.
23. Greary, W. L., and Weed, J. C. Congenital atresia of the uterine cervix. *Obstet. Gynecol.* 42:213, 1973.
24. Gros, A., David, A., and Serr, D. M. Management of congenital malformation of the uterus: Fetal salvage. *Acta Eur. Fertil.* 5:301, 1974.
25. Gruenwald, P. Relationships of the growing müllerian duct to the wolffian duct and its importance for the genesis of malformations. *Anat. Rec.* 81:1, 1941.
26. Haney, A. F., Hammond, C. B., Soules, M. R., and Creasman, W. T. Diethylstilbestrol-induced upper genital tract abnormalities. *Fertil. Steril.* 31:142, 1979.
27. Herbst, A. L., Hubby, M. M., Blough, R. R., and Azizi, F. A comparison of pregnancy experience in DES-exposed and DES-unexposed daughters. *J. Reprod. Med.* 24:62, 1980.
28. Herbst, A. L., Ulfelder, H., and Puskanzer, D. C. Adenocarcinoma of the vagina: Association of maternal stilbestrol therapy with tumor appearance in young women. *N. Engl. J. Med.* 284:878, 1971.
29. Ingersoll, F. M. Fertility following myomectomy. *Fertil. Steril.* 14:596, 1963.
30. Israel, S. L., and Mutch, J. C. Myomectomy. *Clin. Obstet. Gynecol.* 1:455, 1958.
31. Jarcho, J. Malformation of the uterus. *Am. J. Surg.* 71:106, 1946.
32. Jones, H. W., and Baramki, T. A. Congenital Anomalies. In S. J. Behrman and R. W. Kistner (eds.) *Progress in Infertility* (1st ed.). Boston: Little, Brown, 1968. P. 63.
33. Jones, H. W., Delfs, E., and Jones, G. E. S. Reproductive difficulties in double uterus. *Am. J. Obstet. Gynecol.* 72:865, 1956.
34. Jones, H. W., and Jones, G. E. S. Double uterus as an etiological factor in repeated abortion: Indications for surgical repair. *Am. J. Obstet. Gynecol.* 65:325, 1953.
35. Jones, H. W., and Wheeless, C. R. Salvage of the reproductive potential of women with anomalous development of the müllerian ducts: 1868-1968-2068. *Am. J. Obstet. Gynecol.* 104:348, 1969.
36. Jones, W. S. Obstetric significance of female genital anomalies. *Obstet. Gynecol.* 10:113, 1957.
37. Kaufman, E. *Lehrbuch der Speziellen Pathologischen Anatomie fur Studierende und Arzte.* Berlin: Walter de Gruyter, 1922. P. 1151.
38. Kaufman, R. H., Binder, G. L., Gray, P. M., and Adam, E. Upper genital tract changes associated with exposure in utero to diethylstilbestrol. *Am. J. Obstet. Gynecol.* 128:51, 1977.
39. Keetle, W. C. Comment to Barter et al., Further experiences with the Shirodkar operation. *Am. J. Obstet. Gynecol.* 85:798, 1963.
40. Kelly, H. A., and Cullen, T. S. *Myomata of Uterus.* Philadelphia: Saunders, 1909.
41. MacNaughton-Jones, J. Specimens and cases. *Br. Gynecol. J.* 20:242, 1904.
42. Malone, L. J., and Ingersoll, F. M. Myomectomy in Infertility. In S. J. Behrman and R. W. Kistner (eds.), *Progress in Infertility* (1st ed.). Boston: Little, Brown, 1968. P. 115.
43. Malone, L. J., and Ingersoll, F. M. Myomectomy in Infertility. In S. J. Behrman and R. W. Kistner (eds.), *Progress in Infertility* (2nd ed.). Boston: Little, Brown, 1975. P. 85.

44. Martin, A. Quoted by W. F. Finn and P. F. Muller. Abdominal myomectomy. *Am. J. Obstet. Gynecol.* 60:109, 1950.

45. Michalas, S., Prevedourakis, C., Lolis, D., and Antsaklis, A. Effect of congenital uterine abnormalities on pregnancy. *Int. Surg.* 61:557, 1976.

46. Miller, N. F. Clinical aspects of uterus didelphys. *Am. J. Obstet. Gynecol.* 4:398, 1962.

47. Moore, O. Congenital abnormalities of female genitalia. *South. Med. J.* 34:610, 1941.

48. Musich, J. R., and Behrman, S. J. Obstetric outcome before and after metroplasty in women with uterine anomalies. *Obstet. Gynecol.* 52:63, 1978.

49. Niver, D. H., Barrette, G., and Jewulewicz, R. Congenital atresia of the uterine cervix and vagina: Three cases. *Fertil. Steril.* 33:25, 1980.

50. Novak, E. Editorial comment. *Obstet. Gynecol. Surv.* 6:417, 1951.

51. Phelan, J. T., Counseller, V. S., and Green, L. F. Deformities of the urinary tract with congenital absence of the vagina. *Surg. Gynecol. Obstet.* 97:1, 1953.

52. Pillsbury, S. G. Reproductive significance of changes in the endometrial cavity associated with exposure in utero to diethylstilbestrol. *Am. J. Obstet. Gynecol.* 137:178, 1980.

53. Puddicombe, J. F. Some uterine anomalies due to variations in the fusion of the müllerian ducts. *Surg. Gynecol. Obstet.* 49:799, 1929.

54. Rock, J. Discussion with H. W. Jones, E. D. Delfs, and G. E. S. Jones. Reproductive difficulties in double uterus. *Am. J. Obstet. Gynecol.* 72:882, 1956.

55. Rock, J. A., and Jones, J. W. The clinical management of the double uterus. *Fertil. Steril.* 28:798, 1977.

56. Rubin, I. C. Myomectomy in the treatment of infertility. *CIBA* 6:1977, 1954.

57. Rubin, I. C. Uterine fibromyomas and sterility. *Clin. Obstet. Gynecol.* 1:501, 1958.

58. Ruge, P. Geburtshilfe. *Gynaekologie* 10:141, 1884.

59. Semmens, J. P. Congenital anomalies of female genital tract. *Obstet. Gynecol.* 19:328, 1962.

60. Semmens, J. P. Abdominal contour in the third trimester: An aid to diagnosis of uterine anomalies. *Obstet. Gynecol.* 25:779, 1965.

61. Siegler, A. M., Wang, C. F., and Friberg, J. Fertility of the diethylstilbestrol-exposed offspring. *Fertil. Steril.* 31:601, 1979.

62. Simpson, J. L., and Christakos, A. C. Hereditary factors in obstetrics and gynecology. *Obstet. Gynecol. Surv.* 24:580, 1966.

63. Steinberg, W. Strassman's metroplasty in the management of bipartite uterus causing sterility or habitual abortion. *Obstet. Gynecol. Surv.* 10:400, 1955.

64. Stevenson, C. S. Myomectomy for improvement of fertility. *Fertil. Steril.* 15:367, 1964.

65. Strassman, E. O. Plastic unification of double uterus. *Am. J. Obstet. Gynecol.* 64:25, 1952.

66. Strassman, E. O. Operations for double uterus and endometrial atresia. *Clin. Obstet. Gynecol.* 4:240, 1961.

67. Te Linde, R. W. *Operative Gynecology* (4th ed.). Philadelphia: Lippincott, 1970.

68. Thompson, J. D., Wharton, L. R., and Te Linde, R. W. Congenital absence of the vagina. *Am. J. Obstet. Gynecol.* 74:397, 1957.

69. Tompkins, P. Personal communication to R. Kistner, April 10, 1974.

70. Tompkins, P. Personal communication to R. Kistner, Feb. 9, 1974.

71. Tulandi, T., Arronet, G. H., and McInnes, R. A. Arcuate and bicornuate uterine anomalies and infertility. *Fertil. Steril.* 34:362, 1980.

72. Williams, E. A. Uterovaginal agenesis. *Ann. R. Coll. Surg. Engl.* 58:266, 1976.

73. Woolf, R. B., and Allen, W. M. Concomitant malformations. *Obstet. Gynecol.* 2:236, 1953.

74. Zarou, G. S., Esposito, J. M., and Zarou, D. M. Pregnancy following the surgical correction of genital atresia of the cervix. *Int. J. Gynaecol. Obstet.* 11:143, 1973.

75. Zourlas, P. A. Surgical treatment of malformations of the uterus. *Surg. Gynecol. Obstet.* 141:57, 1975.

# Essential Elements of Microsurgical Technique

Surgery performed under magnification, i.e., microsurgery, represents an outgrowth of the scientist's interest in magnification that may be dated from the invention of the telescope by Roger Bacon in the thirteenth century. The compound microscope was invented in the late sixteenth and early seventeenth centuries. Although Galileo is given credit for this invention in 1610, others in Holland and Naples produced similar instruments during that same time period. By the midseventeenth century many experiments were being performed using the compound microscope. One recalls the paper by J. Marion Sims in which he described his experience visualizing sperm under the microscope, which led to the early description of the Sims's postcoital examination. The onset of microsurgery is usually dated from the work of Nylen, published in 1921 [25]. This ear, nose, and throat surgeon first used a monocular operating microscope and, later, a binocular stereoscopic microscope to perform surgery for otospongiosis. During that decade, only the ENT surgeons adapted the new operating microscope to surgical procedures. Not until 1954, however, when Carl Zeiss introduced the Operating Microscope (OPMI-1) was an instrument of this type commercially available. This microscope was designed for ear surgery and continues to be known in most operating rooms as the ear microscope, although newer models are quite useful in neurosurgery and, occasionally, gynecologic microsurgery.

In fact, the onset of microsurgery might be dated earlier with the work of Von Zehender, an ophthalmologist, published in 1886 [5]. Von Zehender used binocular glasses (loupes) to perform surgery of the eye under magnification. This work was followed by similar studies reported by Von Rohr and Stock in 1913. In spite of the interest in the operating microscope in the 1920s and 1930s, eye surgeons continued to use the loupes during these decades and it was not until the late 1950s, following the work of Baracaquer and, later, Troutman, that the operating microscope became an integral part of eye surgery. Initially, the Zeiss OPMI-2 and later the Zeiss OPMI-6 became known as the eye microscopes [1].

Remarkable advances took place in the field of vascular surgery and constructive plastic surgery during the 1960s. Surgeons demonstrated marked improvement following small vessel anastomosis using the operating microscope. The first reimplantation of a finger was performed in Japan in 1965 [35]; however, it was another ten years before an Australian plastic surgeon reported the first successful skin transplant by microvascular anastomosis. Reconstructive microsurgery has progressed steadily during the last decade, as is shown in the recent texts of O'Brien [26], and Daniel and Terzis [5].

During the 1960s, following the work of House [20], published in 1961, neurosurgeons began to use magnification for resection of acoustic neuromas, as well as transsphenoidal hypophysectomy.

Kurt Swolin, in 1967 [33], was the first gynecologist to publish an application of microsurgical technique in the field of infertility surgery. Salpingostomy performed by this surgeon under the operating microscope resulted in improved, but not dramatic, pregnancy results. In 1969, David, Brackett, and Garcia [7] reported improved patency and pregnancy results using a microsurgical approach for uterotubal reanastomosis in rabbits. Although, in 1972, Garcia [12] also reported improved pregnancy results in females after tubal reanastomosis following prior sterilization, enthusiasm for this procedure did not arise until Gomel's presentation at the American Laparoscopic Society meeting in 1976 [13a]. Gomel's meticulous surgical technique and excellent pregnancy results following midtubal reanastomosis and uterotubal reanastomosis were supported and enhanced by the work of Winston and Diamond [8, 39]. At that point, the place of microsurgery in the field of surgery of the fallopian tube was clearly established.

## Definitions

Microsurgery has been described in a limited sense as a surgical technique that employs the operating microscope and, in broader terms, as a surgical approach in which the improved ability to visualize a structure influences the surgeon's approach to reconstruction of that structure. The use of magnification is, however, the essential feature in all definitions of microsurgery.

Regardless of the specific definition of microsurgery one favors, it is clear that the use of magnification in the area of infertility surgery has markedly altered the surgical approach to the oviduct. The ability to visualize microscopic details of the tubal lumen and fimbria has improved the gentleness with which the surgeon handles these structures and the accuracy of repair. Accordingly, instruments with finer tips and sharper blades have been incorporated into the surgeon's armamentarium. Suture material that is almost invisible to the naked eye is now routinely employed to hold structures in place during healing. Lastly, the approach to hemostasis has changed completely. Visualization of small vessels is a simple matter under magnifications of 10 to $20\times$, permitting identification of the bleeding site and accurate hemostasis by either electrocoagulation (bipolar) or by a laser beam. This technique termed *microelectrosurgery* has been a major advance in this field. The recently introduced carbon dioxide laser appears to be an even more accurate tool for cutting and hemostasis.

In this chapter, the authors have described the fundamentals of microsurgical technique for the infertility surgeon. The essential features of microsurgery, an overview of levels of magnification, and specific details of this author's (G.W.P.) operating room are presented first. Next, optical principles and operating microscopes, the various microscopic aids available to the microsurgeon are described. Elements of lighting and photography are also included. The section that follows discusses microelectrosurgery. The selection of an electrosurgical generator is of utmost importance in microsurgery and some understanding of the differences between cutting, coagulating, and bipolar currents is necessary. In Chapter 6, Dr. Joseph Bellina describes the principles and physical properties of the carbon dioxide laser. Use of these principles permits the surgeon to select the proper spot, size, and power output of the laser during a microsurgical procedure. Comparisons between microelectrosurgery and the carbon dioxide laser technique will undoubtedly become increasingly sophisticated and will require the surgeon to understand the principles of each method. In the last section, instruments used by this author (G.W.P.) and other instruments available for gynecologic microsurgical procedures are described. Important aspects of suture materials and needles are also discussed in this section.

## Essential Features of Microsurgery

### Levels of Microsurgical Technique

The term *microsurgery* has been employed in the broader sense in this text to imply an overall surgical technique, i.e., "microsurgical technique." There are, however, different levels or degrees of application of these microsurgical principles. As is described below, there is a range of optical and technical instrumentation presently available to the gynecologic microsurgeon, and it is the instrumentation that dictates the level of microsurgical technique to be employed. The question as to whether the four levels described here, from loupe to OPMI-7-P/H, are, in fact, microsurgical procedures is unsettled but appears to be answered in the affirmative, because all of them employ magnification. Whether all are suitable for gynecologic microsurgery is a separate issue.

#### LOUPE AND HEADLAMP

Ocular loupes presently available provide magnifications from 2.5 to $8.0\times$ with fields of view quite comparable to those available with the operating microscope. A comparison of the loupe and the operating microscope will be presented on page 145. As will be discussed later, the combination of loupe and accessory fiberoptical lighting is essential for proper use of this technique. Although this approach offers considerably improved visual fields, it fails to provide the convenient range of magnification available with the Zeiss OPMI-6S and OPMI-7-P/H microscopes. The degrees of magnification available to the surgeon are limited to the specific loupes in his possession. Also, it is impossible to increase magnification (with this technique) for careful evaluation of a structure. This deficiency was found to be particularly significant during evaluation of tubal fimbria and the use of an operating microscope is thought, by this author (G.W.P.), to be essential for proper microsurgical salpingostomy. This author (G.W.P.) has used the loupe technique in a standing position; however, variable focal distances are available that permit its use in the sitting position.

The headache and vertigo that occur commonly when using the ocular loupes disappear after a period of adaptation to this technique. Lighting provided by the fiberoptical headlamp was quite adequate and comparable to that available with the newer operating microscopes.

The limitation on maximal magnification and the difficulty in changing magnification restrict this technique to the excision of ovarian adhesions extending into the cul-de-sac, which are inaccessible to the operating microscope. As will be discussed later, this author (G.W.P.) used the loupe technique on 23 patients who underwent microsurgical fimbrioplasty during 1978, changing from 2.5 to 4.5× loupes when additional magnification was thought to be necessary. Although the results of this fimbrioplasty technique were satisfactory, the results of salpingostomy were not. The authors have not used loupe magnification during total reanastomosis, although it is significant that Jones and Rock [21] have reported excellent pregnancy results following end-to-end tubal reanastomosis performed with the aid of 4.5× loupes.

ZEISS OPMI-1 MICROSCOPE

This microscope uses a manual magnification changer and requires manual change of focus. The OPMI-1 is discussed on page 135. This optimal system, quite useful in ENT surgery, does not permit the rapid temporary use of high magnification for inspection of tissue surfaces. The necessity of manual change in magnification or focus makes this instrument impractical in the field of infertility surgery. The light available with this instrument is often inadequate (see page 135), but may be improved by an addition of the Vertalux fiberoptical system. A House-Urban quadrascope head permits the assistant to see the operative field, although some difference in magnification is present. Again, this microscope (like the loupe) is often used with the surgeon in the standing position, although it can be employed equally well in the sitting position. This author (G.W.P.) initially used this instrument during end-to-end anastomosis while standing, and although a pregnancy rate of 7/10 patients was achieved, the resulting fatigue and eye strain made conversion to a sitting position while using the OPMI-6 and, later, the OPMI-7-P/H and OPMI-6S a welcome relief.

ZEISS OPMI-6 MICROSCOPE

For the first time, variable (zoom) magnification and the ability to vary focus by foot-pedal control are available, representing a great improvement for the surgeon who must keep both hands in the operative field. Once the surgeon has used this system it is almost impossible to return to the OPMI-1 microscope. The incandescent bulb light-source on older models is inconvenient (see page 137), but conversion to fiberoptic lighting is quite practical. Again, as with the OPMI-1, the House-Urban quadrascope head is necessary if one uses an assistant, although the modified OPMI-6S discussed below provides an improved alternative. Finally, the X-Y axis, of great use on the OPMI-7-P/H is usually not available in the standard OPMI-6 models but can be added if desired. Coarse focus obtained through a motorized stand is also a rarity on this model, but, again, can be added as it has been on the OPMI-6S (modified) and OPMI-7-P/H. Parenthetically, it is convenient to sit when using the OPMI-6 if the operating table permits.

ZEISS OPMI-7-P/H, OPMI-6S, AND WECK MICROSCOPES

These three microscopes offer most of the essential features of a magnifying system that are useful to the infertility surgeon, and they have been discussed at length on pages 138–140. The essential features are

1. Variable magnification with foot-pedal control.
2. Motorized focus under foot-pedal control; both fine and coarse focus are important.
3. X-Y axis: The ability to move the microscope head in all directions under foot-pedal control.
4. Assistant head: Optimal surgery is possible when the assistant can sit or stand opposite the surgeon and see the operative field clearly.
5. High intensity lighting: Variable intensity control with fiberoptic system.
6. Photographic capability: The ability to record the surgical procedure on 35 mm film and video when desired.

It is apparent that the four magnification levels discussed above offer a few of these essential features, but in no instance are all available unless one uses Zeiss OPMI-7-P/H or OPMI-6S, or the Weck operating microscope. The benefits of variable magnification become increasingly useful as the surgeon's experience increases. Variable focus and the X-Y axis permit the surgeon to inspect portions of the fallopian tube with ease and to operate in a larger area without breaking concentration. Under these conditions, sitting does not increase the time of surgery but, rather, will be found to shorten the time required for a procedure. Also, end-to-end reanastomosis can be accomplished comfortably on both tubes within 3 hours and, often, within a 2½ hour interval. Few microsurgical procedures will be found to last longer than 3 hours if proper preoperative preparation has been made.

*To Sit or Stand*

In addition to choosing one of these four magnification systems, the surgeon must decide whether to operate in the sitting or the standing position. This is not a decision readily made, because all other gynecologic surgery is performed while standing (some surgeons do sit during vaginal procedures), and one has the preconception that sitting is for weaklings who wish to dabble over their work. Finally, the operating tables presently in use in most operating rooms make sitting at the patient's side with one's legs straddling the center console and knees hitting metal supports an uncomfortable experience.

This author (G.W.P.) used a combination of the loupe and the headlamp technique as well as the OPMI-1 and OPMI-6 microscopes in the standing position for approximately 2 years before discovering that sitting was the only way to comfortably perform microsurgery. One must laugh at the thought of operating under magnification while standing on one foot and using the opposite foot to adjust focus or magnification. However, sitting was equally difficult during the initial phase.

Special adaption of the operating table must be made to permit the surgeon to sit comfortably with both knees under the table.* The table shown in Figure 5-1 was intended for orthopedic use but was found to be ideal for gynecologic microsurgery. Note the thin metal frame supported by a console at its distal end. This frame slides along the console, which is fixed securely to the operating room floor. No side motion of the table is possible, and it also can be placed in the Trendelenburg position.

An operating room table of this type permits the surgeon to sit comfortably. He is able to place his wrists or lower forearms on the edge of the Kirshner retractor and to use fine finger motion to its fullest degree. Foot pedals are conveniently arranged on the floor and manipulated by a stockinged foot. Rapid and accurate foot movement to the proper pedal is accomplished most easily without shoes, as suggested by Seigler.

*Operating Room Layout*

Gomel has emphasized that preparation for microsurgery represents 75 percent of the microsurgical procedure, and certainly all surgeons will find this a valid comment. The positioning the microscope and the patient on the operating room table should be worked out before surgery. Similarly, it is essential that each member of the operating room team be familiar with his role and be able to perform it efficiently. Figure 5-2 depicts the floor plan presently used by the author (Patton), and includes the following features:

1. Operating room table, electrically controlled
2. Soft stool
3. Operating microscope
4. Foot pedal to control microscope
5. Cart containing headlamp, microelectrosurgical generator, special sutures, and extra instruments
6. Operating room electrosurgical generator
7. Stereo
8. Mayo stand and instrument table (not shown)
9. Four-way plugs (not shown)
10. Anesthesia equipment (not shown)

*This may be accomplished on existing operating room tables by reversing the patient's usual position on the table or by extending the foot end of the table approximately 2 feet by use of arm boards or other makeshift apparatus. This arrangement should be carefully worked out prior to the day of surgery.

**Figure 5-1.** Kifa table system: flat table top—type P; Kifa, Stockholm, Sweden.

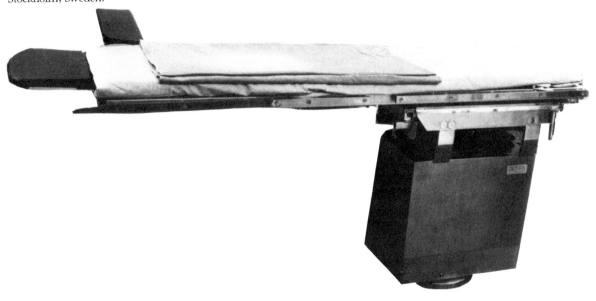

**Figure 5-2.** Operating room floor plan used by this author (G.W.P.) includes special table, operating microscope, suture and instrument cart, electrosurgical generator, and stereo.

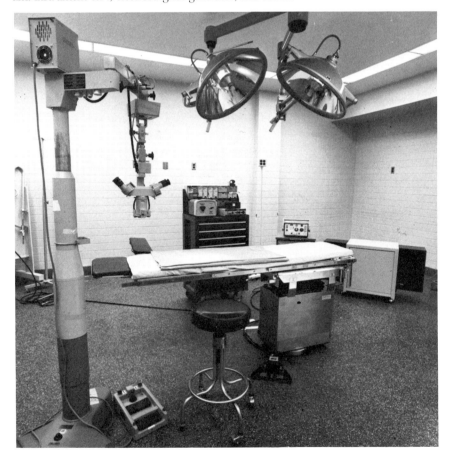

**Table 5-1.** Operating room arrangement for microsurgery*

| Equipment | Medications and solutions | Set-up for extra Mayo† |
|---|---|---|
| Operating microscope: OPMI-7-P/H or OPMI-6S with 250 mm lens; if beam splitter is used, place 225 mm or 200 mm lens on microscope | Lactated Ringer's solution (plain) 1000 ml in bowl with Asepto (#2137) | Hanks dilators |
| Use flat, nonbreakaway table top (Kifa) | 5000 units (5 cc) heparin in 500 ml lactated Ringer's solution for irrigation (washes blood off tissue and helps prevent adhesions); this is to be connected to sterile single cysto tubing and hung on IV pole by anesthesia | Single-toothed tenaculum |
| Valley Lab SSE electrosurgical generator (recently changed to Davol System 5000); hand switch for monopolar current, foot switch for bipolar current | | Sponge stick |
| | | Small preparation bowl with Betadine |
| | | 4 × 4 sponges, extra-large package (uncounted sponges) |
| Elektrotom MC/MS hand control unit | 5 ml methylene blue in 500 ml IV NaCl | Duck-billed speculum |
| Soft black-top rolling stand | | Harris uterine cannula (HUI #2954) |
| Basic infertility instrument set (hospital) | 1 ampule Pitressin in 100 ml IV NaCl; if used, will need a 3 cc syringe and a 30 g needle; used for vasoconstriction | #16 Foley catheter with drainage bag (#2851 and 2858) |
| Surgeon's microsurgical instrument set | | Towels (2) |
| Mayo stands (2) | 100 ml Hyskon (have in room); used to prevent adhesions | Size 7½ gloves and glove powder |
| Surgeon's suture cart | | K-Y jelly |
| Surgeon's headlamp and loupes | | K-52 tubing (1) |
| Four-way plugs (2) | | 10 cc syringe filled with saline for cannula |
| Surgeon's stereo | | 5 cc syringe with water for Foley catheter |

*Used by this author (G.W.P.).

†Patient will be frog-legged with feet taped; surgeon will wear gloves only (no gown); this procedure is to insert the HUI uterine cannula and the Foley catheter.

## Summary of Essential Features of Microsurgical Technique

Four types of magnification and lighting systems have been discussed, as well as the great convenience of an operating room table that permits the surgeon to work in a sitting position. The basic features of gynecologic microsurgery are as follows:

1. Magnification system: Loupe, OPMI-1, OPMI-6, OPMI-6S (modified), OPMI-7-P/H, and Weck microscopes
2. Lighting: Fiberoptic
3. Microelectrosurgical generator and microelectrodes
4. Special microsurgical instruments, medications, and solutions
5. Sitting position
6. Assistant

A final note relating to the use of an assistant seems pertinent. Diamond recommends using an operating room assistant, yet he operated for two years without an assistant who could see the magnified field. The use of an experienced assistant permits the surgeon to move quickly through a difficult anastomosis or salpingostomy procedure and is absolutely essential for optimal results.

Some other equipment and supplies, together with some suggestions for convenient working conditions are as follows:

1. Special instruments of personal choice (e.g., glass rods)
2. Irrigating solution, heparin, and Hartman's solution
3. Uterine cannula (HUI)
4. Kirschner retractor
5. Use of technique of packing cul-de-sac
6. Removal of shoes to use foot pedals
7. Positioning of patient on operating room table with right arm tucked in

Each of these aids has been found useful by this author (G.W.P.) and will be discussed at greater length in Chapter 7. A list of operating room equipment, medication, and solutions used by this author (G.W.P.) is presented in Table 5-1. Other surgeons use additional aids during surgery, such as Winston's use of the technique of packing the vagina [39]. Each surgeon must establish a routine with which he is comfortable and must follow it faithfully (Fig. 5-3).

All four levels of microsurgical technique employ some degree of magnification and accessory lighting. The disadvantage of changing the level of magnification when using the loupe technique and the disadvantage of manual magnification and the focus change required with the Zeiss OPMI-1 microscope have been pointed out. Neither of these two systems appears to the authors to be satisfactory for fimbrial surgery or cornual anastomosis. Certainly the Zeiss OPMI-6S and OPMI-7-P/H and Weck microscopes are so convenient that the authors feel they will become standard instruments in gynecologic microsurgery. The loupe and headlamp, however, may continue to be used for resection of adhesions that are difficult to reach. It is this author's (G.W.P.) present practice to begin a microsurgical procedure with lysis of tubal or ovarian adhesions that are deep in the cul-de-sac, aided by loupe magnification and a fiberoptic headlamp. It may be necessary for the surgeon to change sides of the table during this phase of adhesions resection, a procedure that is usually performed in the standing position. Having accomplished this preliminary dissection with the microelectrode (see page 145) the Zeiss OPMI-6S microscope is now moved into the operating field and the surgeon assumes a sitting position, usually at the patient's left side. Further surgery, whether it be resection of minor tubal adhesions, tubal anastomosis, or fimbrial surgery is performed in this sitting position. The ability to tilt the head of the operating microscope permits the surgeon to work comfortably on either adnexa, as does the use of a

motorized X-Y axis on the microscope. Specific aspects of the author's microsurgical technique are presented in Chapter 7.

An essential element of microsurgery often overlooked is the necessity for a dependable, experienced operating team. This team includes an assistant who is familiar with microsurgical techniques and comfortable using the operating microscope and an instrument technician and circulating nurse who are experienced at microsurgical procedures. It is necessary to be able to move quickly from macrosurgery to microsurgery. The process of draping the operating microscope and quickly moving it into the field without confusion takes practice but is highly rewarding. Lastly, the anesthesiologist must enjoy microsurgery to achieve optimal results. Excessive ventilatory volumes move the pelvic structures enough to make a delicate procedure difficult. Certainly a compatible operating team and a pleasant environment contribute to a successful microsurgical procedure.

**Figure 5-3.** Surgeon with assistant in surgical suite. Note comfort and simplicity of the sitting position.

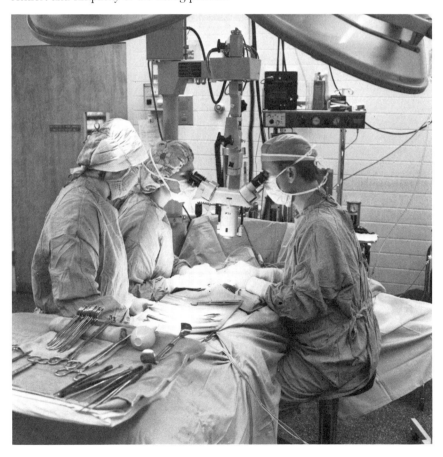

## Optical Principles and Operating Microscopes

### Optical Principles

The gynecologist must be capable of assembling and disassembling the operating microscope when necessary before and after its use in the operating room. Surgeons in other specialities will be using the same microscope and may use various objective lenses, eyepieces and beam-splitting accessories. The concept of a building-block assembly championed by Zeiss has been particularly useful for the gynecologic surgeon who shares the OPMI-1 (ENT) and OPMI-6 (eye) operating microscopes. Hand surgeons and plastic surgeons also will change objective lenses and eyepieces on the OPMI-7-P/H and OPMI-6S, but, usually, fewer variations are encountered with these microscopes and the Weck microscope. The goal of this assembly is to achieve the required levels of magnification with the operating microscope placed at a suitable distance above the operative field, thereby permitting the gynecologist to both visualize and work on selected portions of the fallopian tube with ease.

The optical principles of the various operating microscopes are similar and will be discussed later in this section. These instruments, referred to as Galilean-type microscopes, are constructed so that parallel imaging occurs between the components of the microscope (Fig. 5-4). As the surgeon looks through the eyepiece of the microscope, the image seen by each eye is carried in parallel fashion to the objective lens, at which point the images of the left and right eyes merge at the focal point of the lens, i.e., 200 mm (8 inches). In this manner, the binocular system achieves a three dimensional quality. Additional benefits of this parallel viewing system include markedly decreased eye fatigue, because accommodation of the eye is not necessary, and the ability to insert a beam-splitting attachment in one visual path of the other permits easy focusing of this system with photographic accessories. These principles have been discussed at length by Mr. Hoerenz [15, 16, 17, 18, 19].

**Figure 5-4.** Pathway of visual image following insertion of a beam-splitting device into the operating microscope. Notice the parallel image beams and diversion of image from a single (right) path to the camera. (Courtesy of Carl Zeiss, Inc., Thornwood, N.Y.)

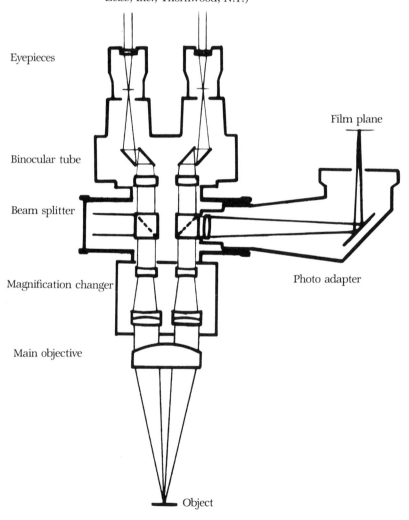

Eyepieces

Binocular tube

Beam splitter

Magnification changer

Main objective

Film plane

Photo adapter

Object

## EYEPIECES (OCULARS)

Eyepieces are simple magnifying lenses that provide stereoscopic vision and are available in magnifications of 10, 12.5, 16, or 20×, although 16× is rarely available in most operating rooms. Obviously, the difference between 10 and 12.5× is minimal; however, the increase of 20× will make a significant difference, doubling the total magnification. Eyepieces are equipped with diopter settings that permit the surgeon to eliminate his personal eyeglasses and place his refractive correction on the microscope eyepiece, if he so wishes. The surgeon must wear his glasses if he has astigmatism or needs a correction not in the range of the diopter setting. Rubber attachments, called *high-point oculars*, are available for the eyepieces; when folded over they permit one to wear eyeglasses comfortably. A cross-hair or other-shaped figure, termed a *reticule*, may be included in the base of the eyepiece to assist with focusing during photography.

## BINOCULAR TUBES

The binocular tube holds the eyepiece and conveys the magnified image to the eyepiece in parallel and stereoscopic fashion from the magnification changer on the body of the microscope. This tube also has an optical system in which magnification is determined by the focal length of the binocular, either 125 or 160 mm, which is in addition to that provided by the eyepiece. The eyepiece and binocular tube together provide a fixed magnification that cannot easily be altered during surgery, and constitute the optical components of the assembly and binocular. The binocular is either straight or inclined, as is noted in the diagram in Figure 5-5. Most OPMI-1 microscopes outfitted for otolaryngology have a straight binocular and, therefore, require conversion of this component to an inclined binocular for use by the gynecologist. All ophthalmologic surgeons use an inclined binocular on the OPMI-6. The OPMI-7-P/H and OPMI-6S have a straight binocular; however, it is placed on the beam-splitting attachment at an angle that makes it ideal for gynecologic surgery.

**Figure 5-5.** Three interchangeable binocular systems. On the left is a short (125 mm), straight tube; in the center a long (160 mm), straight binocular. The straight binoculars are currently used by ENT and neurologic surgeons. On the right is an inclined binocular that is available with a short tube (125 mm) and a long tube (160 mm). The inclined binocular is convenient for gynecologic microsurgery with the Zeiss OPMI-1 and OPMI-6 microscopes. A short, straight (125 mm) binocular is used with the Zeiss OPMI-7-P/H and OPMI-6S. (Courtesy of Carl Zeiss, Inc., Thornwood, N.Y.)

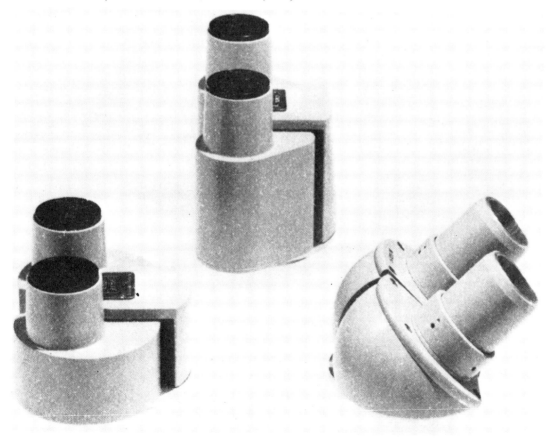

The third component of the magnification system that can be altered prior to surgery is the objective lens. This round lens screws easily into the lower part of the microscope body (magnification changer) and is available in focal lengths from 100 mm to 400 mm in 25 mm increments representing a change of 2.5 cm, or 1 inch, in focal distance. The objective lens is constructed with the object toward infinity so that the distance between the lens and the object is equal to the focal length. This means that if one uses a 300 mm lens to visualize the fallopian tube, the distance between the lens and the site visualized will be 300 mm, or 30 cm, or 12 inches. This represents the distance between the fallopian tube and bottom-most portion of the microscope, which is the area of hand movement of the surgeon and his assistant. A 200 mm lens would reduce the distance to 20 cm, or 8 inches. Other distances are convenient for various other surgical specialities. The eye surgeon usually employs the 175 mm lens, the hand surgeon a 200 mm, and the ENT surgeon a 400 mm. Most gynecologists use an objective lens between 250 and 300 mm, although when using the OPMI-7PH and OPMI-6S with the beam-splitter attached, the 250 mm lens is convenient.

The choice of an objective lens is dependent on the distance the surgeon wishes to be from the operative field and the level of magnification required or both, because the greater the focal length of the objective lens, the lower the magnification available. In the equation for magnification, the focal length of the objective lens is the entire denominator. Therefore, an increase in focal length from 150 to 300 mm will reduce by one-half all magnifications available with this system. This disadvantage can be overcome by the gynecologist, however, if he uses higher levels in the magnification changer or increases the eyepiece or focal distance of the binocular tube, because maximum magnification is rarely used in infertility surgery.

A third characteristic of the objective lens that is significant in gynecologic surgery, is the property of increasing field size with increased focal length. As the focal length of the objective lens increases, the size of the field seen through the microscope also increases, and magnification decreases. This ability to vary the size of the field is particularly relevant in working on adhesions that encompass a significant portion of the ovary and fallopian tube. Increased field size is also convenient during photography and, in fact, the 400 mm lens is the only one that permits inclusion of all pelvic structures. Using an eyepiece of $12.5 \times$ and a binocular tube with a 125 mm focal length, the field sizes obtained are as follows:

| Objective lens (mm) | 200 | 250 | 300 | 400 |
|---|---|---|---|---|
| Field size (mm) | 26 | 31.5 | 38.8 | 52.5 |

The eyepiece, binocular tube, and objective lens are all selected by the surgeon and placed on the microscope prior to the start of surgery. Together they result in the *base magnification*, according to the formula:

$$\text{Base magnification} = \frac{\text{eyepiece} \times \text{binocular tube}}{\text{objective lens}}$$

MAGNIFICATION CHANGERS

The body of the operating microscope contains the magnification changer. The Zeiss OPMI-1 microscope was the first operating microscope that provided variable magnification. This is accomplished by a manual turret, or drum assembly, composed of three channels. One is a clear channel equal at each end that does not magnify. Therefore, the factor, or magnification, is 1 at this setting, which happens to be number 16 on the OPMI-1. Two settings labeled 16 are present, representing the two ends of this channel. The second channel, containing optical components, has a very high magnification when viewed through one end and a very low magnification when viewed through the other end, thereby providing the highest magnification factor, $2.5 \times$ at setting 40, and the lowest magnification factor, $0.4 \times$ at setting 6. The third channel, also containing optical components, provides two intermediate magnification levels, $1.6 \times$ at setting 25 and $0.6 \times$ at setting 10. Figure 5-6 depicts the concept of the turret assembly.

Manual change of magnification is inconvenient for the surgeon, who has both hands occupied. It seriously interrupts the operative technique and, therefore, forces one to select an average level of magnification, which may be slightly too high or slightly too low for much of the time. One tends to select a middle level of magnification and to use this level for long periods of time. In fact, microsurgery with this microscope is often not significantly different than that performed using the operative loupe and headlamp, a point that will be discussed further in the section titled Loupes (surgical telescopes). The need for a motorized zoom system was emphasized by Troutman and other ophthalmologists and resulted in the design of the Zeiss OPMI-2 operating microscope. Later, the OPMI-6 operating microscope became the primary instrument used by ophthalmologists, and it is present in the operating rooms of most general hospitals today.

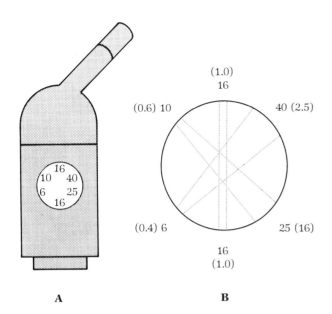

A

(1.0)
16

(0.6) 10          40 (2.5)

(0.4) 6          25 (16)

16
(1.0)

B

**Figure 5-6.** Turret assembly of the Zeiss OPMI-1 microscope. **A.** Side view of the manual turret assembly on the OPMI-1. **B.** The levels of magnification and the association between the numbers 6, 10, 16, 25, and 40, on the exterior of the microscope body, and the respective magnification factors, 0.4, 16, 1.0, 1.6, and 2.5, that are used to calculate actual magnification.

**Figure 5-7.** Components of Zeiss OPMI-6, OPMI-6S, and OPMI-7-P/H microscopes. The four basic components are shown, and next to each section those specific components used in gynecologic microsurgery are given.

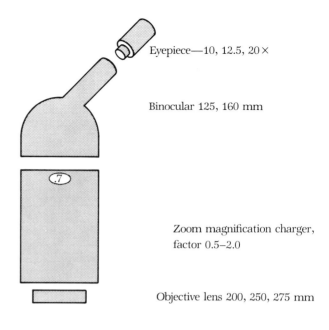

Eyepiece—10, 12.5, 20×

Binocular 125, 160 mm

Zoom magnification charger, factor 0.5–2.0

Objective lens 200, 250, 275 mm

The OPMI-6 and, later, the OPMI-7-P/H, the OPMI-6S (modified), and the Weck microscopes, having introduced the motorized zoom magnification system, brought about a dramatic change in microsurgery. It became possible with this technical change to vary magnification smoothly by foot-pedal control. This was accomplished by the introduction of a double-lens system that moved in such a manner as to provide a gradual change in magnification. The lowest magnification available increased slightly to a factor of 0.5. The lowest factor on the OPMI-1 at setting 6 was 0.4. The early models of the OPMI-6 and the present OPMI-7-P/H contain a magnification system that varies from factors 0.5 to 2.5. This is termed a *1:5 magnification system*. Since 1977 the highest level has been reduced to factor 2.0 in the OPMI-6 and 6S, achieving a 1:4 zoom system. The factor can easily be found on these two microscopes by observing the number in the small window just beneath the binocular tube on the microscope body. The components of the variable zoom microscope are shown in Figure 5-7.

SIZE AND DEPTH OF FIELD

Selection of a level of magnification also involves a selection of the size of the field being visualized and the depth of field that remains in focus. The observation by this author (G.W.P.) that comfortable magnification for tubal reanastomosis is found to exist between 4.2 and 10.7×, reflects not only the fact the the fallopian tube can comfortably be seen at these levels, but also that the size of the fields of vision at these magnifications is 47.5 and 18.7 mm, respectively, thereby providing areas of comfortable size in which to operate. Representative

**Table 5-2.** Fields of view at various magnifications

| Magnification (Mv) | 2.7 | 3.4 | 5.4 | 6.7 | 10.7 | 12.3 | 16.8 | 27 |
|---|---|---|---|---|---|---|---|---|
| Field of view (mm)* | 74 | 59 | 37 | 30 | 19 | 15 | 12 | 8 |

*Calculated by equation F (field of view) = $\frac{200}{Mv}$.

comparisons of level of magnification and size of field area are shown in Table 5-2. The equation for calculating the diameter of this field is

$$F = \frac{200}{Mv}$$

where   F = field
        Mv = visual magnification

Although the size of field available at various magnifications is immediately obvious to the surgeon, the depth of field is not. An understanding of this concept of depth of field is essential when focusing the operating microscope. This optical principle leads the microsurgeon to focus at high power and then to move to a lower power to operate. As is shown in Figure 5-8, an object in focus at 20× will be in excellent focus at all lower levels of magnification. A dramatic change in depth of field occurs between 4 and 10×, because at 4× there is a depth of field of 2.5 cm, compared to slightly more than 0.5 cm at 10×.

**Figure 5-8.** Depth of field at magnification 20, 10, and 4×. Note that object in focus at 20× must be in focus at all lower levels of magnification.

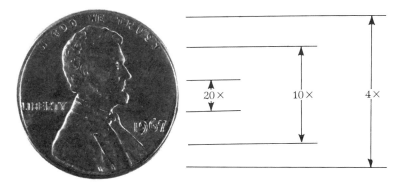

**Table 5-3.** Magnifications available with the 200 mm objective lens

| Eyepiece | Binocular | Base magnification | Factor | | | | | |
| --- | --- | --- | --- | --- | --- | --- | --- | --- |
| | | | 0.4 | 0.5 | 0.63 | 1.0 | 1.6 | 2.5 |
| 10 | 125 | 6.25 | 2.5× | 3.1× | 3.9× | 6.25× | 10.0× | 15.6× |
| 10 | 160 | 8.0 | 3.2 | 4.0 | 5.0 | 8.0 | 12.8 | 20.0 |
| 12.5 | 125 | 7.8 | 3.1 | 3.9 | 4.9 | 7.8 | 12.5 | 19.5 |
| 12.5 | 160 | 10.0 | 4.0 | 5.0 | 6.3 | 10.0 | 16.0 | 25.0 |
| 20 | 125 | 12.5 | 5.0 | 6.3 | 7.9 | 12.5 | 20.0 | 31.3 |
| 20 | 160 | 16 | 6.4 | 8.0 | 10.1 | 16 | 26.0 | 40.0 |

**Table 5-4.** Magnifications available with the 250 mm lens

| Eyepiece | Binocular | Base magnification | Factor | | | | | |
| --- | --- | --- | --- | --- | --- | --- | --- | --- |
| | | | 0.4 | 0.5 | .63 | 1.0 | 1.6 | 2.5 |
| 10 | 125 | 5 | 2× | 2.5× | 3.2× | 5× | 8× | 12.5× |
| | 160 | 6.4 | 2.6 | 3.2 | 4.0 | 6.4 | 10 | 16 |
| 12.5 | 125 | 6.25 | 2.5 | 3.1 | 3.3 | 6.3 | 10 | 15.6 |
| | 160 | 8 | 3.2 | 4 | 5 | 8 | 12.8 | 20 |
| 20 | 125 | 10 | 4 | 5 | 6 | 10 | 16 | 25 |
| | 160 | 12.8 | 5.1 | 6.4 | 8 | 12.0 | 20.5 | 32 |

**Table 5-5.** Magnifications available with the 300 mm objective lens[a]

| Eyepiece | Binocular | Base magnification | Factor[b] | | | | | |
| --- | --- | --- | --- | --- | --- | --- | --- | --- |
| | | | 0.4 | 0.5 | .63 | 1.0 | 1.6 | 2.5 |
| 10 | 125 | 4.2 | 1.7× | 2.1× | 2.7× | 4.2× | 6.7× | 10.5× |
| 10 | 160 | 5.3 | 2.1 | 2.7 | 3.3 | 5.3 | 8.5 | 13.3 |
| 12.5 | 125 | 5.2 | 2.1 | 2.6 | 3.3 | 5.2 | 8.3 | 13.0 |
| 12.5 | 160 | 6.7 | 2.7 | 3.4 | 4.2 | 6.7 | 10.7 | 16.8 |
| 20 | 125 | 8.3 | 3.3 | 4.2 | 5.3 | 8.3 | 13.3 | 20.8 |
| 20 | 160 | 10.7 | 4.3 | 5.4 | 6.7 | 10.7 | 17.1 | 26.8 |

[a]The lowest magnification on the Zeiss OPMI-6 and OPMI-7 is factor 0.5, slightly higher than the 0.4 on the Zeiss OPMI-1 microscope.

[b]Calculations based on equation: Magnification $= \dfrac{\text{eyepiece} \times \text{focal distance of binocular}}{\text{objective} \times \text{factor}}$

CALCULATING MAGNIFICATION

The principle of the magnification systems in the Zeiss and the Weck operating microscopes is twofold. First, it consists of those elements of magnification that are fixed and termed the *base magnification*. These components, the eyepiece, binocular tube, and objective lens, have been placed on the microscope prior to surgery and cannot be changed easily. Second, the magnification changer can vary the levels of magnification at the surgeon's will during the operating procedure. The equation of visual magnification (Mv) is

$$\text{Mv} = \text{base magnification} \times \text{factor}$$
$$\text{Mv} = \frac{\text{eyepiece} \times \text{binocular}}{\text{objective} \times \text{factor}}$$

Magnification is therefore increased by increasing the eyepiece, the binocular, or the magnification factor. Increases in focal distance of the objective lens result in decreased magnification. The various magnifications available when using the 200, 250, and 300 mm objective lenses have been recorded in Tables 5-3, 5-4, and 5-5. It is important to realize when using photography or videotape that the magnification recorded on film or video cassette is not the same as that seen through the eyepiece of the operating microscope. The formula for magnification during photography (Mp), to be discussed further in the section titled Photography and Videotape, is

$$\text{Mp} = \frac{\text{focal length of photo adapter}}{\text{objective} \times \text{factor}}$$

As an exercise in calculating magnification it is of interest to calculate those magnification components necessary to make the number settings on the OPMI-1 equal to actual magnification levels. One can see that three possibilities exist:

$$\frac{\text{Eyepiece } 20\times \ \times \text{ binocular } 160}{\text{Objective } 200} = 16$$

$$\frac{\text{Eyepiece } 12.5\times \ \times \text{ binocular } 160}{\text{Objective } 125} = 16$$

$$\frac{\text{Eyepiece } 10\times \ \times \text{ binocular } 160}{\text{Objective } 100} = 16$$

In all three cases the base magnification is 16. Recall that at setting 16 on the OPMI-1 the factor is 1. Therefore base magnification equals total magnification at that setting, and because both also are equal at all other settings, the number listed on the dial (setting) will equal the magnification present under the microscope.

**Figure 5-9.** Conversion of OPMI-1 for gynecologic microsurgery requires three steps. First, the coupling of the microscope body to the stand must be changed from angled fitting to the parallel coupling shown. Second, the straight binocular must be changed to an angled binocular. Third, (not shown) the objective lens must be changed to 250 or 275 mm to achieve the proper focal distance. A fourth consideration, to be discussed later (see Fig. 5-11), involves the addition of fiberoptic lighting and use of the House-Urban Quadrascope head. (Courtesy of Carl Zeiss, Inc., Thornwood, N.Y.)

Obviously, these objective lenses are not adequate for the gynecologist, and therefore, under conditions of gynecologic microsurgery, the turret settings will not equal visual magnification.

### Operating Microscopes

ZEISS OPMI-1

The first operating microscope with variable magnification was introduced by Carl Zeiss in 1954. This new microscope was designed by Dr. H. Littman for surgery of the ear. The major advance in this operating microscope was its ability to alter magnification without altering the working distance, or focal distance, termed *parafocality*. This microscope also provided coaxial illumination, adjustable eyepieces, binocular tubes, and objective lens in the typical building-block type assembly pioneered by Zeiss. Twenty-five years later this microscope remains a workhorse in most operating rooms. It is still used by ENT surgeons and, often, by gynecologists. This is the microscope that the author first used experimentally and, later, in a few clinical patients undergoing end-to-end reanastomosis following Pomeroy-type sterilization procedures.

Conversion of the Zeiss OPMI-1 microscope for use in infertility microsurgery is shown in Figure 5-9. It is pos-

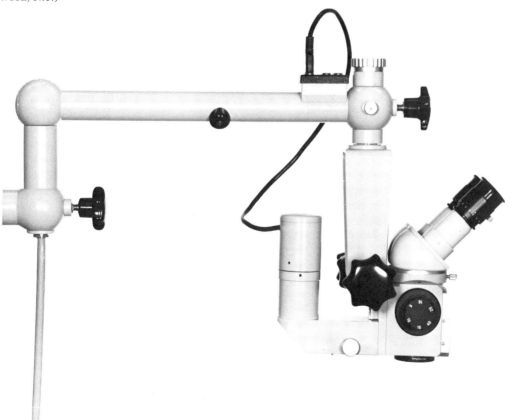

sible to place a Zeiss beam-splitter between the microscope body and the binocular tube of the OPMI-1. This attachment permits the use of monocular and binocular observation accessories as well as 35 mm photography and a video capability. Figure 5-10 shows the beam-splitter used with this operating microscope.

**Figure 5-10.** The beam-splitting device used with the Zeiss OPMI-1 and OPMI-6 microscopes to divert either the right or the left visual image to that side of the microscope body. (Courtesy of Carl Zeiss, Inc., Thornwood, N.Y.)

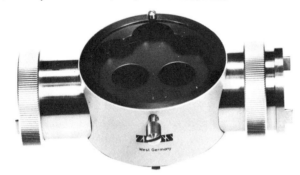

A House-Urban quadrascope head is an alternative type of beam-splitter that may be attached to this microscope to permit the surgical assistant to stand directly opposite the surgeon during the operative procedure (Fig. 5-11).

In spite of the major breakthrough represented by the design of the OPMI-1, many limitations existed. The major disadvantage of the manual magnification changer on the OPMI-1 is that its levels of magnification are fixed and difficult to change during surgery. In fact, microsurgical technique with this microscope may approach the level of that with the ocular loupe and head-lamp.

Photography through the Zeiss beam-splitter is often inadequate because of insufficient lighting at high magnification. A 50-watt bulb may be substituted for the usual 30-watt bulb and used on overload to produce maximum light. This lighting system is the same as that used in the OPMI-6 microscope discussed later. The actual candlepower and a comparison with fiberoptic

**Figure 5-11.** A House-Urban Quadrascope head is an alternative to the Zeiss beam splitter shown in Figure 5-10. This attachment permits an assistant to view the surgical field while standing 180 degrees from the surgeon (applies to OPMI-1 and OPMI-6 only). Fiberoptic lighting is also shown. (Courtesy of Carl Zeiss, Inc., Thornwood, N.Y.)

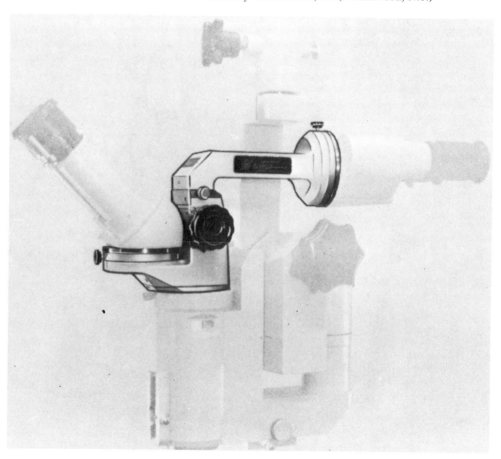

illumination are presented in the section titled Light Sources. A strobe flash attachment is available from Zeiss and produces excellent 35 mm photography.

Another disadvantage of the OPMI-1 relates to the optics used in the quadrascope head. The magnification and field of view seen by the surgical assistant differs from that seen by the surgeon and is a real inconvenience. The same quadrascope attachment can be used with the OPMI-6 microscope, and as we will discuss later, the same disadvantages apply. A camera attachment is available with the House-Urban attachment, but, again, insufficient light is a problem.

**Figure 5-12.** Zeiss operating microscope OPMI-6 adapted for gynecologic surgery. (Courtesy of Carl Zeiss, Inc., Thornwood, N.Y.)

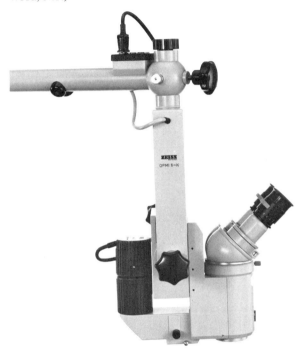

As was noted previously, the introduction of a motorized zoom magnification system increased the applicability of the operating microscope. Pioneered by Troutman and others, the ophthalmologists incorporated the operating microscope into their surgical technique in the early 1960s. Microsurgery became the standard of practice in surgery of the eye and the OPMI-6, the standard microscope used by these surgeons. Most operating rooms also have at least one of these models available. At first glance the OPMI-6 looks much different from the OPMI-1. The difference is the slit lamp and side arm, oblique light accessory used by the ophthalmologist to avoid the glare of direct light focused on the curved surface of the eye. These accessory pieces are easily removed by the gynecologist who must also change the objective lens from the 175 mm focal distance to the usual 250 mm lens. This change is depicted in Figure 5-12.

The eyepieces, binocular tube, and objective lens are identical to those used with the OPMI-1. The coaxial light source with incandescent bulb is also similar. The difference is in the magnification changer. In place of the round dial and turret, the OPMI-1 has a small window in which appears a number indicating the magnification factor.

As was noted in the discussion of the OPMI-1 microscope, the Zeiss beam-splitter attaches easily to the OPMI-6, providing access to 35 mm photography, a binocular viewer, and video. Again, inadequate light is a problem; however, the 50-watt bulb on overload is optimal.

A major drawback of this microscope, as with the OPMI-1, is the inability of the assistant to visualize the operating field. This is partially overcome by the House-Urban quadrascope beam-splitting accessory, but, again, the difference in magnification makes this an impractical attachment. As will be discussed later, the larger size of the OPMI-6 head is an additional problem, as is the difficulty in moving the head 180 degrees to permit the surgeon to change sides of the table, if that appears necessary.

ZEISS OPMI-7-P/H AND OPMI-6S

The two most convenient Zeiss operating microscopes available for gynecologic microsurgery are the OPMI-7-P/H and OPMI-6S. The magnification changer used on these instruments is similar to that employed on the OPMI-6; however, a beam-splitting attachment has been placed on the microscope body, dividing light and vision equally. Similar straight binocular tubes and eyepieces on either side of the beam-splitter produce identical views of the operating field for both the surgeon and his assistant (Fig. 5-13).

A convenience of these microscopes, in addition to the beam-splitter and zoom magnification system, is the easy mobility of the microscope head. Much more flexible than the OPMI-6 head, the OPMI-7-P/H and the OPMI-6S can be moved into the operating field and quickly adjusted owing to its smaller size and extremely convenient coupling arrangement. It is easily tilted to visualize the left and right adnexal areas.

**Figure 5-13.** Zeiss operating microscope OPMI-7-P/H with beam-splitting attachment. (Courtesy of Carl Zeiss, Inc., Thornwood, N.Y.)

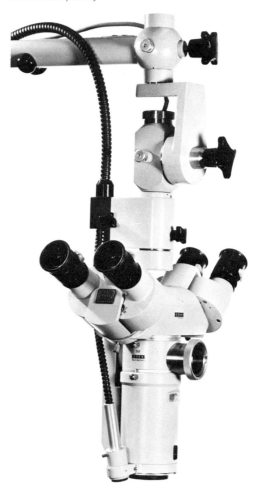

Three accessories add greatly to the use of these two microscopes. The first is a heavy-duty stand equipped with rapid coarse focus. This permits rapid adjustment of focus when working on tubal fimbria or adhesions. Both situations require more than the average amount of microscope mobility and require variations in depth that tend to make focus difficult. A disadvantage of the OPMI-7-P/H microscope that was corrected on the OPMI-6S is the lack of fine focus. The second accessory is the attachment for automatic X-Y axis motion (Fig. 5-14), controlled by a foot pedal (see Fig. 5-15). The X-Y axis attachment permits automatic movement of the microscope body in a forward-back, left-right direction under foot-pedal control. The convenience for the gynecologist is the ability to move along the fallopian tube or from fallopian tube to ovary without breaking concentration. Finally, fiberoptic illumination by the Vertalux fiberoptic system permits greatly increased lighting, thereby improving vision as well as photography.

**Figure 5-15.** Foot pedal used with Zeiss OPMI-7-P/H and OPMI-6S operating microscope. Both fine focus and zoom are controlled by a pedal. The joy stick controls the X-Y axis, and the buttons control coarse focus by moving the stand. (Courtesy of Carl Zeiss, Inc., Thornwood, N.Y.)

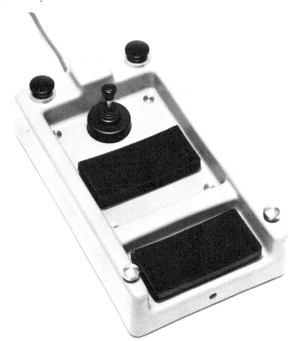

**Figure 5-14.** The X-Y axis permits the surgeon to move the microscope body forward and back as well as left and right; it is an essential feature of the operating microscope used in gynecologic microsurgery. (Courtesy of Carl Zeiss, Inc., Thornwood, N.Y.)

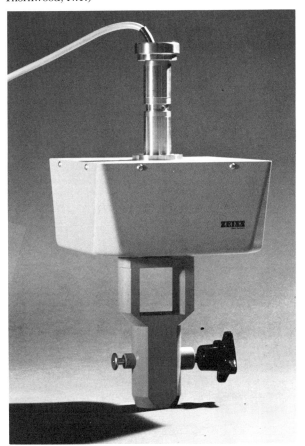

5. Essential Elements of Microsurgical Technique

The single deficiency of the OPMI-7-P/H was the lack of fine focus. This microscope can only be focused by moving the stand, i.e., it has only coarse focus. The OPMI-6S provides all the features of the OPMI-7-P/H noted above, in addition to fine focus. This author (G.W.P.) prefers the OPMI-6S for gynecologic microsurgery (Fig. 5-16).

**Figure 5-16.** Zeiss operating microscope OPMI-6S arranged for gynecologic microsurgery. (Courtesy of Carl Zeiss, Inc., Thornwood, N.Y.)

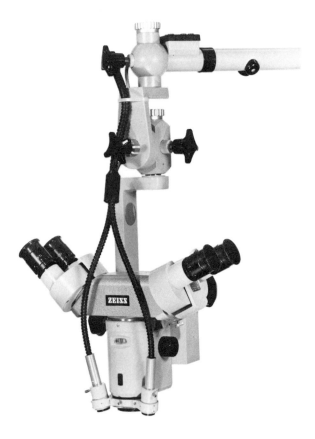

WECK-TROUTMAN OPERATING MICROSCOPE

Dr. Richard Troutman, a pioneer in microsurgical techniques in eye surgery, worked with Weck Instrument Company in the 1960s to attempt the design of an "ideal" operating microscope [36]. The resulting instrument, although by Troutman's admission not completely ideal, was first designed for ophthalmology but has also been employed in plastic and gynecologic microsurgery. It has all the features one looks for in an operating microscope; namely, adjustable lenses, easy mobility, foot-controlled zoom magnification in a 1:5 ratio, adjustable focus, and fiberoptic lighting. The most significant feature relates to dual head pieces permitting the surgeon and his assistant to control the focus and tilt while viewing the identical field (Fig. 5-17).

**Figure 5-17.** Weck-Troutman microscope arranged for gynecologic microsurgery.

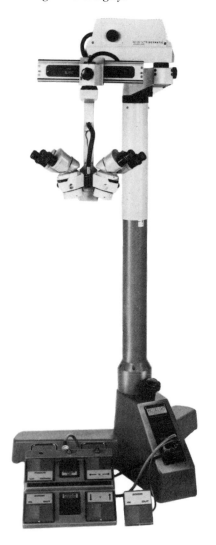

In spite of these excellent features, few gynecologic microsurgeons use this microscope, nor do the hand or eye surgeons use it extensively. Zeiss microscopes are far more prevalent in most operating rooms, and this author (G.W.P.) has had no personal experience with the Weck microscope.

Opinions vary on the usefulness of the Weck-Troutman microscope. Daniel and Terzis, in their recent text on reconstructive surgery, commented that in their personal experience the limitations of this microscope included "limited reach, lack of balance of the suspension system, and inadequate fiberoptic illumination at or above 15×." These authors also commented that "the two microscopes we used had multiple mechanical malfunctions unavailable to routine service" [5]. On the positive side, Diamond has performed hundreds of gynecologic microsurgical procedures with the Weck-Troutman microscope and recommended it highly. This is apparently the primary microscope used by this gynecologic microsurgeon [8].

FLOOR STANDS

Operating microscopes in most operating rooms are attached to a type of floor stand. Ceiling mounts are available and convenient but very expensive, in need of a high degree of ceiling support, and prone to vibration. The floor models used most often will be discussed.

The preceding discussion of various types of microscopes, including the Zeiss OPMI-1, OPMI-6, OPMI-7-P/H, OPMI-6S and Weck-Troutman microscopes have in essence referred to the microscope head. In general, any microscope head produced by Zeiss can be attached to any Zeiss floor stand. Obviously, a larger, heavier stand will provide increased stability for a heavy microscope head, such as the OPMI-6, OPMI-6S, and OPMI-7-P/H. In addition, the electrical connections required by these particular heads must be installed on the individual stand. Weight is a particular problem when accessory parts, such as the beam-splitter and photographic equipment, are being used with the OPMI-7-P/H or OPMI-6S, and a heavy-duty floor stand with leg extensions has been found optimal. Whenever possible, this author (G.W.P.) recommends a ceiling mount, which reduces handling of the microscope body and markedly reduces damage to the instrument. The added cost of the ceiling mount will quickly be recovered by decreased maintenance cost.

*Light Sources*

Excellent lighting is almost as important to the microsurgeon as magnification. An integral part of the increased ability to see the operative field through the operating microscope is owing to the increase in light on this field. As one increases magnification, the light required to see adequately also increases, and significantly more light is required at high magnification than low. A detailed discussion of optical principles and types of

microscopes has preceded this section on lighting; however, the surgeon must not underestimate the importance of this essential component of his system of visualizing the operative field that, unfortunately, is often compared with the simple act of turning on the light switch in one's living room.

It is necessary to understand the concept of coaxial illumination. The microsurgeon realizes that when he turns on the microscope light source, he is able to see the operative field clearly and without shadows. To achieve this effect, Zeiss and others have directed the light downward from the microscope body in the same plane as the rays of observation. This type of lighting system is termed *coaxial illumination* and is diagrammed in Figure 5-18. If one looks carefully at the drawing, it is apparent that a prism placed above the objective lens is designed so as to disperse the light from either a bulb or fiberoptic source directly into the field of view.

**Figure 5-18.** Coaxial illumination. The drawing outlines the path of visual image and the light source that illuminates the object. The prism arrangement permits both paths to be parallel, thereby eliminating shadows.

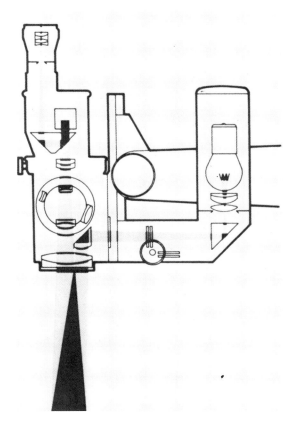

The two sources of light available in the various operating microscopes and headlamps are the incandescent bulb and fiberoptic illumination (Fig. 5-19). Early models of the OPMI-1 and OPMI-6 microscopes used a standard 6-volt, 30-watt incandescent tungsten bulb. A 50-watt tungsten bulb was also available but had a shorter life span and produced too much heat for the usual bulb housing on these microscopes. Illumination with the 300 mm objective lens combined with the 30-watt bulb at 6 volts is 1,000 footcandles and with the 50-watt bulb at this voltage is 1,400 footcandles. It is possible to increase the voltage to 7.2 volts by placing the foot switch on overload, thereby increasing the 30-watt bulb system to 1,900 footcandles and the 50-watt system to 2,500 footcandles. Increasing the voltage on overload, however, markedly shortens the life of the incandescent bulb and produces excessive heat. It is interesting to note the difference in light available when using various objective lenses. Decreasing the focal length of an objective lens increases the available light and, conversely, an increase in focal length decreases available light. This is demonstrated vividly in Table 5-6.

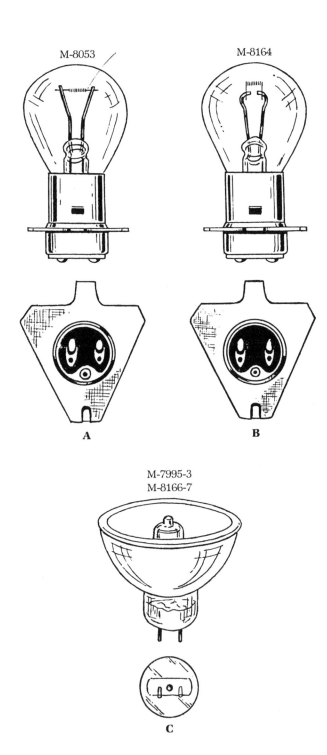

**Figure 5-19. A.** Tungsten 6-volt, 30-watt lamp. **B.** Tungsten 6-volt, 50-watt lamp. **C.** Halogen bulb. This is a 12-volt, 100-watt lamp for use with fiberoptic lighting.

**Table 5-6.** Association between the focal length of an objective lens and the light available

| | Objective lens | | | |
| --- | --- | --- | --- | --- |
| | 300 mm | | 200 mm | |
| Bulb (watts) | 30 | 50 | 30 | 50 |
| Operating microscope[a] | | | | |
| 6-volt | 1,000[b] | 1,400 | 2,200 | 3,100 |
| 7.2-volt | 1,900 | 2,500 | 3,100 | 4,300 |

[a]OPMI-1 and OPMI-6 equipped with 30- or 50-watt incandescent bulb.
[b]Light available in operating field in footcandles.

In the 1970s, Zeiss and other manufacturers introduced fiberoptic lighting on their newer microscope models and also designed fiberoptic illumination systems that would adapt to existing operating microscopes (Fig. 5-20). Markedly increased illumination is possible with fiberoptics, as the gynecologist has already experienced during diagnostic laparoscopy. One notices the intense white light bursting from the ends of the fiber bundle, compared to the yellow, less intense quality of the incandescent tungsten bulb. A detailed description of fiberoptic lighting was presented in Chapter 2. A drawing of the 12-volt, 100-watt halogen bulb used in fiberoptic systems was presented in Figure 5-19C.

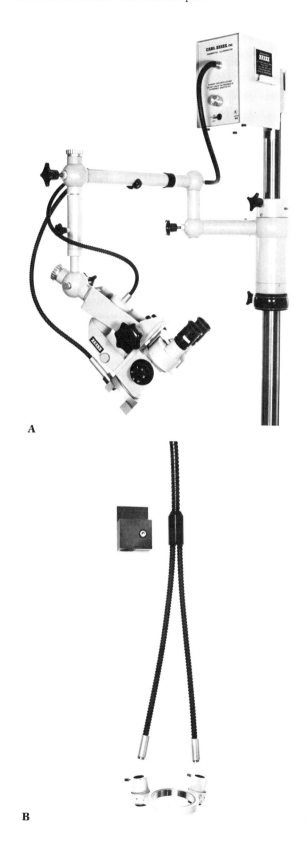

**Figure 5-20. A.** Fiberoptic lighting adapted to Zeiss OPMI-1 microscope. **B.** Vertalux fiberoptic lighting attachment for OPMI-6S and OPMI-7-P/H microscopes.

A

B

**Table 5-7.** Lighting available with operating microscopes*

| Lighting | 300 mm objective | |
|---|---|---|
| | 300-watt (footcandles) | 50-watt (footcandles) |
| Incandescent tungsten bulb, 6 volts | 1,000 | 1,400 |
| OPMI-1, OPMI-6 (tungsten), overload 7.2 volts | 1,900 | 2,500 |
| | Footcandles | Comment |
| Fiberoptic with halogen bulb (OPMI-7, OPMI-6) monolox | 1,000 | Fiberoptic in bulb housing |
| Vertalux 1 (halogen) | 2,300 | Fiberoptic adjacent to lens |
| Vertalux 1, 6 volts plus 30-watt bulb, 7.2 volts | 3,400 | Fiberoptic next to lens plus tungsten bulb |
| plus 50-watt bulb, | 4,400 | |
| 6 volts | 3,900 | |
| 7.2 volts | 5,000 | |
| Vertalux 2 | 3,200 | OPMI-1, OPMI-6 |
| OPMI-7-P/H (vertalux) | 4,000 | OPMI-7-P/H |
| Fiberoptic headlight | 4,000 | Used with loupes |

*The tungsten bulb is used in coaxial systems and the halogen bulb in fiberoptic systems.

A summary of the light available in the lighting systems used by the gynecologist is presented in Table 5-7. Because the lighting source available on most OPMI-1 and OPMI-6 operating microscopes is the 30-watt bulb, the light available when using the 300 mm objective lens is close to 1,000 footcandles and may be increased to 1,900 footcandles on overload for occasional use. In contrast, the fiberoptic system on the standard OPMI-7-P/H and OPMI-6S produces about 4,000 footcandles, an increase of 2 to 4 times that of earlier microscope illumination. If one intends to use the OPMI-1 or OPMI-6 operating microscope for gynecologic microsurgery, the addition of accessory lighting by utilization of the Vertalux I fiberoptic system increases to 3,400 to 4,400 footcandles the light available, which is quite comparable with that available on the OPMI-7-P/H. As will be further discussed later in this chapter, the fiberoptic headlamp marketed recently as an accessory when using loupes provides 4,000 footcandles at 16 inches, which is identical to that available with the OPMI-7-P/H and much better than the incandescent system on existing OPMI-1 and OPMI-6 models.

*Loupes (surgical telescopes)*

The report by Rock and Jones [21] that tubal reanastomosis using a 4.5× loupe produced an 80 percent pregnancy success rate clearly demonstrated the usefulness of this form of magnification in infertility surgery. This author (G.W.P.) has used both 2.5 and 4.5× loupes for lysis of adhesions, fimbrioplasty, and salpingostomy, as will be discussed in a later section. The comments by other gynecologists that loupes produce vertigo, headache, and increased muscle strain during surgery are not well founded if one learns to use these instruments as he has had to learn to use the operating microscope. The second major criticism, that the use of loupes presents difficulty in obtaining high intensity light, has been overcome by the use of the fiberoptic headlamp. Although loupes force one to use fixed magnification, a place for this type of magnification may exist in the field of infertility surgery and certainly deserves further study.

Two types of ocular loupes are available, simple and compound. The first type, rarely used and termed "simple," consists of a pair of simple magnifying lenses, usually 2×, mounted on an eyeglass frame. Because this is a simple lens system, 2× magnification will have a focal distance of 125 mm, which is 5 inches, obviously too short for comfortable surgical work. Most loupes in use today use a 14 to 16-inch focal distance. The alteration in focal distance is provided by the compound lens, which is a multiple lens system and is referred to as an operating telescope. These compact multiple lens systems can be ground into eyeglasses that are the surgeon's personal refractive correction. Vision around the lens is, therefore, quite comfortable. The lens system in the compound loupe is subdivided into doublets and, by adjusting the combination of these lenses, the focal distance and magnification can be altered. Therefore, the manufacturer can offer 2.5× loupes with a choice of focal distance from 12 to 20 inches (Fig. 5-21A). Recently, one manufacturer* introduced a loupe system with an expanded field of view that makes these instruments quite comparable to the operating microscope at a fixed magnification (Fig. 5-21B). A comparison of field of view and magnification is shown in Table 5-8.

*Designs for Vision, New York.

**Table 5-8.** Field of view in ocular loupe and operating microscope

| Operating microscope | Magnification | 2.1 | 3.3 | 5.2 | 8.3 | 13 |
|---|---|---|---|---|---|---|
| | Field (mm) | 77 | 61 | 40 | 25 | 15 |
| Loupe | Magnification | 2.5 | 3.5 | 4.5 | 6.0 | 8.0 |
| | Field (mm) | 80 | 73 | 55 | 45 | 35 |

**Figure 5-21. A.** Operating loupe; magnification 2.5× and focal distance, 16 inches. **B.** Operating loupe; expanded field 4.5× and focal distance, 16 inches. (Courtesy of Designs for Vision, New York, N.Y.)

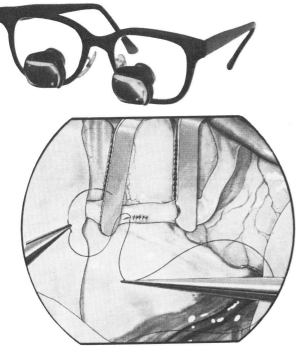

**A**    Anastomosis—magnified 2.5×    Focal distance—16″

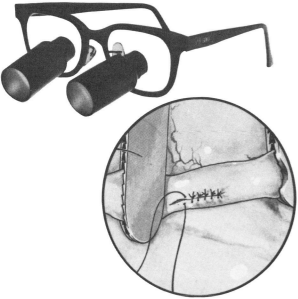

Anastomosis—magnified 4.5×
Focal distance—16″

**B**

5. Essential Elements of Microsurgical Technique

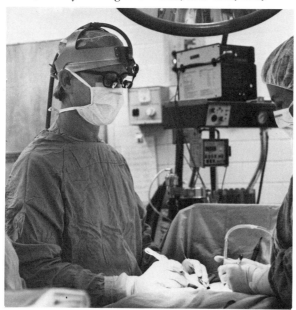

**Figure 5-22.** Accessory fiberoptic lighting provided by this headlamp is an essential adjunct when ocular loupes are used. (Courtesy of Designs for Vision, New York, N.Y.)

This table also compares the field of view available with the operating telescope (loupe) and operating microscope. It is apparent that the field of view is slightly larger with the loupes at similar magnifications. This is particularly true at 3.5× and at 8×, the highest point available in the loupe system. The ability to alter magnification easily has already been noted.

High intensity light is available by using a fiberoptic headlamp (Fig. 5-22). As was noted in the section on light sources (see Table 5-7), the headlamp produces 4,000 footcandles at 16 inches. The comparison with the operating microscope has revealed that this level of light is higher than that on the standard models of the Zeiss OPMI-1 and OPMI-6 microscopes and is equal to the advanced fiberoptic system available on the OPMI-6S and OPMI-7-P/H microscopes.

The loupe and headlamp should therefore be used together for optimal results (see Fig. 5-22). This has the disadvantage of added weight on the surgeon's head as well as the limited vision dictated by the fixed magnification of the operating telescope (loupe). However, this inconvenience is certainly no greater than that of moving the operating microscope into the surgical field. The major advantage of the loupe and headlamp system is the markedly improved mobility it provides, enabling the surgeon to dissect under the magnification of 2.5 to 3.5× adhesions that are difficult to reach in the cul-de-sac. This is an impossibility for those surgeons whose surgical technique is restricted to the use of the operating microscope.

*Photography and Videotape*
The ability to record all or portions of a microsurgical procedure on either film or videotape is available on all the operating microscopes discussed above. The simplest of these procedures involves 35 mm photography. Videotaping is also quite simple; however, picture quality is difficult to maintain, and splicing and editing are extremely complex. Lastly, Super 8 and 16 mm photography require dedication as well as assistance but offer the reward of well done "moving pictures."

During a microsurgical procedure, 35 mm photographs can be taken by attaching a 35 mm single-lens reflex (SLR) camera to the Zeiss photoadapter. This photographic arrangement also requires a beam-splitting attachment to direct a portion of the light and a portion of one of the parallel image-beams to the camera. "The parallel beams in the operating microscope are ideal for the insertion of optical beam-splitters" [15, 16, 17, 18, 19]. We have noted earlier that the Zeiss operating microscope is built on the Galilean principle of parallel image-beams diagrammed below (see Fig. 5-4).

**Figure 5-23.** Photo adapters. **A.** Zeiss standard f-220 mm adaptation for 35 mm photography. In contrast, the Zeiss-Urban attachment, **B,** is a dual photo adaption, permitting use of a 35 mm camera, f-300 and cine, or television with f-137 mm. (Courtesy of Carl Zeiss, Inc., Thornwood, N.Y.)

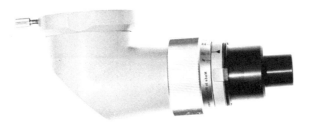

**A**

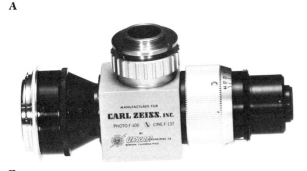

**B**

The beam splitter is a device that contains two small beam-splitting glass cubes (one for each of the parallel light paths), each of which deflects fixed portions of the light of the observer path, 90 degrees to the right. The beam splitter in Figure 5-10 is used with the Zeiss OPMI-1 and OPMI-6 operating microscopes. The parallel images seen through the right and left eyes are separate. Thus, diversion of light and image to the right of the microscope would be accomplished by diverting the image seen by the right eye. In contrast, diversion to the left would be accomplished by reflecting the light and the image from the path seen by the left eye. The beam splitter in the OPMI-6S and OPMI-7-P/H, in contrast, is a modification in which one of the side segments has been removed, thereby adapting it for use with these two operating microscopes. The operating principle of this modified beam splitter is the same as that discussed above; however, the image and light from only one visual field is reflected 90 degrees for use during photography or videotaping.

5. Essential Elements of Microsurgical Technique

**147**

As was pointed out earlier, the beam splitter on the Zeiss OPMI-1 and OPMI-6 microscopes has been modified for use on the OPMI-7-P/H. The f-220 photo adapter may be used with either beam-splitting attachment and is interposed between the camera and the beam splitter. Two units are available for 35 mm photography, both of which have been used by this author (G.W.P.) (see Fig. 5-23). The first is the 35 mm photo adapter with a focal length of 220 mm. As shown in Figure 5-24, the camera body rests on top of the photo adapter. Adjustments (f-stops) can be made on the photo adapter, although this author (G.W.P.) used either f-11 or f-8 in all cases. In contrast is the dual photo adapter produced by Urban and Zeiss (see Fig. 5-23B). This photo adapter permits 35 mm photography and video recording concurrently. The surgeon can also use this attachment for 35 mm photography, videotaping, or 16 mm photography alone. This combination adapter permits flexibility in these three realms of photography for a modest increase in cost. At this writing, the 35 mm photo adapter f-220 costs $750 compared to $1,295 for the dual adapter produced by Urban and Zeiss.

The surgeon should note that the focal distance of the 35 mm camera attachment is 300 mm on the dual adapter, compared to 220 mm on the single 35 mm adapter. If one refers to the equation for magnification at photography, it is clear that the focal distance of the adapter is the numerator in this equation, thereby indicating that an increase in focal distance will increase magnification on the film. Likewise, this would decrease the field size somewhat, and also increase the light requirement. This author (G.W.P.) has not found a significant difference in the 35 mm photographs obtained with these two adapters. In summary, the basic components of 35 mm photography are:

1. Reticule in eyepiece
2. Beam-splitting attachment: Zeiss f-220 or House-Urban dual adapter
3. Photo adapter: Zeiss f-220
4. 2× magnifier (not used by the author)
5. Camera adapter permitting use of any 35 mm camera body

The camera adapter shown in Figure 5-24 can be used with virtually any 35 mm SLR camera. The important features of a 35 mm camera are

1. Automatic light-sensing mechanism
2. Automatic film advance
3. Mechanism for triggering the film advance
   a. Infra red
   b. Foot pedal and cable

Two additional Zeiss photo adapters are of interest—first, a single video adapter with f-107. This provides a lower magnification and a larger field of view than is obtained with the dual adapter with cine f-137 shown in Figure 5-23B. Secondly, a dual adapter with photo f-250 and cine/video f-107 has a similar advantage, although it divides the available light into two segments, thus reducing light intensity at each port.

**Figure 5-24.** Assembly for 35 mm photography. Included are the **A.** beam splitter (use modified beam splitter with OPMI-6S and OPMI-7-P/H; **B.** photo adapter f-220; **C.** 2× magnification (not necessary); **D.** camera adapter; **E.** camera body (OM-II or Contax RTS). (Courtesy of Carl Zeiss, Inc., Thornwood, N.Y.)

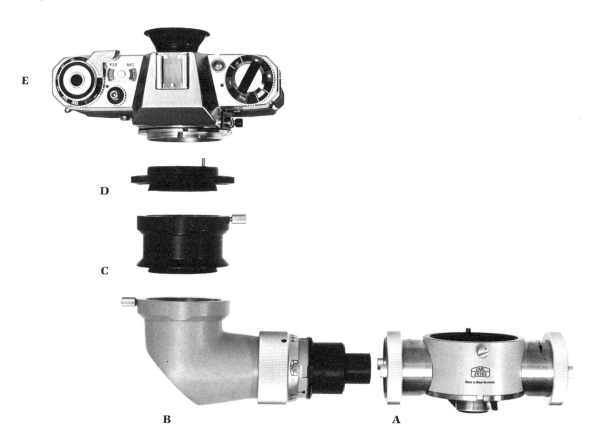

Most modern SLR cameras provide both a manual and an automatic built-in light-sensing mechanism. The automatic system is exceedingly helpful during microsurgical procedures, because it adjusts the time of exposure to fit the amount of available light. On manual setting, the photographer can set the exposure time as needed, but this is awkward during surgery. This author's (G.W.P.) personal experience has involved the Olympus OM-II and the Zeiss Contax RTS cameras. Figure 5-25 depicts the system presently used by this author.

Adequate light and accurate focus, important features in microsurgical technique, become even more vital when 35 mm photography is used. Zeiss offers a number of focusing aides, termed *reticules* to improve focus through the operating microscope. These crosshair patterns fit on the lower portion of the eyepiece and are focused at infinity to provide a sharp image for comparison with the image in the operating field that is being brought into focus for photography. As was noted earlier, the low light-intensity available with 30- and 50-watt incandescent bulbs on the OPMI-1 and OPMI-6 operating microscopes makes photography difficult. The use of overload current is an improvement but shortens the life span of the bulb and produces excessive heat. The Vertalux fiberoptic attachments are a great advantage for photography and, finally, a strobe attachment (Zeiss) coordinated with the camera produces excellent lighting.

**Figure 5-25.** Camera assembly used with OPMI-6S (also suitable for OPMI-7-P/H) includes the special beam splitter, Zeiss Urban dual photo adapter and Contax RTS camera body with automatic film advance. A Zeiss video camera has also been included. (Courtesy of Carl Zeiss, Inc., Thornwood, N.Y.)

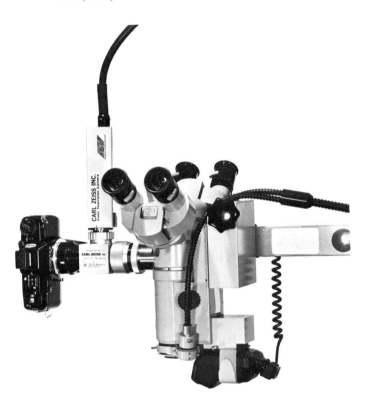

This author (G.W.P.) used three types of film. Kodacolor 400 film and recently ASA 1000 produce excellent prints and color negatives that can be made into slides, and, of course the high ASA film provides real assistance when using less than optimal light sources. Ektachrome 200 (daylight) and Ektachrome 160 (tungsten), both produce excellent 35 mm slides. The lower ASA setting does not appear to be significant under normal light conditions, and, in fact, this film can be pushed to ASA 400. At present, the author uses Ektachrome 200 film and records portions of each microsurgical procedure. The film is easily developed within twenty-four hours, and may be kept in the patient's office record.

Three attachments are, therefore, of great use when one takes 35 mm photographs during microsurgery. The automatic light-sensing device already noted is available on both the Olympus OM-II and Contax RTS cameras. The Yashica Company in cooperation with Zeiss has recently introduced a quartz sensing-device that may represent an improvement in this field. A motor drive that provides automatic film advance is also necessary, because one cannot advance the film by lever action when the camera is completely draped; nor is this practical during an operative procedure, because all hands are occupied. The Olympus OM-II provides a mechanical film advance (Winder I) that compares to the electronic system on the Contax RTS. Both the OM-II, Winder I and the Realtime Winder available on the Contax RTS camera have been used successfully by this author (G.W.P.).

Finally, some type of remote control of camera firing is necessary, because vibration of the microscope is produced when anyone touches the camera button. Initially the infra red with control attachment provided by Yashica for the Contax RTS seemed to be an answer; however, a slight delay always occurred between the verbal command and the nurse's movement to fire the camera. This author (G.W.P.), therefore, has found a foot-pedal control of this camera very convenient and, in fact, uses a special arrangement made for him by Yashica.

The magnification actually recorded on film is not that visualized by the surgeon, because the image being photographed does not travel through the binocular or the eyepiece of the microscope, both of which are included in the calculation for magnification. The image being photographed travels through the objective lens, the magnification changer, the beam splitter, and, finally, the photo adapter, which directs it to the camera body. The equation for calculating magnification is

$$Mp = \frac{\text{focal length of photo adapter}}{\text{objective lens} \times \text{factor}}$$

where Mp = magnification on photograph

The focal length of the photo adapter is printed on the instrument. Auxiliary magnification is available by adding a $2\times$ magnifier that fits between the camera adapter and the photo adapter. This change enlarges the film image so that it fills the entire frame and eliminates the circle seen on photographs taken at high magnifications. This author (G.W.P.) has not found the $2\times$ magnifier to be helpful.

*Videotape and Cinematography*

The process of recording an operative procedure on videotape is uncomplicated. The dual Zeiss-Urban photo adapter permits the attachment of a television camera by means of an attachment called a C-mount. The camera is then attached to a television monitor for observation during surgery and to a recording device similar to that used in home television recording. A unit that records a one-half-inch videotape is used by this author (G.W.P.). The greatest drawback to this system is the expense of a high quality television camera. Accessory lighting may also be required. The author has used a medium-grade television camera and has found the color and detail of this process to be disappointing. A typical unit for video recording during microsurgery is shown in Figure 5-25. Recently Sony introduced a color video camera model DXC-1850 that provides horizontal resolution of 400 lines and light sensitivity at 200 foot candles. This advanced system provides excellent quality videotapes with the standard Vertalux light system of the Zeiss OPMI-6S microscope.

Super 8 and 16 mm photography is possible through the operating microscope. These photographs are sharper than video and preferable when they are to be used for teaching. A 16 mm camera assembly is shown in Figure 5-26.

**Figure 5-26.** A 16 mm camera may also be used with the Zeiss OPMI-6S or OPMI-7-P/H microscopes. (Courtesy of Carl Zeiss, Inc., Thornwood, N.Y.)

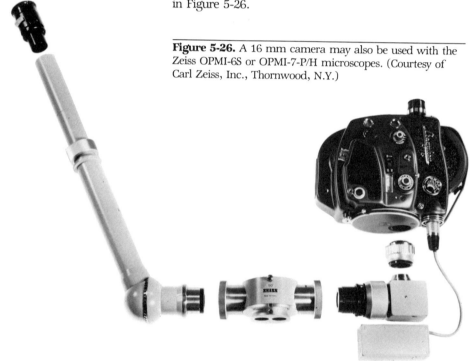

## Essentials of Microelectrosurgery

*If the incision is to be made in delicate tissue only, a fine needle electrode is used. . . with a fine needle as the active electrode, the endotherm knife is capable of cutting so fine a line as to heal almost without scar formation.*

HOWARD KELLY, 1925

The infertility surgeon uses electrosurgery during operative laparoscopic procedures and at laparotomy during a microsurgical approach to the repair of tubal disease. The gross technique of electrocoagulation used during laparoscopic tubal sterilization procedures in the early 1970s has given way to a careful monopolar and bipolar operative laparoscopic technique that permits the cutting of tubal and ovarian adhesions and occasional salpingoneostomy. A more dramatic change in electrosurgery has been associated with those surgical procedures performed under magnification and has led to the term *microelectrosurgery* [34]. The ability to carefully excise a filmy adhesion or coagulate a small bleeding vessel with a fine monopolar or bipolar electrode while working on a section of oviduct at magnifications of 5 to 15 × has helped to make the microsurgical approach possible. Electrical principles that distinguish the cutting and coagulating currents described later in this chapter apply to both laparoscopic and infertility microsurgical procedures. The discussion below will attempt to relate these principles to the actual uses of these currents. The recently introduced carbon dioxide laser is designed to achieve a surgical result similar to microelectrosurgery and is discussed in Chapters 6 and 7.

### Definitions

The terminology associated with electrosurgery is both confusing and unfamiliar to the gynecologist. However, one must understand these principles to follow the discussion of their clinical application. To begin this orientation, electrosurgery is really a form of diathermy (dia-, through; therme, heat). There are two divisions of diathermy, medical and surgical. Both involve the same electrical principles demonstrated in 1893 by D'Arsonval [6], namely, that high frequency current can be passed through an individual with no effect other than the production of heat (Fig. 5-27).

Medical diathermy employs this principle by using two large electrodes of equal size placed on the patient. High frequency electrical current can then be passed through the part of the body interposed between the electrodes, and a mild degree of heat is produced. The heat produced by this technique is a direct result of the resistance that living tissue offers to the passage of high frequency electrical current.

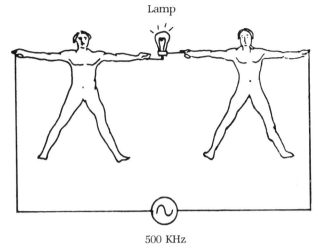

**Figure 5-27.** D'Arsonval's experiment (1893) in which he passed 1 to 3 amps of high frequency current, 50,000 cycles per second, through human subjects. (From L. A. Geddes, L. F. Silva, D. P. DeWitt, and J. A. Pearce. What's new in electrosurgical instrumentation. *Med. Instrum.* 2:355, 1977.)

Lamp

500 KHz

Surgical diathermy uses a small (needle or ball) electrode, termed the *active electrode*, that concentrates electrical current and, therefore, heat, in a small area, such that this intense heat causes actual tissue destruction. The electrode does not become hot initially but simply conducts high frequency current to the tissue. Only after tissue resistance to the passage of this current is encountered does the temperature of the tissue and then the electrode rise. Heat is a result of tissue resistance known as *impedance* in electrical terminology. Oringer states that ". . .impedance or [tissue] resistance converts high frequency current into heat energy which is then hot enough to 'cook the cells' and coagulate them or to disintegrate or volatize the cells" [28]. A second large electrode, termed the *dispersive electrode* or *patient plate*, is used in surgical diathermy to collect the high frequency electrical current that has been introduced by the active electrode and to return this current to the generator.

Surgical diathermy encompasses all procedures used in electrosurgery*. The subdivisions of electrosurgery are

Monoterminal (use of a single electrode)
    Electrodessication
    Electrofulguration
Biterminal (use of two electrodes)
    Electrocoagulation
        Monopolar
        Bipolar
    Electrosection (cutting)
Electrocautery* (use of a hot wire)

## Electrosection and Electrocoagulation

The electrosurgical current utilized during operative laparoscopy and during tubal microsurgery is a high frequency current that is passed between two electrodes, one large (dispersive) and one small (active), in a circuit termed biterminal.† Although the discussion that follows focuses primarily on the active electrode, one must not ignore the dispersive electrode (patient plate). Painful, disfiguring burns will occur at this site if proper contact between the plate and the patient is not achieved. These electrodes are available as metal plates that require conductive jelly and as prelubricated disposable units that attach easily to the patient's leg. The operating room nurse must remember to check each prepackaged patient plate carefully before attaching it to ascertain that the conductive liquid has not evaporated.

*The inclusion of electrocautery (thermocoagulation, Semm) as a form of electrosurgery is controversial, because it does not involve the use of high frequency current, but uses low voltage current to heat the electrode directly and to sear or cauterize the involved tissue [31].
†The thermocoagulation current used by Semm employs a low frequency current to heat the cutting instrument and then to sear or cook the tissue directly.

### Electrosection (cutting)

The cutting is not done by the electrode, which has no sharpened edge, but actually by the current which forms ahead of the electrode, and an electrical arc which by volatizing the tissue, separates them as though they were cut.

W. T. BOVIE, 1928

The discussion of electrical principles (page 159) describes the waveforms of partially rectified and fully rectified currents that produce a tissue cutting effect. Oringer [28] has summarized the character of cutting current in his statement that

when damped, fully rectified high frequency current is applied to the tissue by biterminal application and the surgical electrode is moved along the surface of the tissue. As it makes contact the current density becomes so concentrated along the line of contact that individual cells in the line of cleavage undergo molecular disintegration and volatization creating a precise incision.

The quotes by Bovie (1928) and Oringer (1975) are remarkably similar in content and appear to summarize the basic concept of cutting current. Remarkably little insight into the actual cellular effect of a cutting current has been gained since the reports by Bovie (4) and McLean [24] in 1928. Solid state circuits have produced pure cutting currents that simulate the earlier vacuum tube circuit responsible for the endotherm knife of Wyeth [37]. The major advance in the recent application of cutting current to microelectrosurgery has involved the use of a finer needle electrode and use of lower voltage pure cutting current. The ability to see the tissue more clearly through the operating microscope forces the surgeon to perfect this technique and to avoid charring and dessication. Cutting occurs at the tip of the electrode, which must be held directly above the tissue at a 90-degree angle and should be moved quickly to avoid coagulation.

Cutting technique using a microelectrode is as follows:

1. Select intensity setting on the generator as low as possible to avoid charring (sparking), but high enough to permit free movement of the fine active electrode through the tissue.
2. The active electrode should be a fine needle.
3. A hand contact unit is helpful. The surgeon should depress either the fingertip or foot switch to activate the cutting current before making tissue contact.
4. Movement of the electrode is important. Cutting occurs at the very tip of the needle, not on the edge. If the electrode is held stationary, a degree of coagulation will occur at that site.

### Electrocoagulation

This current is similar to a cutting current, because it employs a biterminal high frequency current. The difference relates to the type of high frequency electrical current (the waveform) delivered to the electrode and the speed of movement of the electrode through the tissue. Coagulation employs a damped waveform typically produced by the spark-gap generator of Bovie, and still manufactured as the Ritter Bovie. Solid-state units referred to later in this section simulate this waveform, by a process termed *modulation*, to produce a coagulating current. The electrode employed during monopolar coagulation is usually larger than a cutting electrode. The ball electrode is used for coagulation, because it produces a larger surface area than does the needle, a property that enhances the coagulation effect; however, the ball electrode is too large for use in microelectrosurgery, and a bipolar electrode is usually employed for coagulation with this technique. The electrical current used during bipolar coagulation is the same type of coagulating current as that employed with a monoterminal unit; however, the tissue effect is different, because the path of this current is limited to the space between the two electrodes, with little dispersal. Although an in-depth explanation has not been offered for the coagulation effect, it generally is assumed that a coagulating current produces evaporation of cellular fluids with protein denaturation leading to a congealed tissue effect. It has been theorized that the pause associated with a damped-wave current permits the tissue to cool and, therefore, leads to coagulation rather than to cellular explosion, which occurs with the constant waveform of a cutting type current [27].

In summary, the high frequency currents described above are used to cut tissue (electrosection) or to coagulate small bleeding vessels (electrocoagulation). Electrocoagulation initially applied only to monopolar coagulation but now includes a bipolar coagulation technique. The early spark-gap generators produced a damped electrical current that provided an excellent coagulating effect but resulted in extensive tissue damage during cutting. In contrast, the vacuum tube generator of Wyeth and others was responsible for the radio knife, an instrument that produced excellent cutting with very little tissue coagulation. Unfortunately, the high voltage spark-gap generator of Bovie dominated electrosurgery for many years and undoubtedly was responsible for much of the unfavorable criticism of this technique. Present solid state generators, which will be discussed later, provide variable degrees of coagulating and cutting current that may be altered to fit the needs of the microsurgeon.

*Principles of Electrosurgical Generators*
The electrical differences that characterize coagulating and cutting currents have been discussed earlier. Unfortunately, the simplicity of the early high voltage genera-

tors, such as the Ritter Bovie, lulled the surgeon into complacency, because he needed only to press the foot switch labeled coagulation, or the one next to it, labeled cutting. This approach won't work for the infertility surgeon, however, because a generator that offers a suitable cutting current will not always provide the proper coagulating current for a bipolar forceps, and, in some cases, does not provide adequate monopolar coagulation. One must, therefore, select the proper electrosurgical generator for cutting with the microelectrode and, often, a separate unit for bipolar or monopolar coagulation. An understanding of the types of current that produce the ability of a microelectrode to coagulate or to cut may be grasped from the explanation of the instruments that provide these currents. That instrument, termed a *generator*, converts wall current (110-volt, 60-cycle alternating current) into a high frequency oscillating current that will either coagulate or cut tissue. The frequency of these oscillations is greater than 10,000 cycles per second and is in the range used by radio broadcasting, thus leading to the reference to radio waves or radio frequency current. Two generators, spark-gap and vacuum tube generators, developed during the years 1910 to 1925 produced markedly different forms of current that in the former instance coagulated tissue and in the latter produced a pure cutting effect when applied to animal or human tissue by means of a fine electrode.

To select an electrosurgical generator, the surgeon should understand a few basic electrical principles. The effect desired in electrosurgery, whether it be to cut or to coagulate, ultimately depends on one thing, the transfer of electrical power. The way in which power is transferred distinguishes electrocoagulation from electrosection (cutting). When an electrical current begins to flow, its energy can be stored in a compacitor or coil, or dissipated as light or heat. The flow through a patient is dissipated as heat and avoids muscular stimulation when the frequency is greater than 10,000 cycles per second. The energy dissipated per unit of time is defined by power and is measured in watts. A 600-watt light bulb is both brighter and hotter than a 60-watt bulb, because more energy is delivered to it in the form of current and more power is being dissipated from it in the form of light and heat. Relating this to electrosurgery, it becomes clear that the local tissue effect produced by an electrosurgical unit relates to the amount of energy transferred to the tip of the electrode per unit of time, i.e., power, and the heat it produces when tissue resistance is encountered. The measure of tissue resistance, or impedance, is discussed at length in the following paragraphs.

Electrocoagulation results in cellular dehydration and protein denaturation, which produce a congealed tissue effect several cell layers deep. The cell wall is not grossly ruptured but probably suffers a small perforation during this process of dehydration. This effect is produced by low power delivered in intermittent fashion. In contrast, a cutting effect is associated with a continuous high power current that produces intense heat and results in cellular explosion. In this case, heat is dissipated by vaporization of cellular fluid and does not conduct through the tissue, thereby limiting the tissue destruction associated with cutting current to a few cell layers.

Figure 5-28 demonstrates these two types of power in a form termed *waveform*. A specific waveform exists for each type of electrical current and can be visualized by attaching an oscilliscope to the generator. The transfer of power in a pulsatile mode, depicted in Figure 5-28A, is compared to power being delivered in a continuous fashion, as shown in Figure 5-28B. To understand the differences between these two forms of power output consider the example of boiling a pot of water. The boiling point of the water would be reached sooner if the pot were placed over the heat continuously, rather than moved back and forth, in and out of the flame. This principle demonstrates the difference between coagulating and cutting currents. Under the proper conditions, the waveform demonstrated in Figure 5-28B produces a hotter current and is conducive to cutting tissue, whereas that in Figure 5-28A is intermittent and will result in a coagulation effect. This difference is discussed further in the section that deals with generator types.

**Figure 5-28.** Waveforms associated with (A) coagulation and (B) cutting current. The power output in A is pulsatile, whereas in B it is continuous.

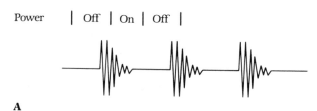

Two terms, damping and modulation, must be explained before discussing generator design. A *damped waveform* is one that decreases in magnitude over an interval of time (see Fig. 5-28A). A guitar string when plucked exhibits damped oscillations as it vibrates back and forth with decreasing amplitude before finally stopping. If one supplied more energy and plucked harder, the string would oscillate longer, delivering more energy in the form of sound, and take longer to come to rest. A coagulating current is characterized by a damped waveform followed by a pause.

The second concept, *modulation*, occurs as a result of superimposing one signal on another signal of different frequency. Voice sounds of 120 Hz are carried on radio waves of roughly 100,000 Hz by the process of modulation (Fig. 5-29). Modulation of sound is encountered in everyday life, as exemplified by the sirens on ambulances. Typically, a 400 Hz signal is modulated with a slow frequency wave producing the gyrating, pulsating effect of the ambulance siren. If one were to continuously increase and decrease the volume of a stereo amplifier, the effect would be termed modulation, because it has combined the sound of music, which is about 5,000 Hz, with the rhythmic 4-cycle per minute oscillation of the knob.

**Figure 5-29.** The two signals of frequency, 120 Hz and 100,000 Hz shown in (A) have been combined into one signal (B) by the process of modulation. This is accomplished by solid-state circuitry.

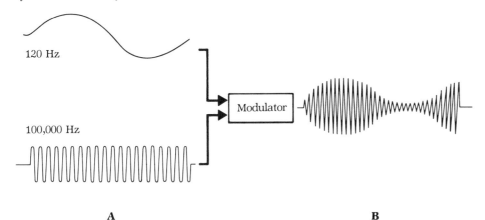

120 Hz

100,000 Hz

Modulator

**A**

**B**

*Basic Types of Generators*

The preliminary discussion of electrical principles can be carried further in an analysis of generator types. The first electrosurgical unit employed in surgery was the spark-gap generator, typified by the unit employed in Boston by Bovie and Cushing [4]. Solid state devices were not available when this design was first introduced in the years 1915 to 1925, although work with the vacuum tube was taking place. The spark-gap generator employed a very simple principle that produced excellent coagulating current and a very satisfactory cutting-coagulation combination effect when it was first introduced. In this design, still in use today, a capacitor (which can store energy) is charged by high frequency current, known as radio frequency, involving oscillations greater than 10,000 cycles per second. When sufficient energy is obtained for a spark to traverse the gap, the capacitor will discharge, and a high frequency current will flow to the surgical electrode. A damped oscillatory output is obtained with this design. As we have discussed, it is this noncontinuous pulsatile current that produces excellent tissue coagulation (Fig. 5-30). By increasing the distance of the spark gap, the unit can be made to charge to high energy levels, thereby producing a more prolonged output, which results in more power being transferred to the surgical electrode. Unrectified current from a spark-gap generator produces a highly damped waveform. "The current flow begins with an initial burst of peak amplitude, then rapidly dwindles to 0, then after a split-second pause, interval, or damping period there is another burst of energy" [27]. Solid-state generators also simulate this waveform by the process of modulation.

During the same interval, 1915 to 1925, work progressed on development of the vacuum tube generator. Early units, termed the *radio knives*, produced an excellent cutting effect with little coagulation, and studies using this technique were reported by Clark [3], Wyeth [14] and others [22, 28]. Although less popular than the spark-gap system for many years, this type of current is far more suitable for microsurgery. The basic principle of the vacuum tube involves a filament and grid. These units employed a vacuum tube oscillating circuit tuned to radio frequency and produced a waveform that was neither damped nor pulsatile but was a continuous sinusoidal wave ideal for cutting.

Addition of a single radio tube to a high frequency generator results in a moderately damped or partially rectified current (Fig. 5-31). Oringer [27, 28] has explained that only the first half of each cycle of alternating current has been converted into high frequency current by this generator. During the second half of the cycle, the high frequency current is at 0 and has, therefore, been damped out. This produces an intermittent flow of high frequency cutting current; however, the pause between bursts permits a coagulation effect during this damped interval. This is also achieved by modulation in a solid-state unit to achieve a blended current.

**Figure 5-31.** Waveform of moderately damped, partially rectified current produced by a vacuum tube or solid-state generator.

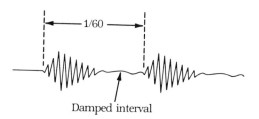

Damped interval

**Figure 5-30.** Waveform of a damped, unrectified pulsatile current used to produce tissue coagulation.

Power interval

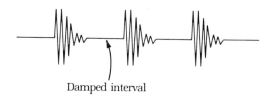

Damped interval

Addition of two vacuum tubes permits the electrosurgical generator to convert both halves of the cycle of alternating current to high frequency current, thus producing a continuous flow of cutting energy. This fully rectified, undamped current is excellent for electrosection (cutting). However, because each individual cycle begins at 0 and ends at 0, there is a minute but perceptible pulsating effect that adds a small element of coagulation to this waveform [27] (Fig. 5-32).

The introduction of transistors and integrated circuits after 1960 markedly increased the sophistication of circuit design and permitted variations of the waveforms used for cutting and coagulating currents. These variations achieved by the concept of modulation discussed above are apparent in the currents provided by modern solid-state electrosurgical generators. It must be stated that vacuum tubes can be used to produce the same circuitry as transistors or integrated circuits; however, they are now seldom used for several reasons. Vacuum tubes have shorter lives than solid-state units and need to be replaced more often. In addition, they cost more and take up considerably more space.

Solid state circuits permitted the elimination of the minimal pulsating effect found in fully rectified circuits by a process of filtration, thereby achieving truly continuous waveform (Fig. 5-33). A pure cutting current is thus achieved, as will be discussed later under specific generator types. The microsurgeon will be surprised at the small amount of bleeding encountered when using this current, because most cutting currents in use today are actually a blend of cutting and coagulation. The settings on the Valley Lab SSE generator demonstrates this point.

**Figure 5-33.** Waveform of an undamped, continuous wave produced by solid-state generators. This current produces a pure cutting effect.

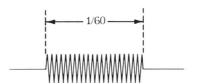

**Figure 5-32.** Waveform of undamped, fully rectified high-frequency current used for cutting. Note the gradual fall of the waveform to the 0 level, indicating a small degree of coagulation effect.

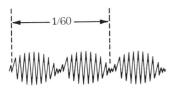

**Figure 5-34.** Modulation permits the combination of waveforms to achieve varying degrees of cutting and coagulation. It is possible to vary the height and the length of **A** and **B** to produce varied blends of cutting and coagulation. Such variation is possible only with solid-state circuits.

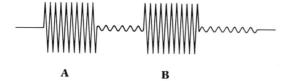

A          B

The new solid-state units allow the surgeon more versatility, because integrated circuits permit the combination of waveforms by modulation to achieve varying levels of cutting and coagulation effects. The so-called blended currents are continuous waves that vary in power output and permit various combinations of cutting and coagulation. Figure 5-34 demonstrates a blended current from a solid-state unit.

A comparison of the four types of high frequency power output is presented in Figure 5-35.

**Figure 5-35.** Types of high frequency power output. **A.** Highly damped (pulsatile) current, which is also termed *unrectified*. This is a coagulating current produced by modulation of a solid-state circuit. **B.** Partially damped current that still has a slight pause. This is also termed *partially rectified* (i.e., by a radio tube) and is used to produce both cutting and coagulation. **C.** Undamped (continuous) current, also termed *fully rectified*, i.e., by two radio grids (rectified). This is a cutting current but provides a very small amount of coagulation. The continuous current shown in (D) is produced by solid-state circuits and is non-modulated.

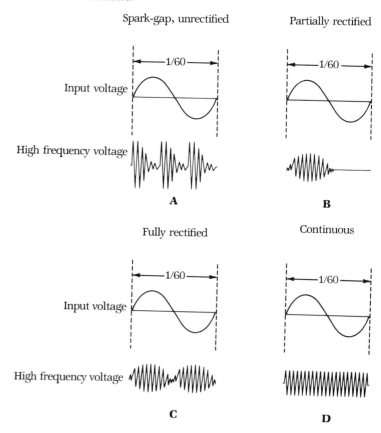

*Tissue Repair*

There are virtually no studies of tissue response to microelectrosurgery as presently practiced by the infertility surgeon. As was pointed out earlier in this chapter, although specific electrical waveforms of high frequency current are associated with specific tissue effect, i.e., cutting and coagulation, ". . .why coagulating requires one type of radio frequency current and cutting another is still a mystery" [13]. Tissue response has been studied following different applications of electrosurgical current. Remarkably, most of the tissue studies on the effect of a cutting current on mucous membranes are in the dental literature [23]. This information certainly should be of immense value in comparing the laser form of microelectrosurgery with the carbon dioxide laser, as is discussed below.

Engle and Harris [11] have studied the response of fallopian tube tissue following electrocoagulation during laparoscopic tubal sterilization and have proposed an interesting progression of events:

When an active electrode is pressed against tissue, the coagulation proceeds in three distinct phases. At first, the tissue is in good electrical contact with the electrode and there is no visible sparking or change in tissue. In effect, the electrode is acting like a patient plate. The tissue begins to heat, and as it heats, its electrical resistance changes. In most moist tissue, the resistance actually drops first. This is reasonable, since hot salt water is a better conductor than cold salt water. As the temperature rises the protein is denatured and the tissue begins to blanch or whiten. This process is accompanied by a rise in tissue resistance as the cells are dehydrated. This could be called the "dessication phase." Soon the resistance rises to the point where the electrical contact with the electrode is poor. When this happens, a spark will jump from the electrode to the nearest moist tissue; how long the spark will continue to jump is directly related to its peak voltage.

These authors have described three phases in tissue response to electrocoagulation and state that "cut and coag waveforms of equal power have a very similar effect during the patient plate and dessication phases prior to sparking." Phases of electrocoagulation are as follows:

1. Patient plate phase
2. Dessication phase
3. Sparking phase

These authors [11] found that these three phases were distinct at low voltage; however, as generator voltage was increased, the process of heating took place so rapidly that the patient plate and dessication phases became quite short. The length of delay in passing through the first two phases was also related to electrode size, the delay being quite short when a fine needle electrode of the type used in microelectrosurgery was employed. The delay in passing through these three stages was also related to the load sensitivity of a particular generator, which means that certain generators put out more power at a low resistance than others. Therefore, if power is more effectively transferred to the tissue at a low resistance than high resistance, the sparking will appear to start immediately, but will cease earlier as tissue resistance increases.

The concept proposed by Engle and Harris [11] describes a progression of events beginning with the warming of tissue; dessication; and, finally, sparking, or a fulguration effect, all of which are individually familiar to the reader. In the operating room the surgeon should employ the surgical electrode to perform electrocoagulation so that he stops at the dessication phase and avoids sparking or fulguration whenever possible. The pure cutting current has a different cellular effect; however, a degree of coagulation is possible with this current and the concept of avoiding sparking by using low voltage and moving the electrode quickly is applicable.

Specific information regarding the depth of tissue damage when a fine microelectrode has been used with a low power generator would be of immense value and permit comparison of the results with results achieved using the carbon dioxide laser. It has been stated that the laser produces tissue destruction by vaporization of cells, and that this destruction is limited to a depth of 100 microns. In fact, this is the same process and would explain the action of a cutting current. It is also significant that various power inputs into the laser are possible, and these variations in power produce variations in heat and, therefore, in various levels of tissue destruction.

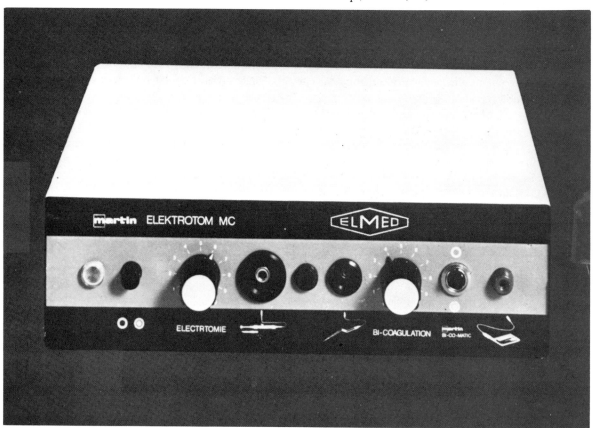

**Figure 5-36.** The Elektrotom MC/MS was specifically designed for surgical specialties employing microsurgical procedures that include bipolar microcoagulation, microsurgical cutting, and delicate contact coagulation. (Courtesy of Elmed Corp., Addison, Ill.)

### Equipment for Microelectrosurgery

*Electrosurgical Generators*

The surgeon must select an electrosurgical generator to provide a pure cutting current suitable for use with a microelectrode. The generator should also provide a suitable current for monopolar coagulation and bipolar coagulation. These three types of current are provided in varying degrees by the generators discussed below.

MARTIN ELEKTROTOM 60GP, MC/MS, 300B

The first solid-state units employed circuits that provided two currents labeled "cold" and "hot" by Martin, and understandable in terms of the principles discussed earlier. Mode I, Elektrotom 60GP was described as radio-frequent (RF) nonmodulated current of low voltage. It was also referred to as a rectified circuit, and finally, as "cold," which was somewhat confusing, but

indicated the lack of sparking. The Elektrotom 60GP delivers a 60-watt output in mode I and has a total power supply of 117 volts. Although this is a small unit not intended for operating room use, this author (G.W.P.) found this pure cutting current exceedingly useful with the Martin microelectrode. In contrast, the model MC/MS has a unipolar generator with a 117-volt power supply and provides a nonmodulated RF current for cutting. This unit also provides an adjustable bipolar circuit. The author has used both the 60GP and MC/MS models in combination with the Martin hand-held microelectrode, which will be described later. An excellent cutting effect with little sparking is noted. Very little coagulation occurs with this cold unit, indicating that tissue heating is lower than with most conventional cutting current (Fig. 5-36). Larger electrosurgical generators, the Elektrotom 170-B and 300-B, are also available from Martin.

**Figure 5-37.** Valley Lab SSE-3. A solid-state unit with variable degrees of blend and a pure cutting current. It has an attachment for bipolar forceps, but bipolar and monopolar circuits cannot be used concurrently.

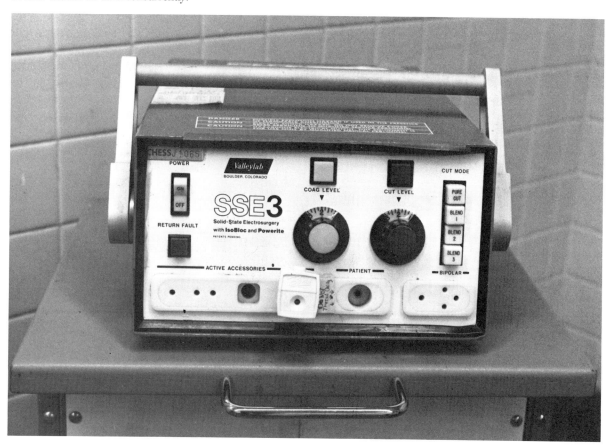

VALLEY LAB GENERATOR

Valley Lab's older solid-state model SSE had a variable control to regulate the amount of coagulation current that was combined with cutting to form a blended current. The new SSE-K, also a solid-state unit, has pure cutting and three additional choices of blended current. This unit also has a bipolar outlet. Maximum voltage of 400 volts is provided. This author (G.W.P.) has used this generator with the Valley Lab microelectrode, which will be described later (Fig. 5-37).

The Malis Bipolar Coagulator is small and extremely convenient to use for bipolar coagulation under the operating microscope if the monopolar generator being used does not have a bipolar attachment. Tissue can be coagulated between the tips of the forceps under irrigation or in a bloody field. A ground plate is not used with this unit. As was noted earlier, the Valley Lab, Birtcher, and Martin Elektrotom MC/MS electrosurgical generators have bipolar attachments in addition to the monopolar cutting and coagulating currents; however, the nurse must manually change from one current to another (Fig. 5-38).

**Figure 5-38.** New Malis bipolar coagulator. This small bipolar unit permits the surgeon to perform bipolar coagulation with foot-pedal control.

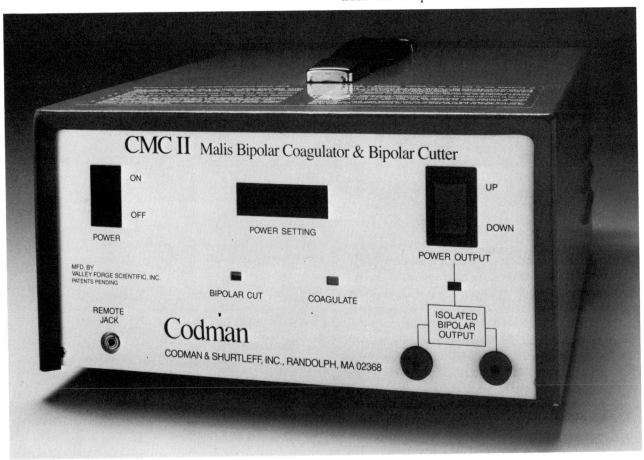

DAVOL SYSTEM 5000

The Davol System 5000 solid-state generator permits the use of both monopolar and bipolar instruments concurrently. At this writing, this capability is not offered by any other generator. All the other units require the nurse to change from monopolar to bipolar. The Davol 5000 unit permits the use of the hand-held electrode for monopolar cutting and coagulation and foot-pedal control of bipolar coagulation. This unit also provides digital readout of power in watts, thus permitting comparison of current from one generator to another. This author (G.W.P.) has found this generator to provide the most up-to-date electrosurgical capability for gynecologic microsurgery (Fig. 5-39).

**Figure 5-39.** Davol System 5000, electrosurgical generator. (Courtesy of Davol Inc., Cranston, R.I.)

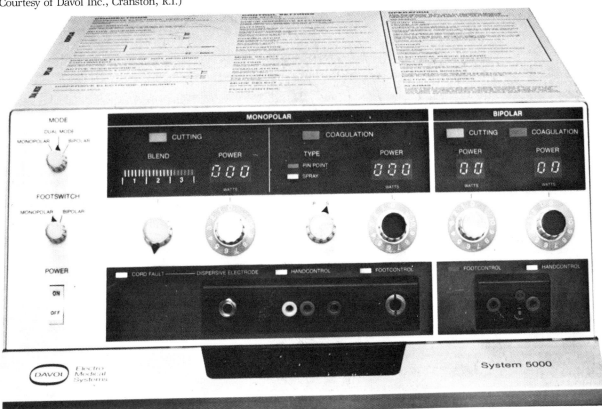

**Table 5-9.** Microsurgical instruments for infertility

| Manufacturer/Distributor* | Designer | Comments |
|---|---|---|
| American V. Mueller | C. R. Garcia | Wide range of instruments, eleven basic microsurgical instruments, teflon rods |
| Codman | E. Diamond | Nonmagnetic titanium forceps, ovary and tube holders |
| Downs Surgical, Inc. | R. M. L. Winston | Many useful microsurgical instruments, excellent needle holder, glass rods |
| Hevesy Medical Instrument | Marik | Basic microsurgical kit |
| Martin, distributed by Elmed, Inc. | V. Gomel | Many useful and innovative microsurgical instruments, excellent tooth and platform forceps, suction irrigation devices |
| S & T Microsurgical Instruments, distributed by ASSI | Multiple designers | Counterbalanced instruments, instruments designed by Acland, Winston, and Gomel; inexpensive, demagnetizer |
| V. Mueller | D. McLaughlen | Coated instruments for use with carbon dioxide laser |

*Each manufacturer offers a basic tubal microsurgical instrument kit.

BIRTCHER CORPORATION, MODEL 737 XL

The Birtcher Model 737 XL, a solid-state unit similar to the Valley Lab unit, the Birtcher generator also provides variable settings to control pure cutting and blended current. This unit has an attachment for the Valley Lab disposable handle, and provides an outlet for a bipolar cord.

RITTER CSV BOVIE

Both the green Bovie and the newer CSV Bovie 2 are classic electrosurgical generators. These units employ spark-gap current for coagulation and vacuum tubes for electrosection (cutting). Maximum voltage is 500 volts; output for cutting is 290 watts and for coagulation 180 watts. Sparking is frequent even at the low settings at which this generator is used. The newer CSV 2 does not include a bipolar attachment. The older CSV Bovie (green) has been discontinued.

RITTER COMPANY, BOVIE 400B

The Bovie 400B is a small solid-state unit highly recommended by Oringer. Maximum voltage is 4000 volts, output with cutting current is 260 watts, and on the coagulation setting is 100 watts. This unit, produced by a separate branch of the Heible-Ritter Corporation in North Carolina, has been employed with a fine-needle electrode during gingivectomy and found to have an excellent pure cutting effect.

## Specialized Instruments and Suture Materials

### Special Instruments for Microsurgery

The need for meticulous care in the surgical procedures for the correction of abnormalities producing infertility in the female requires the use of specialized and delicate instruments. The development of microsurgical procedures for the treatment of tubal and ovarian abnor-

**Table 5-10.** Basic set of microsurgical instruments*

| | |
|---|---|
| 2 | Fine-tipped titanium forceps |
| 1 | Bipolar titanium forceps |
| 1 | Fine-toothed forceps |
| 1 | Platform forceps |
| 1 | Fine-nose, nonlocking needle holder, Winston type |
| 1 | Angled Iris scissors |
| 1 | Sharp straight scissors |
| 1 | Wescott scissor for tissue |
| 1 | Wescott scissor for cutting sutures |
| 1 | Set lacrimal duct probes |
| 1 | Winston probe director to be used as a probe |
| 3 | Glass rods, angled |
| 1 | Fine diamond-blade knife holder with blades |
| 1 | Set of profusion cannulas with straight tips (Stangle) |
| 1 | Bulb irrigation set |
| 1 | Gomel irrigation device |

*Used by this author (G.W.P.) (see p. 167).

malities has necessitated the inclusion of instruments from many sources. Two basic sets of instruments are required during a microsurgical procedure for infertility. The first set contains operating room instruments that are particularly useful during infertility surgery. A second set of microsurgical instruments is also necessary and should be gathered by the surgeon for his personal use only. Six distributors of microsurgical instruments are listed in Table 5-9, and the author's personal set of microsurgical instruments is listed in Table 5-10 and shown in Figures 5-40 and 5-41. Each of these instruments is designed to permit gentle, atraumatic handling of tissue and to prevent abrasions, lacerations, and vascular damage. Needless to say, an excellent operative procedure may be destroyed by subsequent tissue necro-

**Figure 5-40.** Complete instrument case, including metal instrument tray (Downs Surgical).

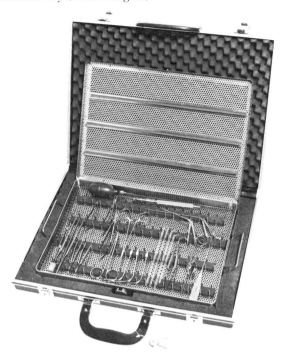

**Figure 5-41.** Metal instrument tray (Downs Surgical).

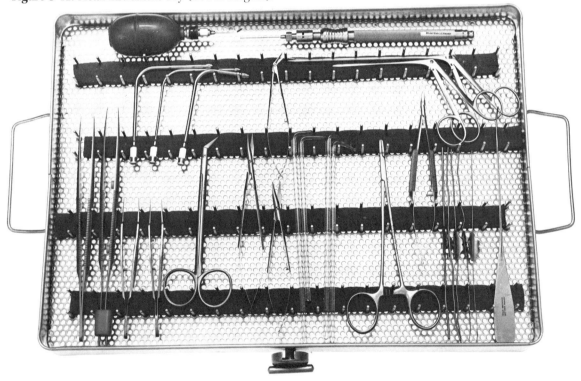

5. Essential Elements of Microsurgical Technique

sis and adhesion formation. In as much as the desired effect of this surgery is the ability to achieve pregnancy, the novice surgeon must be warned that his results will, of course, depend on his experience, but these results will be affected also by his attention to the minutiae of clean dissection, complete hemostasis, and restoration of anatomy, all of which are influenced by the availability of proper surgical instrumentation.

INSTRUMENT CASE

A metal tray that permits storage and sterilization of microsurgical instruments is of great value. All microsurgical instruments can be stored in such a tray and, subsequently, sterilized for each operative procedure without undue effort (Figs. 5-40, 5-41).

RETRACTORS

The Kirschner retractor provides excellent exposure during infertility surgery. This is a flat contour-fitting retractor with shallow blades. The frame of the retractor can be used as a wrist support without exerting undue pressure on the fimbrial vessels and nerves (Fig. 5-42). The O'Connell-O'Sullivan retractor appears similar but should not be used during microsurgical procedures in which wrist pressure is exerted on the lateral blade, because these blades extend deep into the pelvis. Pressure on the lateral aspect of this retractor will cause femoral nerve injury with subsequent quadriceps weakness.

**Figure 5-42.** Kirschner retractor (Downs Surgical).

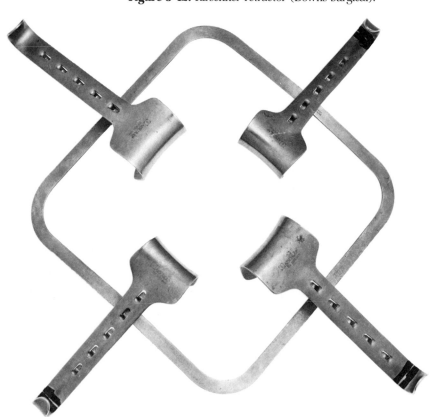

A variety of electrode handles that include fingertip switches are available for microelectrosurgery.

MARTIN ELECTRODE HANDLE AND ELECTRODE (ELMED)

This author (G.W.P.) has used this handle with finger tip switch that is shown in Figure 5-43 (catalog no. 5001). Both the reusable microelectrode and the disposable microelectrode provided by Elmed can be used with this handle. As was noted earlier, the author used the Elektrotom 60GP and MC/MS to provide monopolar nonmodulated current. This handle cord and electrode are gas sterilized with ethylene oxide following each surgical procedure. A surgeon must have additional handles and cords available if more than one surgical procedure is performed during a single 24 hour interval. Recently, Martin introduced a second handle with fingertip control of cutting and coagulation designed by Swolin and distributed by the Elmed Company.

**Figure 5-43.** Electrosurgical handle with finger control and fine needle-tip (Martin-Elmed).

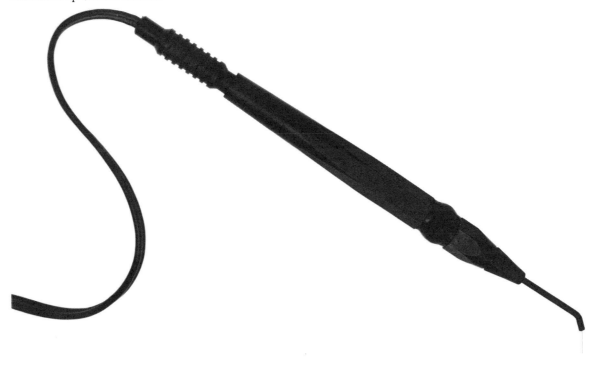

**Figure 5-44.** Disposable yellow electrosurgical handle with removable needle tip (Valley Lab).

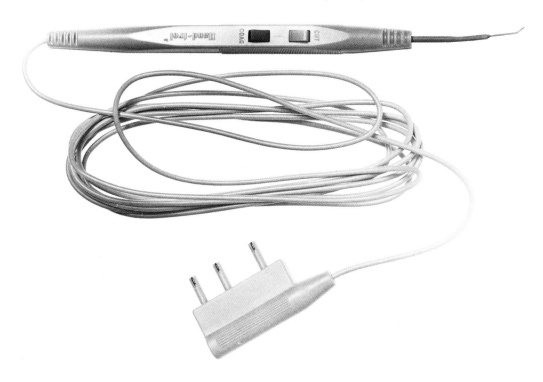

**Figure 5-45.** Buxton clamp. (Courtesy of J. Sklar Mfg. Co., Long Island City, N.Y.)

91-4010

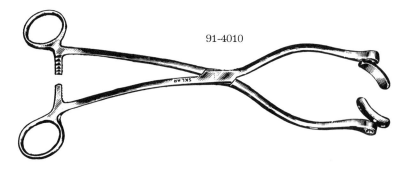

This disposable yellow plastic handle provides fingertip control for cutting and coagulation. The three-pronged cord attaches to the Valley Lab, Birtcher, and other electrosurgical generators. Various tips are available for use with this handle. This handle also incorporates a broad, knife-type tip that is useful for the abdominal incision (Fig. 5-44).

INSTRUMENTS FOR TUBAL LAVAGE (HYDROTUBATION)
The instruments needed for tubal lavage are as follows:

1. Uterine occlusion clamp
   a. Buxton clamp with swivel jaw (Fig. 5-45)
   b. Shirodkar clamp
2. Transcervical cannula (HUI) (Fig. 5-46)

**Figure 5-46. A.** Harris Uterine Injector (HUI); **B.** Harris Uterine Manipulator Injector (HUMI). (Courtesy of Unimar, Canoga Park, Calif.)

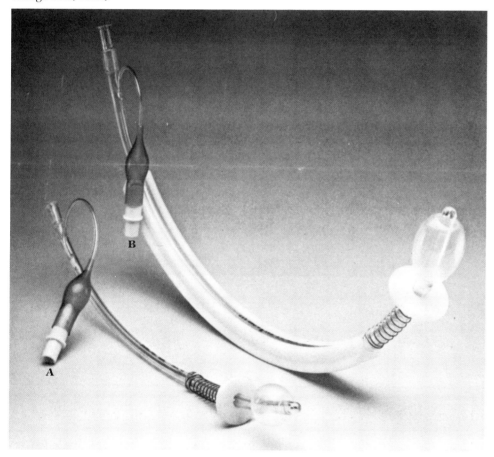

5. Essential Elements of Microsurgical Technique

3. Retrograde (fimbrial) profusion cannulas (Fig. 5-47)

Two techniques of tubal lavage have been demonstrated in Figure 7-14A-D. The Buxton or the Shirodkar clamps are used in transuterine lavage. Transcervical lavage has recently become popular and has been used by this author (G.W.P.) with success. Although pediatric Foley catheters and other instruments have been used during this approach, the HUI transcervical cannula appears to produce the best results, as is shown in Figure 5-46A.

Retrograde profusion of the oviduct shown in Figure 7-14C can be accomplished by placing the angled end of the retrograde cannula (described later) into the fimbriated end of the oviduct. As is shown, four sizes are available (Fig. 5-47).

**Figure 5-47.** Stangle-designed angled perfusion cannulas. (Courtesy of J. Sklar Mfg. Co., Long Island City, N.Y.)

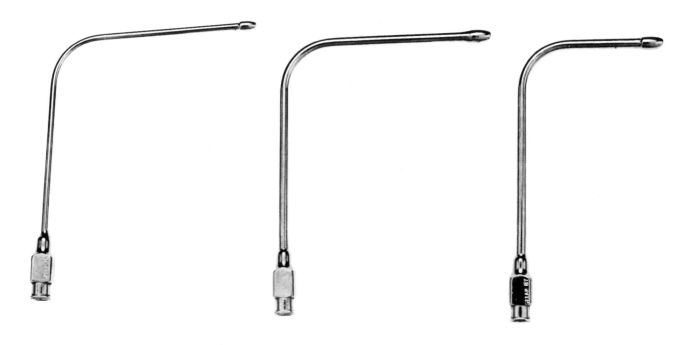

NEEDLE HOLDERS

1. Fine tip for 4-0 sutures (available on macrosurgical tray; Fig. 5-48B)
2. Fine tip for 6-0 sutures (available on macrosurgical tray; Fig. 5-48A)
3. Microsurgical needle holder for 8-0 and 9-0 sutures (Fig. 5-48B)

The fine needles used on sutures, which vary from 4-0 to 9-0 thickness, require special needle holders for each suture. For optimal handling, the needle holder used with 4-0 and 6-0 polyglactin 910 and polyglycolic acid sutures should not be used with larger needles. A very fine-tip microsurgical needle holder without lock is used with 8-0 and 9-0 sutures. A locking mechanism is convenient for the novice and can be used without jerking if the lock release is pressed prior to passing the needle into the tissue. The tip of the popular Castroviejo needle holder is too large for needles smaller than 203 microns but is very useful with 6-0 suture.

---

**Figure 5-48. A.** Winston-type nonlocking microsurgical needle holder. **B.** Fine-nosed needle-holder (Codman).

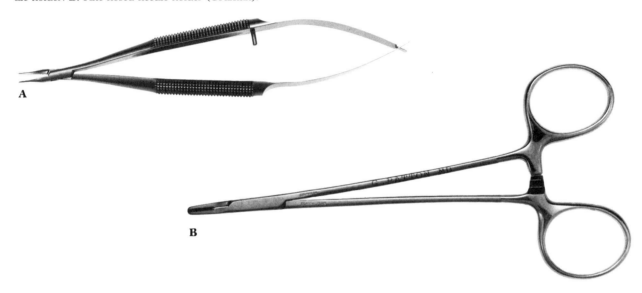

A

B

FORCEPS

1. Debakey, medium and short (available on macro-surgical tray)
2. Cushing's, smooth (available on macrosurgical tray)
3. Microsurgical
   a. Castroviejo with teeth (Fig. 5-49A)
   b. Rhoton; titanium with fine, 0.3 mm smooth tip (Fig. 5-49C)
   c. Platform tip for tying (Fig. 5-49B)
4. Bipolar (Fig. 5-49D)

The microsurgeon will employ various kinds of forceps during surgical procedures of the oviduct, the uterus, and the ovary. Debakey forceps are useful when working deep in the pelvis and when grasping the ovary. Cushing's (brain) forceps, however, are far less traumatic and are useful during the preliminary phase of tissue resection when preparation is being made for use of the operating microscope. Microsurgical forceps with fine tips (Rhoton 7-inch) may be used for handling tissue and for tying. The addition of a bipolar connection to these forceps makes them very useful. Fine-tooth forceps are necessary for cutting the cornual or distal isthmic tube. The muscular wall in this section of oviduct is almost impossible to hold without tooth forceps. The forceps designed by Gomel combines a tying platform with smooth or toothed forceps.

**Figure 5-49.** Forceps: **A.** Fine-toothed (Weck); **B.** Fine-platform forceps (Weck); **C.** Fine-tip titanium (Codman); **D.** Fine-tip bipolar titanium forceps (Codman).

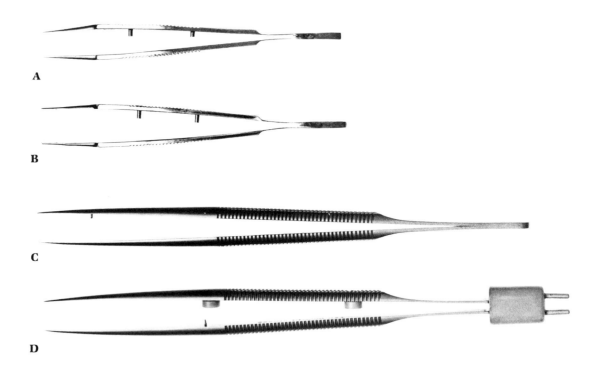

A

B

C

D

1. Church (available on macrosurgical tray; Fig. 5-50A)
   a. straight
   b. curved
2. Angled (Fig. 5-50D)
   a. Potts
   b. angled vascular
   c. angled Iris
3. Wescott (Fig. 5-50B and C)
4. Straight Iris

Fine Iris-type microsurgical scissors of various design are needed for all surgical procedures involving the fallopian tube. The straight Church scissors are used to cut 4-0 and 6-0 sutures, whereas a Wescott scissor is used to cut 8-0 and 9-0 sutures. A Wescott scissor with a curved blade is often used to excise ovarian adhesions. Angled Iris scissors are also employed during fimbrioplasty and salpingostomy in conjunction with a microelectrode. The straight Iris or Vannas scissor is useful when transsecting the fallopian tube prior to anastomosis.

---

**Figure 5-50.** Scissors: **A.** Angled vascular scissors (Codman); **B.** Long, angled Wescott scissors (Storz); **C.** Shorter, blunt-tip Wescott scissors (Storz); **D.** Angled Iris scissors (Storz).

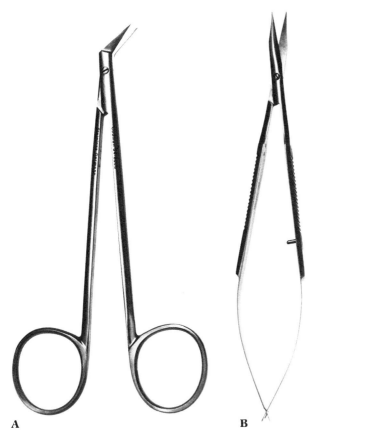
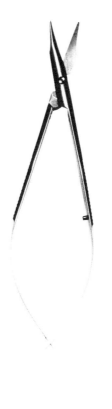
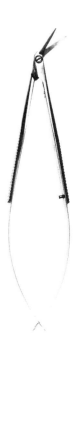

A          B          C          D

Glass rods (Fig. 5-51) do not conduct electricity and, therefore, are used in combination with the microelectrode during resection of adhesions or salpingoneostomy. Rods of various sizes and angles are useful. Although breakage is a theoretical concern during surgery, this has never occurred in our cases. An alternative to the glass rod is the malleable teflon probe shown in Figure 5-52. This was introduced recently and is a good substitute for glass, except when using the carbon dioxide laser. The laser beam has been found to burn completely through the Teflon, creating a noxious odor. Although fine laser beams may etch the glass or splinter a fine glass point, properly designed glass rods are preferred for use with the carbon dioxide laser.

PROBES

1. Lacrimal duct probe (Fig. 5-53)
2. Winston probe director (Fig. 5-54)
3. Malleable cannulated probe
4. Hollow probe with stylet

The lacrimal duct probes of various sizes are useful during tubal anastomosis. The Winston probe director has been used primarily as a probe by this author (G.W.P.). It is a lightweight instrument with a curved tip and is useful during ampullary anastomoses as well as fimbrioplasty and salpingostomy.

The malleable convoluted probe and the hollow probe are instruments designed to assist in passing a 2-0 nylon stent through the isthmic segment during isthmic-uterine or isthmic-isthmic anastomosis. The alligator forceps also can be used for this purpose.

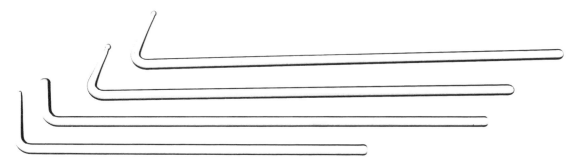

**Figure 5-51.** Variety of glass rods (Downs Surgical).

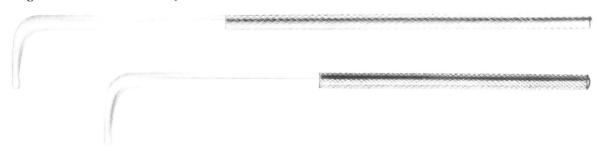

**Figure 5-52.** Malleable Teflon-tip rods (Martin-Elmed).

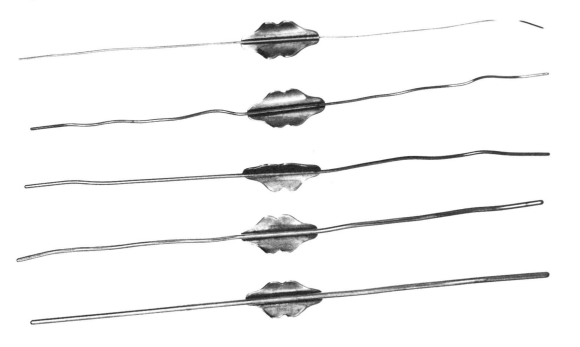

**Figure 5-53.** Variety of lacrimal duct probes (Storz).

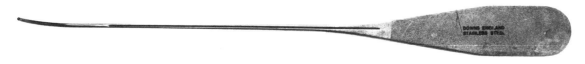

**Figure 5-54.** Winston probe director (Downs Surgical).

1. Gillies and Frazier suction tips
2. Combined irrigation and suction unit
3. Gomel irrigation device (Fig. 5-55A)
4. Bulb irrigation device (Fig. 5-55B)

Suction and irrigation with Ringer's lactate or dilute heparin are essential features of microsurgical technique. Suction is performed with the Gillies or Frazier suction tips. A combination suction and irrigation instrument designed by Diamond has been found useful; it is attached to a dilute heparin solution for use by the assistant. Gomel has designed an irrigation instrument shown in Figure 5-55A. The bulb irrigator shown in Figure 5-55B also is useful.

FINE KNIFE BLADES AND HOLDERS

A microsurgical blade may be employed to cut the cornual segment of the oviduct in preparation for a uterotubal anastomosis. Although scissors may be used occasionally, this muscular wall often requires a sharper, firmer instrument. This author (G.W.P.) has used the micra blade holder during uterotubal anastomosis; however, the Castroviejo razor blade holder and the curved blade designed by Gomel are also useful.

**Figure 5-55. A.** Gomel hand-held irrigation device (Martin-Elmed). **B.** Bulb irrigation device (Storz).

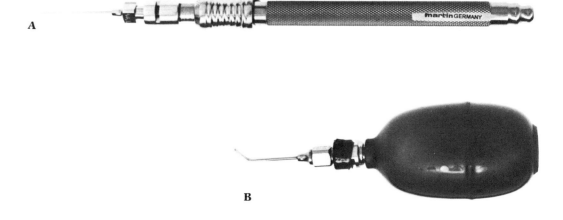

*Alligator Forceps.* This fine-nosed instrument can be passed through the ampullary segment during an anastomosis procedure to identify the occluded end or to assist in passing a stent through this segment (Fig. 5-56).

*Fallopian Tube Forceps.* This forcep will encircle the tube without trauma and is similar in principle to a Babcock forcep.

*Ovary-holding Forceps.* Designed to encircle the ovary, this instrument assists in holding the ovary during excision of adhesions or endometriosis.

*Sutures and Needles Used in Gynecologic Microsurgery*
Synthetic absorbable and permanent suture materials have supplanted the use of chromic catgut sutures in situations where a thread smaller than 2-0 gauge is needed by the gynecologist. The addition of extremely fine suture material in gauges between 6-0 and 10-0 to the armamentarium of the infertility surgeon has been a significant advance since the first edition of the Atlas was published. The choice of a microsurgical suture and needle, however, is an enigma to the beginning microsurgeon. Most well known gynecologic microsurgeons have recommended their personal choices of suture material and needle size, all differing to some degree. This difficult situation has been further confused by the manufacturers' methods of identifying the various needle types that are available with each gauge of suture. The brief discussion here attempts to simplify the surgeon's task of selecting a microsurgical suture and needle.

**Figure 5-56.** Alligator forceps, large and small (Storz).

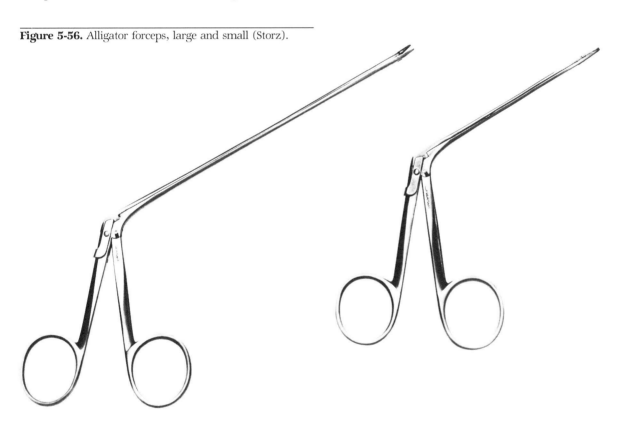

**Table 5-11.** Synthetic absorbable suture

| USP size | Metric size (gauge no.) | Limits on diameter (mm) | | Limit on knot-pull tensile strength (kg) |
|---|---|---|---|---|
| | | Minimum | Maximum | |
| | 0.01 | 0.001 | 0.009 | |
| | 0.1 | 0.010 | 0.019 | |
| 10-0 | 0.2 | 0.020 | 0.029 | |
| 9-0 | 0.3 | 0.030 | 0.039 | |
| 8-0 | 0.4 | 0.040 | 0.049 | |
| 7-0 | 0.5 | 0.050 | 0.069 | 0.14 |
| 6-0 | 0.7 | 0.070 | 0.099 | 0.25 |
| 5-0 | 1 | 0.10 | 0.149 | 0.68 |
| 4-0 | 1.5 | 0.15 | 0.199 | 0.95 |
| 3-0 | 2 | 0.20 | 0.249 | 1.77 |
| 2-0 | 3 | 0.30 | 0.339 | 2.68 |
| 1-0 | 3.5 | 0.35 | 0.399 | 3.90 |
| 1 | 4 | 0.40 | 0.499 | 5.08 |
| 2 | 5 | 0.50 | 0.599 | 6.35 |
| 3 and 4 | 6 | 0.60 | 0.699 | |
| 5 | 7 | 0.70 | 0.799 | |

Source: O. Stroumtsos, *Perspectives on Sutures*. American Cyanamid Co., 1978. Reprinted with permission.

Surgical sutures are classified in three broad categories: absorbable collagen, synthetic absorbable, and nonabsorbable. Collagen sutures are no longer used in surgery of the oviduct. Synthetic absorbable sutures, including polyglycolic acid (Dexon S), polyglactin 910 (Vicryl), and polydioxanone (PDS) are used frequently during infertility surgery, as will be discussed later. The use of nonabsorbable suture is limited to monofilament nylon, although Prolene could also be employed. The diameter of each suture gauge is fixed and must fall within the limits listed in Table 5-11. Metric size designations have been included with USP size.

SYNTHETIC ABSORBABLE SUTURES: POLYGLYCOLIC ACID (DEXON S), POLYGLACTIN 910 (VICRYL), AND POLYDIOXANONE (PDS)
Polyglycolic acid suture (Dexon) was rapidly incorporated into infertility surgery following its production in 1971. Each strand of this suture material consists of braided filaments composed of a homopolymer of glycolic acid. Animal studies have indicated minimal absorption of this material 7 to 15 days postoperatively, significant absorption at 30 days, and maximum absorption after 60 to 90 days. It has been found that polyglycolic acid suture material (Dexon) is absorbed essentially by hydrolysis and not by proteolysis, i.e., digestion of the suture by invading macrophages, as are collagen sutures [29]. In 1975, Davis and Geck introduced Dexon S, a braided suture of smaller strands of polyglycolic acid in a tighter braid than was the earlier Dexon. This change resulted in a stronger suture material that also passed through tissue more easily. A recent modification by Davis and Geck was the introduction of coated Dexon S, termed Dexon Plus. Designed to compete with coated Vicryl, this Dexon suture is coated with polymer of Poloxane 188 that disappears within days. This change was also designed to permit smooth travel through tissues being sutured. Dexon S and Dexon Plus are available in undyed beige and dyed green color. Braided Dexon S and Dexon Plus are available in sizes 8-0 and larger. A monofilament Dexon has recently been introduced in 9-0 and 10-0 gauges.

Ethicon introduced polyglactin 910 (Vicryl) in 1973 to compete with Dexon. This synthetic absorbable suture material is made from a copolymer consisting of 90 percent glycolide and 10 percent lactide, which are derived, respectively, from glycolic and lactic acids. These sutures are also braided and available in natural or violet colors. Resorption of this copolymer in muscular tissue of rats and in rabbit uterine horns has been found to be similar to that observed with polyglycolic acid suture (Dexon). Recently Ethicon introduced coated Vicryl, which was apparently designed to compete with Dexon S. Sutures of 8-0 gauge and larger are now available coated with the copolymer polyglactin 370, composed of 30 percent glycolide and 70 percent lactide, plus calcium steriolate, a lubricant. Polyglactin 910 is available in gauges 8-0, 9-0, 10-0, and larger gauges. At this time Ethicon anticipates that all 9-0 and 10-0 polyglactin 910 sutures will be monofilaments.

Tissue reactions to polyglycolic acid and polyglactin 910 sutures have been reported and compared with reaction to chromic catgut and nylon sutures [14, 30]. Early studies indicated that nylon suture stimulated a milder inflammatory insult than did chromic catgut suture. Two recent studies have suggested that polyglactin 910 may be less reactive than nylon [14, 32]. Gomel compared the histologic reaction of 10-0 polyglactin 910 (Vicryl) and nylon suture in rabbit uterine horn [14]. Both sutures were swaged to a 70 micron taper-needle, making the polyglactin 910 a special order. Tissue reaction was studied at 24 and 80 days. Polyglactin 910 was found in only 2 of 10 specimens studied at 80 days. In both animals a very mild histologic response and absence of giant cell response was noted to be associated with the use of polyglactin 910. The histologic response to nylon at 80 days was significantly greater.

A comparison of the inflammatory response to 3-0 polyglycolic acid (Dexon) and polyglactin 910 (Vicryl) suture in skin and uterine wall of rabbits revealed little difference between the two sutures [30]. A slightly greater inflammatory response to polyglycolic acid at 90 days did not appear to be significant in view of the small number of rabbits in each of the groups at this time interval. In addition, suture material of this large gauge is not presently used in microsurgery.

Recently Ethicon introduced a new type of synthetic absorbable suture material with texture and tying properties similar to Prolene: Polydioxanone (PDS) suture is a monofilament synthetic absorbable suture that appears to retain its tensile strength about twice as long as previous synthetic absorbable suture materials. This suture material is very smooth and appears to stretch slightly when being tied. It requires multiple knots for security. It slides through the ovarian cortex and tubal serosa with virtually no drag and appears to be a significant advance in the area of infertility surgery.

SPECIFIC SUTURES

The sutures used in gynecologic microsurgery include 4-0, 6-0, 8-0, 9-0, and rarely, 10-0 gauge material. This author (G.W.P.) prefers a synthetic absorbable suture for 4-0, 6-0, and 8-0 gauges. Black monofilament nylon is the preferred 9-0 and 10-0 suture material, although this may change if the needle selection available with 9-0 and 10-0 synthetic absorbable suture is expanded to include taper needles of small wire diameters. The introduction of 9-0 and 10-0 monofilament synthetic absorbable suture appears to be a significant advance in this area.

Surgical needles have several characteristics, including the basic shape, size, type of point, and type of suture attachment (Fig. 5-57). The popular shapes for microsurgical use include three-eighths circle and one-half circle. Needle size includes the length and the diameter of the needle, known as wire diameter. Needle points are either taper or cutting. The former, taper needles, are useful in easily penetrated tissue, such as tubal serosa or ampullary mucosa. Cutting-edge needles are used in tough tissue, such as isthmic and cornual muscle. Most microsurgical sutures used by the ophthalmologist employ cutting needles and are not suitable for gynecologic microsurgery. Various types of needle points are shown in Figure 5-58. All microsurgical needles are swaged to the suture material.

The taper-point needle is the least traumatic and most frequently used in microsurgery; however, a cutting needle, such as the spatula or lancet point is occasionally useful. This was particularly true when 8-0 synthetic absorbable suture material was available swaged only on these cutting needles. Until 1981, permanent nylon suture material of fine 8-0, 9-0, and 10-0 gauge was the only stock suture available on a taper needle of smaller diameter. This changed when Ethicon offered 8-0 Vicryl swaged on a 130-micron taper needle as a special order, and in 1981, when Davis and Geck introduced 8-0 Dexon X swaged on a 140-micron taper needle as a stock order. In early 1982, Ethicon converted the two popular 8-0 sutures to stock items.

4-0 SYNTHETIC ABSORBABLE SUTURE: DEXON PLUS, COATED VICRYL, AND POLYDIOXANONE

A beige suture of 4-0 Dexon Plus is used with a T-31 needle. This taper needle is 17 mm long with one-half circle shape. In contrast, 4-0 coated Vicryl is used with an RB-1 taper needle of similar shape. Recently, 4-0 PDS has been found extremely useful on an RB-1 taper needle.

6-0 SYNTHETIC ABSORBABLE SUTURE: DEXON PLUS, COATED VICRYL, AND POLYDIOXANONE

A green Dexon S suture is swaged on a T-30 needle. This is a 13 mm taper needle with a one-half circle shape. The 6-0 coated Vicryl is a violet suture swaged on a TF needle. The recently introduced 6-0 polydioxanone suture on a taper TF needle has replaced Dexon and Vicryl in most instances.

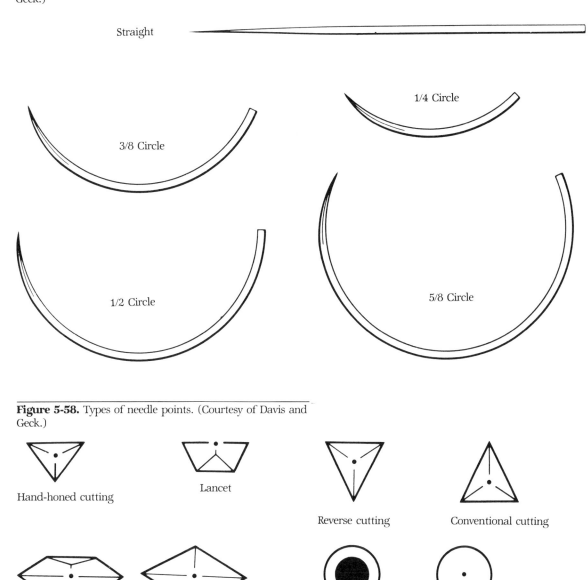

**Figure 5-57.** Various needle designs. (Courtesy of Davis and Geck.)

Straight

1/4 Circle

3/8 Circle

1/2 Circle

5/8 Circle

**Figure 5-58.** Types of needle points. (Courtesy of Davis and Geck.)

Hand-honed cutting

Lancet

Reverse cutting

Conventional cutting

Spatula

Diamond Point

Blunt

Taper

The 8-0 polyglycolic acid suture is a 45 mm braided thread of green color. It is available swaged to needles of several lengths and points.

| TIP | WIRE DIAMETER (MICRONS) | CIRCLE (DEGREES) | NEEDLE NO. |
|---|---|---|---|
| Lancet (cutting) | 203 | 137 | LE-2 |
| Lancet (cutting) | 203 | 175 | LE-2 |
| Reverse cutting | 229 | 115 | CE-30 |
| Taper | 145 | 3/8 | TE-145 Green (7117-18) |

This author (G.W.P.) often uses 8-0 polyglycolic acid sutures (Dexon-S) swaged to a taper TE-145 needle during microsurgical procedures. Rarely, 8-0 suture swaged to an LE-2 (203 micron) lancet needle is employed when a cutting needle is thought necessary.

## 9-0 MONOFILAMENT POLYGLYCOLIC ACID SUTURE: DEXON

A monofilament 9-0 Dexon suture dyed green is available swaged to a LA-2 needle. This is a 160-degree lancet needle with wire diameter of 203 microns. It is essentially the same as an LE-2 needle, with the exception of the curve. This author (G.W.P.) has not employed this suture, because the needles available are not suitable for gynecologic microsurgery. The average size of the 9-0 suture material is 35 microns, and, unfortunately, the smallest stock is 203 microns. A second disadvantage is the absence of a taper needle. At present, both requirements are best met with 9-0 nylon suture material.

## 8-0 POLYGLACTIN 910: VICRYL

This Ethicon product is a violet thread 45 microns in diameter. It is commercially available swaged on needles of several sizes, all of which have spatula side-cutting points. A smaller taper needle has just become available as a stock item. Needles now available are the following:

| TIP | WIRE DIAMETER (MICRONS) | CIRCLE | NEEDLE NO. |
|---|---|---|---|
| Spatula | 203 | 3/8 | GS-9 |
| Spatula | 203 | 1/2 | GS-14 |
| Taper | 130 | 3/8 | BV-130-5 (J-401-G) |
| | | | BV-130-4 (J-405-G) |

Among the stock cutting needles available, this author (G.W.P.) prefers the GS-9 with 3/8 circle and spatula point. A spatula needle is a somewhat flattened side-cutting needle designed for ophthalmology. This needle and the lancet needle noted above produce too much tissue damage for routine use in infertility surgery. A smaller, 130 micron, taper needle is now available swaged on 8-0 polyglactin 910. Traditionally, 8-0 was the largest gauge available in synthetic absorbable suture; however, in 1978 Ethicon introduced 9-0 and 10-0 braided polyglactin 910 swaged on a GS-9 or GS-14 needle. The small gauge of these sutures, 35 and 25 microns, respectively, was in marked contrast to the 203-micron wire diameter of these needles. Recently, 9-0 and 10-0 monofilament polyglactin 910 has replaced the braided sutures, although the GS-9 and GS-14, 203-micron needles are the only stock needles available.

As was stated earlier, the author frequently uses an 8-0 synthetic absorbable suture during tubal anastomosis as well as fimbrioplasty and salpingoneostomy procedures. The 8-0 polyglactin 910 (Vicryl) on a BV-130-5 taper needle provides a 5-inch suture with a single needle that is excellent for tubal surgery. In contrast, 8-0 Vicryl on a BV-130-4 taper needle is an 18-inch double-ended suture that is excellent for tubal anastomosis, permitting a double layer anastomosis of both tubes, often with a single suture.

## 9-0 MONOFILAMENT POLYGLACTIN 910

Polyglactin 910 was first manufactured as a monofilament; however, the stiffness associated with monofilament suture made it unpopular. Braided suture, therefore, replaced the monofilament form and became the popular stock Ethicon product. Recently the company has reintroduced monofilament polyglactin 910 in finer gauges.

| SUTURE | DIAMETER (MICRONS) | KNOT STRENGTH (GRAMS) |
|---|---|---|
| 9-0 monofilament (polyglactin 910) | 38 | 76 |
| 9-0 braided | 38 | 95 |
| 9-0 ethilon | 33 | 50 |

A comparison of 9-0 monofilament and 9-0 braided polyglactin 910 during cataract surgery revealed the following observations [2]. All 9-0 monofilament sutures disappeared in 35 to 37 days, compared to 29 to 31 days for braided suture. Tissue reaction was minimal with both 9-0 sutures; however, the monofilament suture was slightly less reactive. Less tissue drag was noted when tying with the monofilament suture.

The 9-0 monofilament polyglactin 910 is available on the following stock needles.

| TIP | WIRE DIAMETER (MICRONS) | NEEDLE NO. |
|-----|------------------------|------------|
| Spatula | 203 | GS-9 |
| Spatula | 200 | GS-14 |

This author (G.W.P.) recommends that a smaller taper point needle of wire diameter 75 to 130 microns be used with this suture. It is anticipated that needles of this type will soon be available as stock products from Ethicon. Product number V-402G will refer to a BV-130-3 needle with a special taper-cut needle point.

### 9-0 MONOFILAMENT NYLON

Black monofilament nylon has been widely used during tubal anastomosis in animals and in humans (Winston, Diamond) [38, 9]. Available in 8-0, 9-0, and 10-0 gauges on various needles, some as small as 50 microns, this suture provides more choice in stock needle size and type than do the synthetic absorbable sutures at this time. The disadvantage of large needle size and the prior absence of a taper needle point on the synthetic absorbable suture was noted earlier. The 35-micron monofilament nylon (9-0) is often used by this author (G.W.P.) during the suturing of the first layer in a utero-tubal anastomosis procedure. This suture material is available from Davis and Geck, Ethicon, and other manufacturers.

The following needles are available on 9-0 Dermalon from Davis and Geck.

| TIP | WIRE DIAMETER (MICRONS) | NEEDLE NO. |
|-----|------------------------|------------|
| Lancet | 203 | L-2 |
| Lancet | 203 | LE-2 |
| Lancet | 150 | LO-1 |
| Lancet | 150 | LE-1 |
| Lancet | 150 | L-1 |
| Taper | 145 | TE-145 |
| Taper | 145 | TE-143 |
| Taper | 100 | TE-100 |

The following needles are available swaged on 9-0 Ethilon, an Ethicon product.

| TIP | WIRE DIAMETER (MICRONS) | CIRCLE | NEEDLE NO. |
|-----|------------------------|--------|------------|
| Spatula | 203 | | GS-9, 10, 14 |
| Spatula | 145 | | GS-15, 16 |
| Spatula | 150 | | GS-17, 18, 19 |
| Taper | 130 | | BV-130-5, 4, 3 (old #BV-2, 3, 4) |
| Taper | 100 | 3/8 | BV-100-4 (old #BV-5) |

This author (G.W.P.) uses the TE-100 needle (100-micron taper) with 9-0 Dermalon and BV-130-4 needle when using 9-0 Ethilon. This 35-micron nylon suture is also available on a lancet or spatula-cutting needle, either of which is very useful when attempting to pass the needle through the muscular cornual layer. A GS-15 (150-micron spatula) needle by Ethicon or an LE-1 (150-micron lancet) needle by Davis and Geck are useful cutting needles.

### 10-0 MONOFILAMENT NYLON

This 25-micron suture is rarely required in microsurgery of the human oviduct, although it is occasionally useful during an isthmic-isthmic tubal anastomosis. Both 10-0 and 11-0 nylon sutures have been found useful during microsurgical tubal anastomosis in rabbits [10]. Taper needles available on this suture are:

| TIP | WIRE DIAMETER (MICRONS) | NEEDLE NO. |
|-----|------------------------|------------|
| Taper (Davis and Geck) | 143 | TE-143 |
| | 100 | T-100 |
| | 100 | TE-100 |
| | 70 | TE-70 |
| Taper (Ethicon) | 75 | BV75-4, 3 |
| | 50 | BV50-3 |

In summary, the sutures usually employed in gynecologic microsurgery involve synthetic absorbable material in 4-0, 6-0, and 8-0 gauge. The choice between Dexon and Vicryl has now been complicated by the addition of the new monofilament Polydioxanone (PDS) suture. The choice between synthetic absorbable material and nylon has not been resolved, although at present this author (G.W.P.) prefers the former material in most instances of tubal anastomosis or fimbrial repair. A taper needle is an essential feature of a gynecologic microsurgical suture. The smallest diameter needle suitable for the operative procedure should also be employed. The recent introduction by Davis and Geck and by Ethicon of a small diameter needle on 8-0 synthetic absorbable suture is a significant advance in the field of gynecologic microsurgery. When a smaller gauge suture is required, 9-0 nylon on a small diameter needle (100 microns) is employed.

## References

1. Baracaquer, J., Ruttlan, J., and Troutman, R. C. *Surgery of the Anterior Segment of the Eye, Vol. 1.* New York: McGraw-Hill, 1964.

2. Blaydes, J. E., and Berry, J. A comparative evaluation of 9-0 monofilament and 9-0 braid polyglactin 910 in cataract surgery (intracapsular, extracapsular, and phacolmulsification). *Ophthalmic Surg.* 10:49, 1979.

3. Clark, W. L., Cancer of the oral cavity, jaw & throat. *J.A.M.A.* 71:1365, 1918.

4. Cushing, H. Electrosurgery as an aid to the removal of intracranial tumors. *Surg. Gynecol. Obstet.* 47:751, 1928.

5. Daniel, R. K., and Terzis, J. K. *Reconstructive Microsurgery* (1st ed.). Boston: Little, Brown, 1977.

6. D'Arsonval, A. Action physiologique des courants alternatifs a grand frequence. *Arch. Physiol. Norm. Path.* 5:401, 789, 1893.

7. David, A., Brackett, B. G., and Garcia, C. R. Effects of microsurgical removal of the rabbit interotubal junction. *Fertil. Steril.* 20:250, 1969.

8. Diamond, E. Microsurgery in Infertility: Instrumentation and Technique. In J. M. Phillips (ed.), Microsurgery in Gynecology. Downey, Calif.: American Association of Gynecologic Laparoscopists, 1977.

9. Diamond, E. Microsurgical reconstruction of the uterine tube in sterilized patients. *Fertil. Steril.* 28:1203, 1977.

10. Eddy, C. A., Antonini, R., and Pauerstein, C. J. Fertility following microsurgical removal of the ampullary-isthmic junction in rabbits. *Fertil. Steril.* 28:1090, 1977.

11. Engle, T., and Harris, F. W. The electrical dynamics of laparoscopic sterilization. *J. Reprod. Med.* 15:33, 1975.

12. Garcia, C. R. Reconstruction of previously ligated fallopian tubes. Presented at the 11th Annual Meeting of the American Fertility Society, New York, April 1972.

13. Geddes, L. A., Silva, L. F., DeWitt, D. P., and Pearce, J. A. What's new in electrosurgical instrumentation. *Med. Instrum.* 11:355, 1977.

13a. Gomel, V. Tubal reanastomosis by microsurgery. *Fertil. Steril.* 28:59, 1977.

14. Gomel, V., McComb, P., and Boer-Meisel, M. Histologic reactions to polyglactin 910, polyethylene, and nylon microsuture. *J. Reprod. Med.* 25:56, 1980.

15. Hoerenz, Peter. The design of the surgical microscope, Part I. *Ophthalmic Surg.* 46:40, 1973.

16. Hoerenz, Peter. The design of the surgical microscope, Part II. *Ophthalmic Surg.* 4(Suppl. 2):89, 1973.

17. Hoerenz, Peter. The operating microscope. I: Optical principles, illumination systems, and support systems. *J of Microsurg.* 1:364, 1980.

18. Hoerenz, Peter. The operating microscope. II: Individual parts, handling, assembling, focusing, and balancing. *J. Microsurg.* 1:419, 1980.

19. Hoerenz, Peter. The operating microscope. III: Accessories. *J. Microsurg.* 2:22, 1980.

20. House, W. F. Surgical exposure of the interstitial auditory canal and its contents through the middle cranial fossa. *Laryngoscope* 71:1363, 1961.

21. Jones, H. W., and Rock, J. A. On the anastomosis of fallopian tubes after surgical sterilization. *Fertil. Steril.* 29:702, 1978.

22. Kelly, A. Endothermy, the new surgery. *Med. J. Rec.* 1925.

23. Malone, W. F., and Manning, J. L. Electrosurgery in restorative dentistry. *J. Prosthet. Dent.* 20:417, 1968.

24. McLean, A. J. The Bovie electrosurgical current generator. *Arch Surg.*

25. Nylen, C. O. The microscope in aural surgery; Its first use and later development. *Acta Otolaryngol.* (Stockholm) 116[Suppl.]:226, 1954.

26. O'Brien, B. M., and Hayhurst, J. W. Principles and Techniques of Microvascular Surgery. In J. M. Converse (ed.), *Reconstructive Plastic Surgery (2nd ed.).* Philadelphia: Saunders, 1977.

27. Oringer, M. J. *Electrosurgery in Dentistry* (2nd ed.). Philadelphia: Saunders, 1968.

28. Oringer, M. J. Electrosurgery for definitive conservative modern periodontal therapy. *Dent. Clin. North Am.* 13:53, 1969.

29. Rahman, M. S., and Way, S. Polyglycolic acid surgery sutures in gynaecological surgery. *J. Obstet. Gynecol. Br. Comm.* 79:849, 1972.

30. Riddick, D. H., DeGrazia, C. T., and Maenza, R. M. Comparison of polyglactic and polyglycolic acid sutures in reproductive tissue. *Fertil. Steril.* 28:1220, 1977.

31. Semm, K. Endocoagulation: A new field of endoscopic surgery. *J. Reprod. Med.* 16:195, 1976.

32. Smith, D. C. Paper presented at microsurgery seminar, Third International Congress of Gynecologic Endoscopy, San Francisco, Dec. 1977. In V. Gomel (ed.), Recent advances in surgical correction of tubal disease producing infertility. *Curr. Probl. Obstet. Gynecol.* 1 (10), 1978.

33. Swolin, K. Fifty fertility operations: I. Literature and methods. *Acta Obstet. Gynecol. Scand.* 46:234, 1967.

34. Swolin, K. Electromicrosurgery and salpingostomy: Long term results. *Am. J. Obstet. Gynecol.* 121:418, 1975.

35. Tamai, S. Digit replantation: An analysis of 163 replantations in an eleven-year period. *Clin. Plast. Surg.* 5:209, 1978.

36. Troutman, R. C. *Microsurgery of the Anterior Segment of the Eye,* vol. 1. St. Louis: Mosby, 1974.

37. Wyeth, G. A. *Surgery of Neoplastic Diseases by Electrothermic Methods.* New York: Paul B. Hoeber, 1926.

38. Winston, R. M. L. Microsurgical reanastomosis of the rabbit oviduct and its functional and pathological sequelae. *Br. J. Obstet. Gynecol.* 82:513, 1975.

39. Winston, R. M. L. Tuboplasty. In D. W. T. Roberts (ed.), *Operative Surgery.* Woburn, Mass.: Butterworth, 1977.

# 6

# Infertility Surgery and the Laser

Joseph H. Bellina

Modern gynecologists use a number of surgical tools, the most recent of which is the carbon dioxide laser. The scalpel and scissors were among the earliest cutting instruments used in medical treatment. Modern surgical cutting instruments, including those that employ high frequency monopolar and bipolar electrosurgical current as well as cryosurgical instruments, sometimes lack the precision of application achieved in earlier times when the scalpel was employed. The need for precise tissue removal during gynecological surgery became apparent during the 1970s as infertility surgeons used magnification to repair damaged oviducts. Microelectrosurgery initially appeared to fill this need, and the microelectrode used with a low voltage pure cutting current remains a useful technique (see Chap. 5). The recent introduction of the carbon dioxide laser (molecular gas laser system) appears to permit the microsurgeon to incise tissue with even greater accuracy and to expect minimal bleeding or other postoperative sequelae.

It has not been surprising to find healthy skepticism on the part of many gynecologists concerning laser therapy. This feeling is nurtured by a lack of familiarity with the concept of laser technology and an inadequate understanding of the role the carbon dioxide laser can play during a microsurgical procedure. The discussion presented in this chapter tries to satisfy both these questions by first acquainting the gynecologist with concepts that assist in understanding how the laser actually works and then applying this technology to the practice of infertility microsurgery.

Patel, in 1961 [19], working at Bell Laboratories, investigated molecular gas lasers for communication purposes and used monoatomic, diatomic, and other molecular media for a laser effect. His discovery of the carbon dioxide laser led to further investigations by a team of scientists at the American Optical Company. After many modifications, Polanyi and associates [21], working with Jako, developed a micromanipulator that coupled the carbon dioxide laser to the operating microscope and permitted the surgeon to visually control, with great accuracy, the cutting of tissues.

The laser destroys tissue by evaporating the water content of each cell. Hall and colleagues [11], using ultra high-speed color cine photography, demonstrated that tissue was incised by the boiling of intracellular and extracellular water, forming steam that expanded and caused cellular explosion. This instantaneous process appeared to disrupt the tissue architecture and carry cellular debris out of the wound. Some of the debris was charred as it passed through the beam, whereas other tissue was ignited and burned, producing a white glow. The actual area of laser impact did not demonstrate signs of tissue combustion in this study, thus leading one to the conclusion that the carbon dioxide laser destroyed tissue by vaporization of cellular water [9].

Investigation of the use of the carbon dioxide laser as a new surgical mode has been underway since 1967. This instrument has demonstrated unique capabilities for specific surgical procedures and with excellent results. Following completion of the experimental research phase in 1972 [8, 11, 19, 21, 24] the carbon dioxide laser beam was introduced into clinical practice and is now routinely used throughout the world for a number of surgical procedures. The carbon dioxide laser can cauterize, vaporize, or excise diseased tissue. The development of surgical applications has been extremely rapid, considering the short period of time the instrument has been available. There are presently more than 20,000 clinically documented cases in which the laser was the primary mode of treatment.

A number of disciplines and the variety of procedures now embracing the laser are many. In otolaryngology, excellent results have been obtained in the treatment of laryngeal papillomas and tumor tissue resections of the pharynx, oral cavity, nose, and sinuses [13, 15, 25, 26, 28], including microsurgical procedures [12]. In thoracic surgery, the carbon dioxide laser has been used to perform thoracotomies and has provided an atraumatic and efficient mode of treating benign tumors of the trachea and bronchi. Benign and malignant dermatologic tumors [10], hyperplastic scars, keloids, burns [7, 14], and tattoos have been successfully treated with the carbon dioxide laser [23, 24]. Additionally, several authors have reported advantages of using the carbon dioxide laser in other microsurgical procedures [5, 9, 27]. Since 1974, several authors have described the surgical application of the carbon dioxide laser in intraabdominal disease and in the treatment of lower genital tract pathology [1, 2]. In gynecologic surgery, the laser has been attached to a hand unit, or directly to an operating microscope, for microsurgical procedures on the oviduct, or to a colposcope for use during the excision of cervical pathology. It has recently been attached to the laparoscope for use during operative laparoscopy.

## Types of Lasers

At least three lasers are used in medical and surgical treatment today; argon, neodymium yttrium aluminum garnet (Nd.YaG), and carbon dioxide. Each laser system uses a different material that may be solid (neodymium YaG) or a gas (carbon dioxide, argon) to produce a unique type of laser beam. The wavelength and other characteristics of this beam determine the tissue effect and, thus, the surgical application.

The argon laser is a gas laser that produces a beam of visible yellow-green light, wavelength 488–515 $\mu$m. This laser beam seeks red in the form of red pigment or blood and is not well absorbed in water. Therefore, it can be fired into the eye without damaging the cornea or lens and will affect tissue only in the retinal layer. Because of its visible wavelength, fiber optic systems are available for its use by the gastroenterologist, permitting control of bleeding through this telescope.

The neodymium YaG laser uses a solid material to produce an invisible beam of wavelength 1.06 $\mu$m. It is not well absorbed by water and is also attracted to red pigment. It has been used in neurosurgery and gastroenterology.

The carbon dioxide laser is used in infertility surgery, in combination with the operating microscope and with the laparoscope. It uses carbon dioxide gas to produce a laser beam in the infrared spectrum of wavelength 10.6 $\mu$m. Its most significant property is the high degree of absorption of its laser energy by water, which is the major component of soft tissues. This property permits sharp excision of tissue with little damage to surrounding cells.

## Theoretical Background

The laser is an instrument that produces a beam of light with specific characteristics and focuses this beam on a small area. The result of this concentration of laser light is to produce a cutting or coagulating effect on the involved tissue. The discussion that follows attempts to assist the surgeon in understanding how this light beam is produced and what it does to the tissue.

Light is really energy and a beam of light is a collection of photons that carry this energy. The laser generator produces a specific type of light that results in a specific tissue effect. The carbon dioxide laser uses an electric current to initiate a molecular reaction involving molecules of carbon dioxide gas. These molecules of carbon dioxide become highly charged and give off photons containing energy. A large collection of photons comprises the laser beam. The beam thus contains a high degree of energy and is extremely uniform, permitting it to be focused in an exceptionally small area. The energy and small spot size make the effect of the laser beam on soft tissue very useful for the gynecologic surgeon.

The acronym LASER refers to Light Amplification by Stimulating Emission of Radiation, which describes the system used in the development of laser energy. These terms are foreign to the gynecologist, but in brief refer to the development of a laser light beam. The laser unit produces a molecular change in the molecules of carbon dioxide gas that causes these molecules to give off (emit) a highly charged particle called a photon. Radiation in this case refers to the collection of photons that form a light beam of specific wavelength. All electromagnetic waves including radio, television, visible light, and x-rays are referred to as radiation. Only x-rays emit ionizing radiation and are known to be potentially dangerous.

The theoretical basis of laser action, or stimulated emission of radiation, was first proposed by Einstein in 1917 [6]. Early in his career this scientist noted that light and color were the result of wave properties and interaction with photons. The photon is the "other" property given to light when the wave theory fails. Interestingly, scientists still discuss whether light is a wave or a particle. It can be assumed that both are correct under given circumstances. This basic assumption is important when considering the physics of the carbon dioxide laser.

The concept of light can be further understood by discussing the following physical principles. First, consider a single atom in which the electron cloud and nucleus of the atom are in harmony at the resting state. Physicists have named this resting state of the electron cloud *ground zero*, and assigned it a quantum number to indicate that the system, nucleus and electron, is resting or at its lowest energy level.

Second, consider what occurs when the electron orbit becomes disturbed and shifts "away from the nucleus." To achieve this new suborbit, energy (often in the form of heat) must be supplied to overcome the nuclear pull on the electron by stimulating the atom's electrical cloud. This phenomenon is easily demonstrated by heating an iron skillet. The resting "cold" skillet appears black and somewhat cool, because it contains molecules at rest. As the skillet is heated, it becomes red in color, demonstrating that the electrons have gained energy from the fire so that they are no longer resting and black, but now move at "red-hot speed." Further heating or stimulation results in "white-hot" electrons, demonstrating that the electron energy has shifted to yield all visible wave lengths (i.e., white spectrum). This phenomenon can be used to demonstrate the electron orbit shift during heating and cooling. As the skillet cools, the stimulated orbits return to a resting state, and the black color returns. This example of energy shifts can be viewed directly. The colors described were produced by the photons or a symphony of wavelengths released in the process of heating.

It is possible to take this example a step further. Each color observed while heating the skillet (i.e., the stimulating process) represented the visual detection of the photon emissions whose wavelength ranged from red to white. The mixture of all visible colors occurs between wavelengths of 400 to 700 $\mu$m in length. This means that color is related to wavelength and also changes in energy state. Some colors are detectable, whereas others are invisible. We see, or rather our retina can detect, colors from 390 to 780 $\mu$m in wavelength (as emitted by the argon laser). However, other wavelengths in the electromagnetic spectrum, such as infrared (those emitted by the carbon dioxide laser) and ultraviolet, are not visible. Each wavelength has a particular property and each photon has a predictable color, or effect. For example, x-rays have one effect while radio waves have another; the effect is a function of the wavelength and the energy stored in the photon. It is the wavelength of a particular laser beam that determines its tissue effect. These principles are demonstrated in Figure 6-1.

To clarify this principle, consider the x-ray photon, which has an extremely short wavelength ($1 \times 10^{-4}$ $\mu$m) and the radio wave, whose wavelength is very long ($1 \times 10^6$ $\mu$m). Since all light travels at the same speed ($3 \times 10^{10}$ cm per sec), envision the very small x-ray and the very large radio wave moving in space at the same time. Consider in this example the effect produced when an x-ray traveling at the speed of light meets an atom with many clouds of electrons, such as the iron atom of the skillet. Owing to its extremely small wavelength, the x-ray photon will fly past the outer electron clouds of the iron atom until it approaches the small, compact inner clouds around the nucleus. At this point, a collision occurs and an electron will be dislodged and sent into space. This results in ionization, a phenomenon well known to radiotherapists. Next, consider the effect of the large radio wave. When this long wave approaches large masses of atoms, it gently distorts this sea of atoms, resulting in the production of music or sound. By carefully exploring the electromagnetic spectrum from x-rays to radio waves, it is possible to predict the properties of each based on wavelength and photon energy.

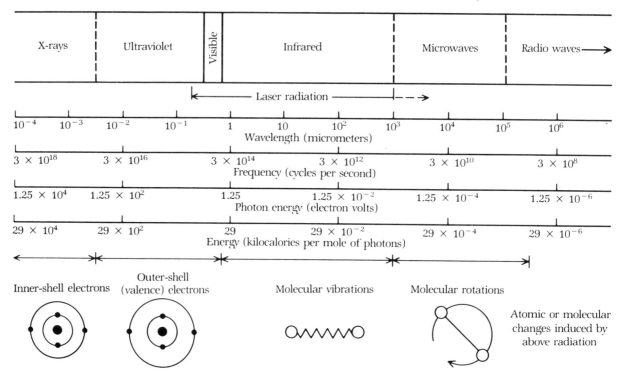

**Figure 6-1.** A segment of the electromagnetic spectrum. Observe that x-rays have a very short wavelength compared to the long wavelength of radiowaves. Notice also, that photon energy decreases as the wavelength increases; however, all photons, regardless of energy move at the same speed of light. (From C. K. N. Patel, High-power carbon dioxide lasers. *Sci. Am.* 219:22, 1968.

One must understand that the stimulation effect involved in laser energy is predictable. In the previous example of the skillet, it took X amount of heat to make the skillet red-hot and Y amount of heat to make it white-hot. The energy needed to produce a predictable property (X or Y) is termed a *quantum* of energy. In the physical world, each atom shift occurs in a predictable fashion and will also reverse in a predictable fashion. The reversability, or release of stored energy, is a major premise in the production of a laser. Assume that if two stimulated atoms collide, each will release its quantity of energy simultaneously and in equal amounts, a property known as *temporal* behavior. This term indicates

that all the photons (waves) are coherent, or moving in parallel fashion, like waves in the ocean, a phenomenon described by Einstein as *stimulated emission of radiation*. Recall that radiation relates to electromagnetic radiation (i.e., from x-ray to radio waves) and is a physical term used to denote movement.

To complete the concept of the laser it is necessary to amplify the light waves discussed earlier. Amplification is accomplished by placing mirrors in the path of the waves of the excited carbon dioxide atoms and adjusting the mirror surfaces to reflect the waves back and forth. This to-and-fro motion causes the light beam to become very intense and is termed *stimulated emission*. The light beam then emerges through a small opening in one end of the optical resonance cavity and travels through the articulating arm of the laser to finally appear as the laser beam.

The process of stimulated emission and amplification produces a light wave with unique properties. This process causes all waves to be in time with each other and equally spaced, a property termed *coherent*. All waves are also parallel to each other, termed *collimated*, and all are of exactly the same wavelength, termed *monochromatic*. These three qualities represent the unique properties of the laser beam.

## The Concept of Generating Laser Energy

A great deal of advanced physics and mathematics would be required to explain in full detail how laser energy is achieved. However, for a qualitative picture, one need only accept some of the results of the advanced theories discussed below. I have said that light can be generated in atomic processes, and laser light is a consequence of these processes. Consider now that an atom consists of a small, positively charged nucleus and negatively charged surrounding electrons. Quantum mechanics explains the interaction of the systems of nuclei and electrons, and the most important concept of this field is that the energy values of an atom are discrete and cannot vary. The specific values or energy levels are characteristic of each atom (quantum energy). Atomic species differ from each other by the number of electrons in the charge of the nucleus. As the number of electrons increases, the structure of the energy levels becomes more and more complex; however, the possible energy of each atom is fixed.

One can demonstrate the concept of energy levels by using the analogy of a ball on a staircase (Fig. 6-2). Raising the ball to a level above the floor requires energy. The potential energy of the ball on the step is determined by the height of the step above the floor. As the ball drops from step to step it loses energy, and when it finally rests on the floor it has lost all energy. This example assists in understanding the changes in energy levels that occur in individual atoms and molecules. The simplified energy level diagrammed in Figure 6-3 demonstrates that an atom gains energy by a process termed *excitation*, which is accomplished by absorbing radiation. It can reach various levels of excitation depending on the amount of radiation absorbed. Loss of energy is referred to as decay. It, too, usually occurs in steps and is referred to as spontaneous emission. When the atom is at its lowest energy level it is termed *ground zero*.

**Figure 6-3.** A simplified energy level diagram. These states are characterized by quantum numbers and are unique for each particular type of atom.

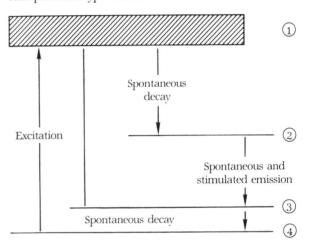

**Figure 6-2.** Potential energy staircase of a ball rolled down the steps.

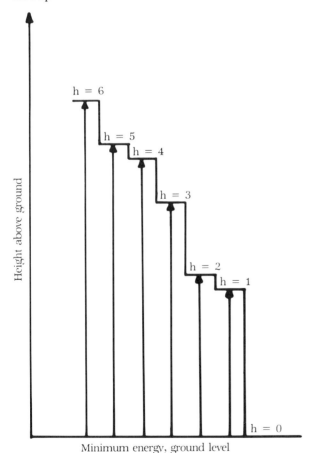

**Table 6-1.** Basic energy levels of carbon dioxide

| Configuration | Designator of energy | Designator of spatial configuration | Relative energy |
|---|---|---|---|
| Asymmetrical mode | 001* | $V_3$ | Highest |
| Bend mode | 100 | $V_2$ | High |
| Symmetrical mode | 020 | $V_1$ | Low |
| Ground state | 000 | $V_0$ | Zero |

*The designator $CO_2$ (001) is the highest energy level.

### The Laser: Molecular Gas Model (Carbon Dioxide Laser)

As with individual atoms, it is possible to change the energy level of molecules, such as carbon dioxide. Following proper excitation, a shift in the rotational and vibrational configuration of molecular gases can produce a shift to higher energy levels. The configurations that the linear carbon dioxide molecule can assume are discussed further on. Basic carbon dioxide energy levels are shown in Table 6-1 [22].

At zero energy level the carbon dioxide molecule is in a resting or ground state. The electron orbits of the $CO_2$ molecule are spaced at equal distances from the carbon nucleus. At the excited level $V_1$, termed *symmetric stretch mode*, the atoms move in a symmetric fashion. As the excitation increases, level $V_2$, or the *bend mode*, is reached. In this arrangement, the interatomic axis is bent or distorted. Finally, the level of excitation $V_3$ is termed the *asymmetric stretch mode*, because the interatomic distances are symmetrically placed in the electron orbit.

To comprehend the photon emission in the various energy levels demonstrated in Table 6-1, an explanation of energy transfer is presented. In quantum mechanics the designations shown in Table 6-1 and discussed above are used to quantitate the energy states. Observations have shown that the carbon dioxide vibrational energy state $V_3$ will decay by spontaneous emission to $CO_2$ (100) or $CO_2$ (020), releasing electromagnetic energy of 10.6 μm and 9.6 μm in wavelength, respectively. This is demonstrated in Figure 6-4 [17, 18].

Addition of nitrogen gas to the optical cavity of the carbon dioxide laser instrument allows the excited vibrational energy of the nitrogen molecule to be transferred directly to $CO_2$. This transfer is a selective $CO_2$ excitation of $CO_2$ $V_0$ (000) to $CO_2$ $V_2$ (001), and produces a high degree of efficiency in generating $CO_2$ (001), because (000) is easily stimulated to $N_2$ (001) in one step. Remember that nitrogen has only one degree of vibration in contrast to carbon dioxide, which has three. Thus, there are two modes of stimulating a $CO_2$ $V_0$ (000) molecule to an excited $CO_2$ $V_3$ (001) molecule, as is shown here.

1. $CO_2$ (00) + electron + kinetic energy = $CO_2$ (001)

   by means of

electrical discharge (low efficiency energy transfer)

2. $N_2$ (000) + electron + kinetic energy = $N_2$ (001)

   then

   $N_2$ (001) + $CO_2$ (001) = (high efficiency energy transfer)

**Figure 6-4.** The energy levels of an excited carbon dioxide molecule and the transfer of energy from excited nitrogen molecules. The high energy $CO_2$ molecule then moves to a lower energy state by releasing energy in the form of photons first at a wavelength of 10.6 μm and then 9.6 μm. The released photons results in laser emission.

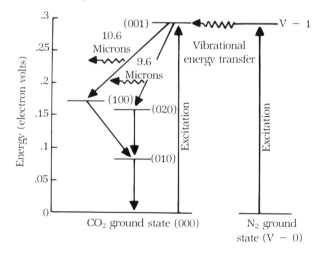

Finally, if the collision per second of kinetic energy is increased, the rate of conversion of $CO_2$ $V_0$ (000) to $CO_2$ $V_3$ (001) will increase, thus achieving greater laser energy by the process termed stimulated emission. Pure $CO_2$ has approximately 100 collisions per second, whereas $N_2$ (under 1 ton of pressure) has 4,000 collisions per second. Thus, with the increased collisions and high efficiency of the $N_2$ transfer of energy to $CO_2$, the system is complete. The final formula requires $N_2$, He, and $CO_2$ for an efficient carbon dioxide laser system.

The element helium (He) is added to the above mixture because of its ability to transfer heat. In the decay process, heat is produced and can be efficiently transferred to the helium atom and then to the wall of the optical cavity of the laser instrument. This, in turn, is the reason the outer laser tube must be added, providing water to conduct heat away from the optical cavity; however, air can also be used for this purpose. It is important to remember that the laser's efficiency is dependent on heat exchange, and thus, a rise in external heat is equivalent to a loss in internal laser efficiency.

*Terminology of Laser Irradiation*

Table 6-2 presents a simple, yet precise outline of the physical parameters used to explain the action of the carbon dioxide laser. Power (P) is related to watts or energy output produced by the laser system and is measured by using a power meter. Most, if not all, laser systems have a power meter built into the system. A rheostat controls the voltage output to the optical cavity, which allows the surgeon to vary output of laser power.

Energy (E) refers to the relationship between time of exposure and power. It is the product of power in watts multiplied by time in seconds. Naturally, if one calculates energy in units of less than 1 second, the level drops, and when it is calculated in time intervals greater than 1 second, it increases, as is shown in Table 6-3. Another way to create the same quality of energy is given in Table 6-4. Tables 6-3 and 6-4 indicate that one can achieve a particular energy level by varying the time of energy exposure or the power. It has been found that tissue injury is not directly related to energy, but rather is influenced by time and power independently. The time of exposure has more influence on tissue effect than does the power of the laser beam. This principle is demonstrated by considering the burn that would be produced if your finger touched the hot skillet mentioned earlier. If the skillet had 40 watts of power and your touch was for 0.5 seconds, or 20 joules of energy exposure, the burn to your finger would be well defined (i.e., a small blister). The extent of the injury would be related to the short time of heat transfer. This can be compared to the tissue damage produced by placing a soldering iron on your finger and turning it on. As the tip of the soldering iron begins to heat from ambient temperature the energy will be gradually increased until

**Table 6-2.** Laser terminology

| Term | Symbol | Unit |
|---|---|---|
| Power | P | W (watt) |
| Time | t | S (second) |
| Energy | $E = P \times t$ | $W \cdot S = J$ (joule) |
| Area | A | $cm^2$ |
| Power density | $I = \dfrac{P}{A}$ | $W/cm^2$ |
| Energy density | $L = \dfrac{E}{A}$ | $\dfrac{W \cdot S}{cm^2} = \dfrac{J}{cm^2}$ |

**Table 6-3.** The relationship of constant power to time and energy

| Power (watts) | Time (seconds) | Energy (joules) |
|---|---|---|
| 20 | 1.0 | 20 |
| 20 | 0.5 | 10 |
| 20 | 2.0 | 40 |

**Table 6-4.** The relationship of constant energy to time and power

| Power (watts) | Time (seconds) | Energy (joules) |
|---|---|---|
| 20 | 1.0 | 20 |
| 40 | 0.5 | 20 |
| 10 | 2.0 | 20 |

20 joules had been transferred. If you kept your finger in place until it received a total energy of 20 joules, a large burn would have occurred, due to the longer time exposure that produced extensive cellular heat (thermal damage) causing tissue destruction. The same energy level can, therefore, result in a markedly different tissue effect, depending on the time during which it is delivered.

## Absorption and Reflection

As discussed earlier in this chapter, the wavelength of a particular laser system determines the effect of the laser beam on tissue. It has been shown that the amount of water required to absorb 90 percent of the laser energy differs at various wavelengths. Thus, the argon laser of wavelength 450 to 515 $\mu$m requires approximately 1,000 mm of water compared to the carbon dioxide laser of wavelength 10.4 $\mu$m, which requires only 0.01 to 0.1 mm of water to reduce its energy by 90 percent of the original amount. The loss, or absorption of energy, is the extinction length and is expressed as the absorption coefficient.

One can appreciate the different effects of the argon, neodymium YaG and carbon dioxide lasers by considering the coefficient of each in a tissue. If one assumes that human tissue is composed of 70 to 90 percent water, the predicted tissue response of various lasers can be considered, since the wavelength of the laser determines this effect. The significance of these observations has been shown in Figure 6-5 and is summarized in the following statements.

**Figure 6-5.** Comparison of tissue damage produced by the carbon dioxide laser, the argon laser, and the neodymium YaG laser. The energy of the carbon dioxide laser is completely absorbed by the superficial layer, while the argon and neodymium YaG lasers penetrate deeply into the tissue. In addition, the argon and neodymium lasers produce notable back scattering.

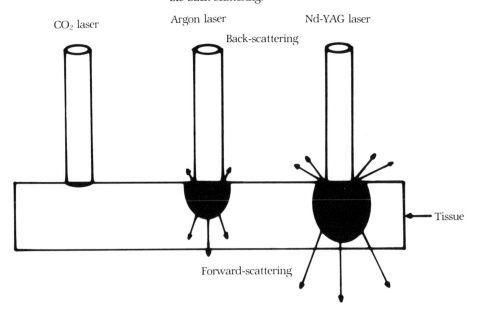

CO$_2$ laser    Argon laser    Nd-YAG laser

Back-scattering

Tissue

Forward-scattering

First, carbon dioxide laser energy is confined to the area where the beam strikes the tissue because it is totally absorbed to within a shallow depth and lateral scattering is negligible. These properties make the carbon dioxide laser suitable for precise surgical removal of soft tissue because typical lesions are less than 2 mm in diameter, and the tissue's water content is high. However, it makes the carbon dioxide laser poorly suited for coagulating deeper broad areas of soft tissue.

Second, the energy of a neodymium YaG laser beam (wavelength 1.06 μm) requires much greater tissue depth for total absorption. Approximately 90 times as much energy is scattered laterally as is absorbed directly along the axis of the beam. These two facts make this laser well suited for deep coagulation of tissue, as in gastrointestinal bleeding, but poorly suited for precise excision of tissue. This laser is also concentrated in red pigmented tissue.

Third, the energy of the argon laser beam at its shortest wavelength also requires a significant tissue depth for total absorption. About 100 times as much energy is scattered laterally as is absorbed directly. It is highly concentrated in red pigmented tissue and is, therefore, well suited to retinal coagulation and control of hemorrhage. The color sensitive absorption in living tissue and inherently deep penetration combined with strong scattering, make it poorly suited for precise surgical procedures.

In summary, the unique properties of the carbon dioxide laser allow for precise vaporization of surface epithelium with a limited zone of cellular injury. The effect of the carbon dioxide laser is precise and can easily be limited to the irradiated surface. By contrast, the argon and neodymium YaG lasers penetrate beyond the target surface, and this forward scattering effect can result in injury to adjacent organs. The back scattering effect seen in argon and neodymium YaG lasers is not a characteristic of the carbon dioxide laser. However, one must also consider reflected energy when considering laser action. Should the irradiated surface be reflective, the laser beam will be deflected in a different direction. Highly polished surfaces, regardless of color, will reflect the carbon dioxide laser and, therefore, instruments of absorptive material must be substituted for the highly polished stainless steel instruments usually employed during microsurgery. Nonflammable plastics, dulled metallic surfaces, or wet surfaces absorb or fail to reflect the carbon dioxide laser wavelengths. Similarly, hard contact lenses or plastic goggles will protect the eyes of the surgeon and his assistant from damage produced by accidentally reflected laser beams. A soft contact lens will absorb the carbon dioxide laser energy owing to its high water content. This is discussed later in the section on laser safety.

## Power Density

Power density is the most important operating parameter of a surgical laser for a given wavelength. The range of power densities employed during surgery determines whether a laser will coagulate, vaporize, cut, or combine these functions when used on living tissue. Various power densities discussed in Chapter 7 have been found to produce the desired effect of cutting adhesions or opening a hydrosalpinx. Actual measurement of the point-to-point power density of a real surgical laser is very difficult, because the focal spots of most lasers used in surgery are less than 2 mm in diameter. However, the beam's total power and average power density are relatively easy to measure. Except in the case of a stationary beam, where peak power density determines the maximum depth of ablation, it is more helpful to know average power density, because this determines both the central depth and the timed rate of mass removal from the furrow made by a moving beam. Average power density can be determined rather easily by measuring the effective spot diameter and the total power of the beam, assuming a Gaussian distribution.

**Figure 6-6.** Two dimensional intensity profile of a laser beam. The Gaussian distribution and beam intensity diminish in a reciprocal exponential function as the distance from the beam axis increases. This is the most fundamental mode TEM 00.

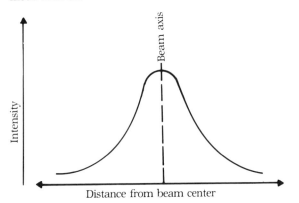

It is important to consider the distribution of laser energy across the entire spot diameter. Fluctuations in cross-sectional energy distribution can readily be demonstrated if one examines the imprint made by short bursts of laser energy on a tongue depressor. Cross sectional energy distribution of the laser beam is referred to as the *transverse electromagnetic mode* (TEM). The most useful is TEM 00 in which a symmetrical crater is formed because of the intense central energy that decreases symmetrically toward the periphery of the beam. The graph in Figure 6-6 demonstrates this symmetry. Other TEM modes include TEM 01, widely used in early carbon dioxide lasers. The uneven power distribution of this mode produces a cold spot in the center of the beam and a distribution of energy referred to as a donut pattern. Other TEM distributions include the multimode. In summary, TEM 00 is the preferred mode because its energy distribution is symmetrical, and because it permits the laser beam to be focused at the smallest spot size.

Power density is related to the beam spot diameter at a given power output, which is a function of the focal length of the operating microscope's objective lens. The longer the focal length of the objective lens, the larger the spot size; that is, at TEM 00 a 400 mm lens produces a 0.8 mm spot, whereas a 50 mm lens produces a 0.1 mm spot. Furthermore, for constant power output, the smaller the spot produced by the laser beam, the higher the power density per unit area. Thus, power density is a function of both spot size and power, and varies inversely with the square of the focal length of the objective lens. The power density and time exposure are the most important parameters of a surgical laser. Because the time exposure depends on the speed of incision, power density is the single most important factor to be considered when choosing a laser apparatus. Thus, the greater the power density of the carbon dioxide laser, the more versatile are its applications in performing surgical procedures.

It should be stressed that the laser beam can have an unequal cross sectional distribution of energy produced by different mirror alignments and geometric patterns within the resonator cavity of various laser units; therefore, the calculated power density describes only an average power density. The total laser beam power required to achieve a desired system can be predetermined. One can measure the spot diameter after firing a test pulse into a wooden tongue depressor or other suitable test target with a laser beam at moderate power level (10 watts for 0.1 seconds), and then viewing the target beside a millimeter scale under the operating microscope. Figure 6-7 demonstrates power densities as a function of focal point diameter. Other power density profiles will yield different average values with a given total power and spot diameter. The surgeon must recognize these variations in the energy distribution of his instrument to predict the degree of tissue damage.

**Figure 6-7.** Diagram of relationship between constant power and laser spot size. Energy delivered to tissue (i.e., power density) will vary in direct proportion to the diameter of the spot as shown by firing the laser beam into a wooden tongue depressor. (Courtesy of Merrimack.)

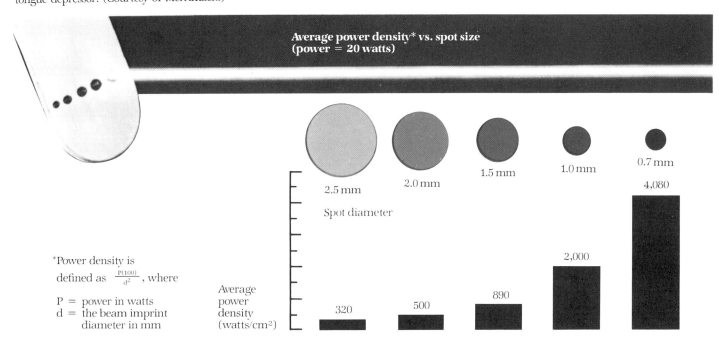

Average power density* vs. spot size (power = 20 watts)

2.5 mm   2.0 mm   1.5 mm   1.0 mm   0.7 mm

Spot diameter

*Power density is defined as $\frac{P(100)}{d^2}$, where

P = power in watts
d = the beam imprint diameter in mm

Average power density (watts/cm²)

320   500   890   2,000   4,080

Power is measured in watts, energy in joules. Energy equals power times duration of exposure in seconds. It follows that power, energy, and tissue destruction are all directly proportional. The time of laser exposure can be controlled by a shutter that is activated by a foot pedal. The great number of combinations of power settings and duration of exposure allow the surgeon great flexibility in the application of laser energy. Different settings are appropriate for different surgical situations and produce different biologic effects. In general, the surgeon may select the continuous beam at various power settings for cutting tissue. In contrast, intermittent laser energy at various time settings produces a different effect, somewhat more useful for tissue coagulation. Naturally, the type of tissue influences this decision. Recently, Cooper Medical introduced a variable super pulse mode that permits greater variation of a laser beam energy at a very high power density. This is similar to the intermittent mode, but produces higher peak voltages with greater intervals of cooling that should permit a purer cutting effect. The depth of tissue destruction is controlled by varying the power density of the beam and the duration in which it is applied. It assumes that all of this energy is used to vaporize tissue, and that laser energy is evenly distributed over the area of the focal spot. In reality, however, some energy may be reflected by the target tissue and by slight variations of the energy distribution within the laser beam. In small, commercially available surgical lasers it would be difficult to eliminate these variations without tremendous expense. Fortunately, the surgeon is usually not hampered by these deviations, but recognizing the characteristics of the beam allows for its optimal use.

**Table 6-5.** Relationship between power setting and power density levels[a]

| Power setting laser dial-watts | Power density[b] (W/cM$^2$) |
|---|---|
| 1 | 400 |
| 2 | 800 |
| 3 | 1,200 |
| 4 | 1,600 |
| 5 | 2,000 |
| 10 | 4,000 |
| 15 | 6,000 |
| 20 | 8,000 |
| 25 | 10,000 |
| 30 | 12,000 |

[a]Power density levels are given for a spot diameter of 0.55 mm, calculated by using standard deviation = 0.5 mm.
[b]Power density (PD) equals power in watts times 100 divided by the square of the spot diameter (in millimeters).

*Practical Measurement for Power Density*
The above discussion of power density is difficult to integrate into a gynecologist's daily working practice. Thus, we have condensed a version of the exponential formula into an algebraic expression:

$$\text{Power density (PD)} = \frac{\text{power in watts} \times 100}{[\text{spot diameter (mm)}]^2}$$

Most early carbon dioxide laser units provided only one spot diameter at a particular working distance, that is 300 mm. In fact, the power density numbers provided in the surgical sections of Chapter 7 assumed a constant spot diameter of 550 $\mu$m (0.55 mm). The variation in power density is achieved by changing the power output of the laser unit or defocusing the operating microscope. This is demonstrated during microsurgical lysis of adhesions when the power density of the laser can range from 2000 W per square centimeter to 10,000 W per square centimeter. These values were obtained by using the equation just given in which spot size remained at 0.55 mm and the laser power was varied from 5 to 25 watts. Naturally, tissue effect will also be influenced by the time interval of laser energy applied. The complete range of power density values is given in Table 6-5.

Recently introduced carbon dioxide laser units provide the availability to vary spot diameter at constant working distances without defocusing the operating microscope. At a 300 mm focal distance, the spot diameter of the Cooper Medical unit can be varied from 0.5 mm to 2.5 mm. Thus, power density can now be varied by a second parameter and one that is at the surgeon's fingertip because the control knob for spot size is located near the joystick. This control knob is also available with new units sold by Sharplan, Xanar, and Merrimack. This is discussed later in the chapter.

**Table 6-6.** Relationships between objective lens and laser spot diameter*

| Objective lens (mm) | Smallest laser spot diameter (mm) |
|---|---|
| 50 | 0.18 |
| 100 | 0.20 |
| 200 | 0.37 |
| 250 | 0.45 |
| 300 | 0.55 |
| 400 | 0.7 |

*The smallest theoretical spot diameter achieved with the carbon dioxide laser in the TEM 00 mode.

Varying the spot size changes the power density and thus, alters the laser effect on the involved tissue. Decreasing spot size increases power density and concentrates this energy on a small area. In contrast, increasing the spot diameter spreads the same power over a larger area and produces a lower power density. The surgeon can, therefore, select a small spot diameter, without defocusing the operating microscope, for cutting adhesions or tubal serosa and a larger spot diameter to provide hemostasis without varying power input. The somewhat similar concept of high frequency cutting and coagulating currents has been discussed at length in Chapter 5 in the section on microelectrosurgery.

The individual microsurgeon must be familiar with the spot size of the laser unit he employs, which is calculated for the objective lens being used. Recall that increasing the working distance of the objective lens also increases the size of the field and comparably increases the spot size of the laser beam employed. Estimated spot diameters available with the carbon dioxide laser used in the TEM 00 mode are presented in Table 6-6. Note that the smallest spot diameter is achieved with the 50 mm hand unit. The 300 mm objective lens commonly used uring infertility microsurgery produces a spot diameter of 0.5 mm as discussed at length above.

### Laser Safety

Lasers are potentially dangerous devices. This instrument is capable of concentrating large amounts of energy into very small, well-collimated beams and, thus, has an enormous potential for therapeutic benefit as well as for injury. As with any medical device, the laser must be used with skill, discretion, and common sense.

When used properly, the laser can be a safe and effective operating room instrument. Those who use medical lasers must always adhere to the following general rules:

1. Never operate any laser until you have read and understood the operator's manual furnished by the manufacturer.
2. Never fire the laser at any target until you know the complete path of the beam and are sure that no unintended targets lie in that path.
3. Never fire a therapeutic laser at a living target until you have been instructed by a competent teacher in both the correct operational procedures of the laser and the proper technique for application of the laser energy to the tissue to be treated.
4. Never use a laser for surgery until you have practiced its use on inanimate targets, and also on cadaver parts or laboratory animals, or both.
5. Always take seriously the safety precautions specified by the manufacturer of the laser whenever you use it for any purpose.
6. Never use a laser on human patients until you have taken a course of instruction on laser surgery.
7. Always request that a qualified instructor representing the manufacturer give you and your operating room service personnel training prior to using the laser on humans. Nursing personnel must be properly prepared for this special surgical instrumentation. The minimum number of people required during surgery should be present in the operating room.
8. Ask for a qualified operating room instructor in laser operation to be present to advise you when you first use the laser on human patients.
9. The laser should be activated only by the surgeon who is responsible for the safety system and who has custody of the master key.

## Carbon Dioxide Instrumentation

The energy of the carbon dioxide laser is supplied by passing an electric current through a mixture of helium, nitrogen, and carbon dioxide gases. These gases, stored in tanks in the laser cabinet, are pumped into a cylinder that has reflective surfaces, referred to as an optical resonance cavity. Mirrors placed at either end of the resonance cavity produce the high energy photons that constitute the laser beam. The beam then travels along an articulating arm to either a hand unit or a micromanipulator, where it is focused on a specific spot. A typical carbon dioxide laser unit is shown in Figure 6-8.

Pumping energy into the laser medium produces a *population inversion*, a situation in which more atoms of carbon dioxide are in the excited state than in the ground state. Once the population has been inverted, the process of amplification by *stimulated emission* can occur as follows. An excited carbon dioxide molecule can release (emit) a photon that strikes another excited atom stimulating emission and producing the release of two identical photons. In this manner, the level of excitation, and therefore, the strength of the laser beam builds rapidly. Those molecules that happen to travel in a direction parallel to the axis of the optical cavity are reflected by the mirrors at either end. They return through the active medium and are amplified. This to-and-fro reflection generates a light beam of high energy.

**Figure 6-8.** A typical carbon dioxide laser unit. From the floor upwards, note the footswitch, the cabinet containing tanks of gas, and the control panel. A central column supports the horizontal optical resonance cavity at one end of which is the articulating arm, and the attached hand unit. (Courtesy of Merrimack.)

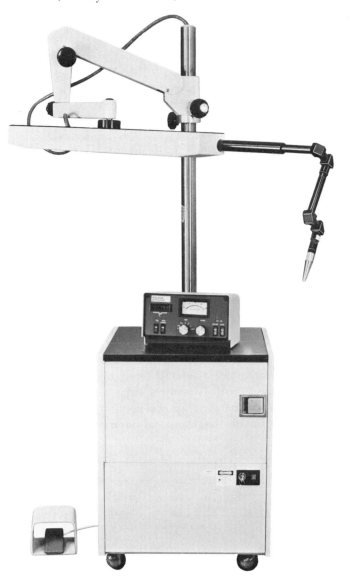

Since the mirror at one end of the optical cavity is semi-transparent, a stream of photons will exit through this opening (Figure 6-9). The process of reflection in the optic cavity produces a photon beam that has three unique properties discussed earlier. It is (1) collimated, (2) coherent, and (3) monochromatic. The cross sectional density of energy is thus exceedingly great. After its release from the optic cavity, the laser energy passes through a system of mirrors and lenses in the articulating arm of the laser unit and is finally focused on a spot termed the *focal point.* The surgical usefulness of the laser is achieved by the ability to focus this high level of energy at a specific point and to move the point in appropriate fashion during selective surgical procedures.

**Figure 6-9.** Optical cavity and the various means of creating the laser effect.

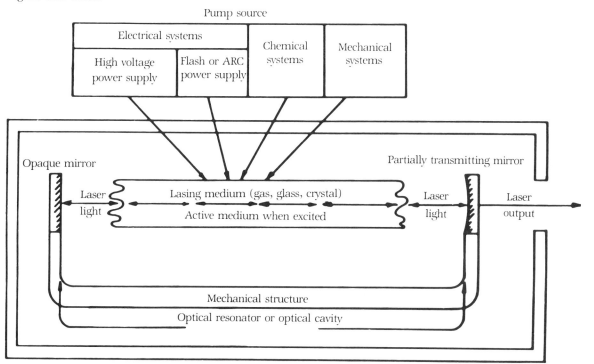

One of the carbon dioxide surgical laser systems used in our studies (manufactured by the American Optical Corp.) has been described in detail by Polanyi and colleagues [20]. Other manufacturers of water-cooled carbon dioxide lasers use a similar mechanical design. A standard electronic cabinet contains the gas supply for the laser, vacuum pump, power pack, operating controls, and safety interlocks. The water-cooling system is self-contained, and only a connection for the electric power source is needed.

The laser beam is issued from the optical cavity and is directed into a beam-manipulating arm that contains a mirror in rotating joints with a focusing lens at the beam exit. This arrangement allows the surgeon to focus the laser beam at any point within a large area. A shutter is opened by a foot switch to allow the laser beam to reach the target, which is pinpointed by a luminous red spot or helium neon laser (target beam). Either continuous exposure or time exposure can be used, and the power can be varied from 0 to 45 watts by adjusting a knob on the control panel. The variable super pulse present on the Cooper Medical laser is a third choice. When not in use, the instrument is placed on standby and the beam is deflected into a heat sink by the reflecting shutter.

When the carbon dioxide laser is used during microsurgery, it is connected to the operating microscope by a micromanipulator that contains a special gimballed mirror. The narrow laser beam entering the micromanipulator strikes this mirror located between the monocular optical axes of the stereomicroscope. The mirror is positioned at 45 degrees to the primary incident laser beam and deflects the energy along the viewing axis of the microscope. This arrangement must be modified if a biheaded stereoscopic operating microscope with recording system is to be substituted. Apertures in the mirror permit normal viewing through the microscope when the laser system is attached. A lens located in the primary incident laser beam focuses the energy on a spot at a distance equal to the working distance of the microscope objective lens. By appropriate lens selection this distance can be varied to suit the surgeon.

The gimbal-mounted mirror permits the laser beam to be directed to any location within plus-or-minus 3 degrees of the central axis of the microscope. The diameter of the working area is therefore about one tenth the working distance. A joystick type of control is provided in a convenient location a few inches to the right or middle of the operating microscope and permits the surgeon to move the mirror about the gimbal axis. The mechanical linkage between the joystick and the gimbal is arranged to make the motion of the beam directly proportional to the same joystick movement with a demagnification ratio of 7 : 1. The sensitivity and naturalness of this adjustment allows the surgeon to position the beam to any preselected location (Fig. 6-10).

A helium neon laser of very low power is used to produce a red marker spot at the site where the focused energy of the carbon dioxide laser beam will strike the tissue. This red marker is visible whenever the laser is in use and it permits the surgeon to see exactly where the carbon dioxide laser beam will strike the tissue. This has also been demonstrated in Fig. 6-10.

### Current Carbon Dioxide Laser Systems for Microsurgery

The current laser models available for microsurgical adaptation in the United States are listed here. Each system has certain advantages and disadvantages: A microsurgeon contemplating a purchase should evaluate each system and decide which one best suits his needs.

1. Sharplan 733, 743
2. Merrimack 840, 850
3. Coherent 450
4. Biophysics Medica
5. Xanar
6. Cooper Medical 250 Z, 500 Z
7. Biolas 40, 80

All of these manufacturers offer a hand unit and a micromanipulator for attachment to the operating microscope, although Zeiss OPMI-6S and 7PH model microscopes present specific attachment problems.

The major points to consider in a laser acquisition are as follows:

1. Power output of 30 watts at the final exit port, *not* at the laser head.
2. Articulation system to allow placement at foot of operating table or other location as desired.
3. Smoothly articulating handpiece assembly.
4. Variable focal lengths.
5. Micromanipulator assembly.
6. Variable spot size adapter.
7. Super pulse—variable or not variable.
8. Service and maintenance contract.
9. In-service training for operating room personnel.

**Figure 6-10.** Schematic diagram of a micromanipulator assembly demonstrating the pathway of the laser beam and helium-neon target beam as they are reflected by a mirror controlled by a lever, termed a *joystick*.

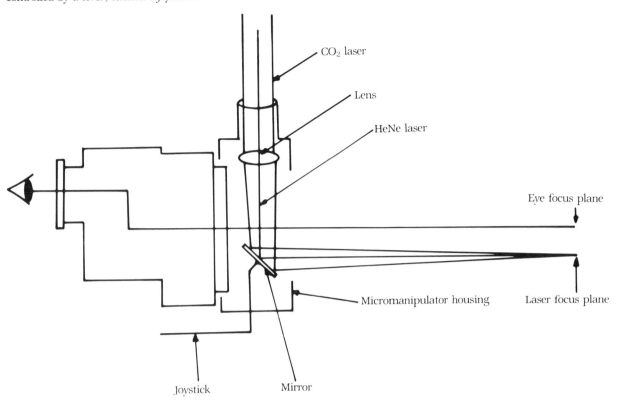

Please note that the carbon dioxide laser has recently been used successfully during operating laparoscopy, and adaptation to the laparoscope should be included with the laser model selected. Sharplan offers a laser laparoscope attachment suitable for its carbon dioxide lasers, and Eder Instrument Co. has marketed a laser laparoscope attachment that appears to attach to all other carbon dioxide laser units.

The operating microscope micromanipulator is an optical platform containing an articulated mirror at 45 degrees to the incipient laser beam and a handle or joystick that moves the mirror (Fig. 6-11). This platform attaches to the lower portion of the microscope body in the area of the objective lens. Most micromanipulators contain a set of fixed focus lenses that allow the surgeon to change his working distance and focal spot size. The major disadvantage of some current models is that the articulated mirror obstructs 30 percent of the surgeon's viewing field when it is attached to a binocular stereoscopic operating microscope. To overcome this problem, one must extend the optical platform and change the articulated mirror from 45 to 49 degrees. This eccentric placement results in a beam-tissue interaction that is 85 degrees, rather than 90 degrees. This slight deviation from the perpendicular axis results in a slight alteration in tissue heat flow that is not thought to be significant. The major gain in this new arrangement is that the surgeon can use video tape to simultaneously record while operating without losing the image to the recording device or to his visual field.

In addition, the surgeon should require the laser manufacturer to provide a working distance of 200 to 300 mm with an appropriate small spot size (see Table 6-6). All laser units which provide the mode TEM 00 should produce identical spot sizes at comparable working distances. A larger spot size at this distance implies the presence of a different mode, such as TEM 01 or multimode. If the surgeon uses a sitting position during microsurgery he should experiment with a convenient objective lens for use with the micromanipulator. Once the micromanipulator has been properly modified it should be fitted to the surgical microscope. Fine adjustments should be made to ensure that all planes are parafocal. In addition, certain microscopes have objective lenses that protrude or retract in the zoom mode, and allowance for this change must be made. Should the operating microscope have a double objective stereoscopic system, the micromanipulator must then be fitted to one side and modified so as not to obstruct the second objective system. Once mounted, the micromanipulator should be marked so that it can be easily removed and replaced in the exact location on the microscope suspension. This allows the manipulator to be removed and cleaned. The reflective articulated mirrors should be cleaned with acetone and lens paper.

---

**Figure 6-11.** Early micromanipulator. Notice the eccentric optical port in relationship to the laser exit port. This eccentricity results in a 40 percent loss of the visual field.

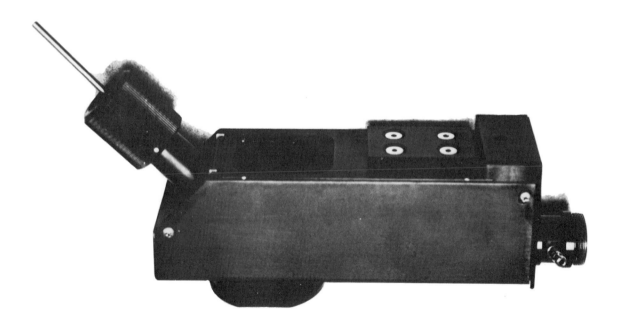

Never use an abrasive material that could scratch the highly polished surface. The gallium arsenide lenses should be cleaned in a similar fashion. These systems should not be gas sterilized, since ethylene oxide can remove or damage the infrared coating on the lens surface. Alcohol or Cidex can be used to clean the outside of the manipulator, but soaking will begin a leaching process from the lens mounting surface into the metallic lens. Leaching will reduce the focal properties of the system, and, eventually, an expensive lens replacement will be required. The variable spot size component could also be damaged during this process.

*Omega Modification of Laser Micromanipulator*

In this modification, the optical platform has been lengthened sufficiently to allow the articulated mirror to be placed beyond the 300 mm objective lens of the OPMI-6 Zeiss microscope (Fig. 6-12). The articulated mirror assembly was repositioned to 85 degrees to replace the infrared focal point within the surgeon's viewing field. A spacer was added to the dovetail to allow use of the rapid on/off assembly. In addition, care was taken to mill the spacer so that it always returned to the exact locus on the microscope attachment assembly. This design makes realignment unnecessary when the micromanipulator is removed for cleaning.

**Figure 6-12.** Omega micromanipulator assembly mounted to the OPMI-6 Zeiss microscope.

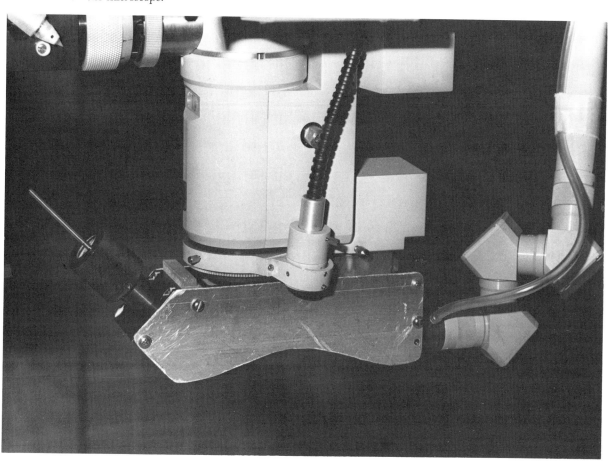

The lens assembly was fitted with three lenses to allow the choice of variable focal points of the infrared laser energy. We selected a 500 μm, 1 mm, and 3 mm focal points spot size at a working distance of 300 mm. This system can be varied by changing to a Zeiss 400 mm objective lens, thereby obtaining three additional focal points. This arrangement gives six discrete focal points of laser energy for microsurgical procedures. Finally, the protective sidewalls of the micromanipulator were sculptured to allow for maximum lumination from the bifid fiber optical light system of the OPMI-6 microscope. Once completed, the assembly was mounted and checked to assure proper alignment of the HeNe pointer to the surgeon's viewing field through the OPMI-6 microscope (Fig. 6-12).

*Variable Spot Size Adapter*

As noted previously, the omega micromanipulator was designed to provide three variations in spot size. At a focal distance of 300 mm (suitable for most gynecologic microsurgeons) and a spot size of 500 μm, 1 mm and 3 mm were available. This concept of varying the spot diameter of the carbon dioxide laser beam has been expanded by most laser manufacturers during the past year, and at present, Merrimack,* Sharplan, Xanar, and Cooper Medical offer such an attachment. At a focal distance of 300 mm the spot size of most units can be changed from 500 μm to 2.5 mm without defocusing the microscope.

Recently, Sharplan has introduced a micromanipulator with an adapter to vary spot diameter. At present this is not totally suitable for use with the OPMI-6S Zeiss microscope, since the Vertalux fiberoptic lighting attachment does not fit comfortably around this unit. A convenience of the Merrimack unit is the special housing for the fiberoptic lighting attachment. The Cooper Medical 250 Z unit also has a suitable adapter.

Xanar offers variable spot size and states that a minimal spot diameter of 0.2 mm can be achieved when using a 300 mm objective lens. In fact, the company states that the minimal 0.2 mm spot diameter can be obtained at focal distances from 250 mm to 400 mm. This is contrary to presently accepted principles relating spot diameter to focal distances (see Table 6-6) and should require a special lens system to compensate for changes in working distances. The minimal spot diameter advertised for this Xanar unit is the smallest available on commercially available carbon dioxide laser units (Fig. 6-13). As noted earlier, all laser units that deliver the laser beam in the mode TEM 00 should produce identical spot diameters at comparable working distances.

*Editor's Note:* Recently, Merrimack introduced a specially designed micromanipulator for the OPMI-6S-D Zeiss microscope. This micromanipulator contains dual joysticks permitting either surgeon to control the laser beam. It does not interfere with the optical path of the dual binocular viewing microscope as did early micromanipulators discussed previously. This unit also provides a variable spot diameter (Fig. 6-14).

**Figure 6-13.** Microscope adapter providing variable spot size. (Courtesy of Xanar.)

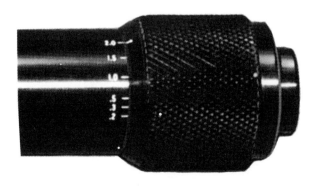

**Figure 6-14.** Micromanipulator for Zeiss OPMI-6S-D and OPMI-7P/H microscopes provides dual binocular viewing without interference in the optical path of the surgeon, permitting visualization of the complete surgical field. The laser beam can be controlled by either of the two joysticks shown. The knob that varies the size of the laser spot size is shown at the end of the fiberoptical light housing. (Courtesy of Merrimack.)

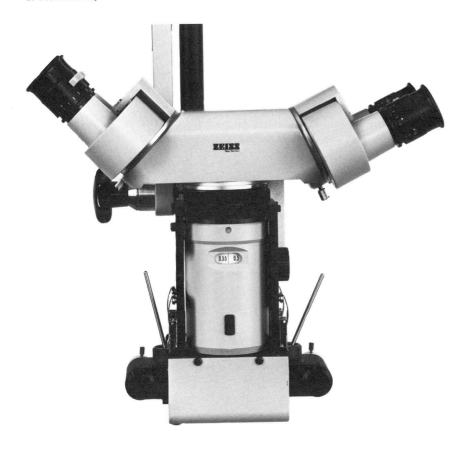

### Laser Scalpel

The laser can be used with a fixed focus hand-held assembly, shown in Figure 6-15. The three focal lengths usually available with this instrument are f:50 mm, f:125 mm, and f:150 mm. Each has a fixed focus, but the surgeon can vary the focal point size by moving his hand. These lenses are able to generate power densities of 1,000,000 W per square centimeter, depending on the laser input and final focus diameter. Great care must be used in handling these laser scalpels. All laser scalpels have a nitrogen input port for laminar flow across the lenses that prevents back scatter from the tissue that could damage the coated lens surface. The laser is used as a scalpel but has the added advantage of limited tissue interaction.

### Laser Accessory Instruments

The major tool used by the laser microsurgeon is the quartz glass rod, because these rods will absorb the incident energy of the laser and can be shaped into any desired configuration by the surgeon. We use these glass rods as elevators and manipulators, as is shown in the procedures demonstrated in Chapter 7. The laser is then fired onto the surface and the tissue severed. A new rod is used if the glass shows pitting or fatigue. The rods are inexpensive and can be fashioned on site by the operating room personnel by using a propane torch that will heat the glass rod to its melting point, allowing for shaping or bending. Bellina has developed a device that allows a fiber optic light to be attached to the glass rod. This assembly allows for excellent transillumination of pelvic structures during infertility surgical procedures.

**Figure 6-15.** Laser hand scalpel with a 50 mm lens. Notice the nitrogen gas port and tubing.

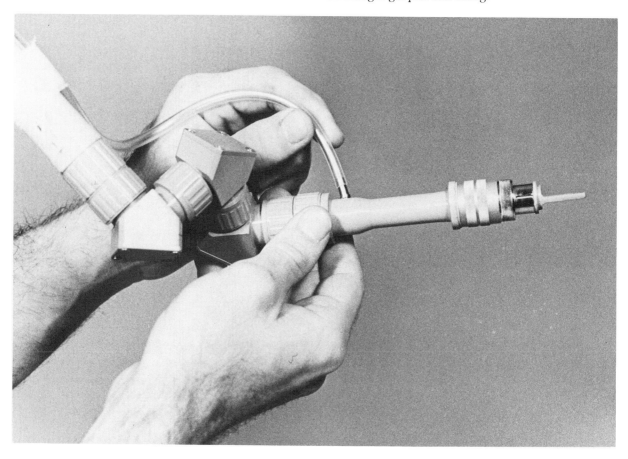

## Laser Laparoscopy

The unique properties of a laser beam permit its energy to be channeled through a laparoscope. An operating laparoscope's outside diameter of 12 mm has been modified to allow for passage of the 10.6 nm carbon dioxide laser beam (Fig. 6-16). Special modification of the operating channel permits the focusing lens and the gas to flow through the same channel. The gallium arsenide lens focuses the laser to a 1 mm spot size, 20 cm beyond the end of the laparoscope. This exact prefocused beam can be used to cut fine adhesions or to vaporize endometrial implants. The laparoscope also has a channel for smoke evacuation.

A recent modification of this system permits a second puncture instrument to carry the laser energy. Again, the lens system focuses the laser to a 1 mm spot size at a distance of 2 cm beyond the probe tip.

In both systems, an HeNe laser is used as a target light. In the combined operating laser laparoscope, the HeNe beam can be adjusted to correspond exactly with the laser focus. This arrangement allows the surgeon to test fire the system and correct the red marker beam for exact carbon dioxide beam alignment.

The laser laparoscope has recently been introduced for clinical use. It is available from both Sharplan and Eder Instrument companies. The advent of flexible fibers capable of transporting the $CO_2$ laser beam is expected to aid in overcoming many of the present difficulties with this system. In addition to these modifications in the telescope, specialized quartz probes are needed to absorb the 10.6 nm laser energy to prevent its deflection onto another surface. Ceramic coated probes are being developed that may solve many problems associated with the use of quartz glass in the abdominal cavity.

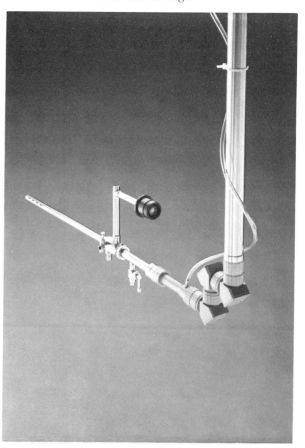

**Figure 6-16.** Laser laparoscope uses the operating channel to beam down the laser onto its target.

## Operating Room Modification

The physical arrangement of a laser equipped operating room requires a large room, approximately 25 by 30 feet. The location of the operating table should allow access to either side of the table without entanglement of electric cords, suction tubing, or gas lines. In our operating room the surgeon stands on the left side of the patient. The laser is placed at the foot of the operating table and the articulating arm elevated to permit maximum clearance. This elevation allows a Mayo stand to be placed at the foot of the table; an additional Mayo stand placed to the right of the surgeon serves as his private tray, and contains his most frequently used instruments. The operating microscope is ceiling mounted and attached to the laser through the articulating arm from the foot of the table. A micro-high-frequency electrosurgical system is placed near the right shoulder of the surgeon.

The anesthesiologist plays an important role at the head of the table and must wear protective glasses at all times during the laser procedure. It is important to note that in the sitting position the anesthesiologist's eyes are usually in a direct line with the exit port of the laser micromanipulator assembly. If a defect exists in the alignment of this unit, it is theoretically possible that a packet of laser photons could hit the eye of the anesthesiologist and result in corneal damage.

The suction apparatus used during laser surgery should be equipped with an in-line filter to remove tars or other substances that tend to foul the hospital vacuum pumps. We have found that a disposable in-line filter together with a semipermeable filter in the vacuum system is most effective. This system is exceedingly cost effective and prevents vacuum pump failures.

In addition, success depends on the mandatory presurgical checking of all equipment. A daily check list includes the following:

1. $CO_2/N_2/He$ gas bottle pressure
2. Visual inspection of lens and reflective mirrors
3. Wall suction semipermeable filter
4. Ground system alarms
5. Test firing of laser to assure proper alignment
6. Video alignment and system parafocal check
7. Luminescence of light pipes

On a weekly basis, the power output of the laser and the vacuum pressure should be checked.

There should also be a chart in the operating room to record the diopter corrections for each surgeon. In addition, the chart should record the diopter correction for the operating assistant. Because a stereoscopic microscope is frequently used, the right lens system can and usually does vary from the left lens system. Thus, each eyepiece must be individually corrected to the surgeon's eyes. This is done in conjunction with focusing the recording system.

In order to properly align the microsurgical system, the following steps must be performed:

1. Place the proper objective lens on the microscope.
2. Place an f:300 focusing reticule in the left eyepiece.
3. Focus the reticule until the two distant crosses appear.
4. Without using the eyepieces, focus the videotape system using the monitor. Adjust the microscope assembly up or down until the left eye is in focus.
5. Check the 16 mm focus camera system and video system if it is used.
6. Lock all systems in place.
7. Correct the right eyepiece by rotating the diopter correcting lens until the proper focus is noted for right eye.
8. Record the diopter correction next to the physician's name and the date. Repeat with all personnel until all diopter corrections are recorded.

The visual system is thus parafocal and corrected to the eyes of each surgeon. The Zeiss OPMI-6 microscope used by our surgical team contains a 50-50 beam splitter with a single exit port. This exit port can receive a teaching arm adapter, a 16 mm camera attachment, a videotape adapter, or a 35 mm camera adapter. Currently, Urban produces a 16 mm–35 mm dual adapter or a videotape 35 mm adapter, as shown in Chapter 5, but not a 16 mm videotaper adapter. However, at this author's (J.H.B) request and design, a 16 mm videotape adapter is now available by special order from Urban.

A Bieleau 16 mm camera is preferred and a Circon video tube used for recording operating procedures. Tungsten ASA 400 positive films are used during cine recording. If a movie is contemplated, negative film is substituted, because this film is felt to produce a better quality 16 mm movie. The surgeon should be aware that a 16 mm movie is very expensive to produce, with current estimates between $500 and $1,000 per minute of edited sound titled film.

### Recording System: Specialized Modification

I have modified my operating room to allow viewing by the patient's family while simultaneously recording the operating procedure on ¾ inch videotape or 16 mm film. One monitor may be viewed by the operating room personnel, the second by the video technicians, and the third by the patient's family. A closed circuit audio system allows the surgeon to communicate with the family and to discuss his findings while operating. It also allows the surgeon to activate the 16 mm camera and to record special or noteworthy events. Should publications require illustrations, the 16 mm frames are analyzed and produced in black and white prints or 35 mm slides. The flexibility of this recording system can be appreciated when one attempts to videorecord and later create a 16 mm movie of the same sequences.

**Figure 6-17.** Zeiss OPMI-6S microscope fitted with a modified micromanipulator. The laser articulated arm assembly is seen to the right of the photograph. Notice the position of the vertalux fiberoptical light attachment.

### Laser Approach to Microsurgery

To effectively use the carbon dioxide laser in microsurgery, one must adhere to strict principles of application. First, the surgeon must be a competent microsurgeon and adhere rigidly to the surgical procedures of proper tissue handling, suturing, and aseptic technique. Having mastered the microsurgical approach to oviduct surgery, a definite knowledge of laser biophysics is necessary to permit the use of the carbon dioxide laser to its maximum advantage. This includes a thorough working knowledge of laser tissue interaction, mechanisms of heat transfer and decay, power density concepts, and the utilization of TEM in tissue [3]. All of the above have been discussed earlier in this chapter. Finally, and of similar importance, is the acquisition of the proper laser equipment. Many types of lasers presently are available, each claiming its own advantage. The microsurgeon must understand his surgical needs and select a suitable system. Figure 6-17 demonstrates an OPMI-6S microscope with a laser attachment, as well as a beam splitter and photo adapter holding a 35 mm camera.

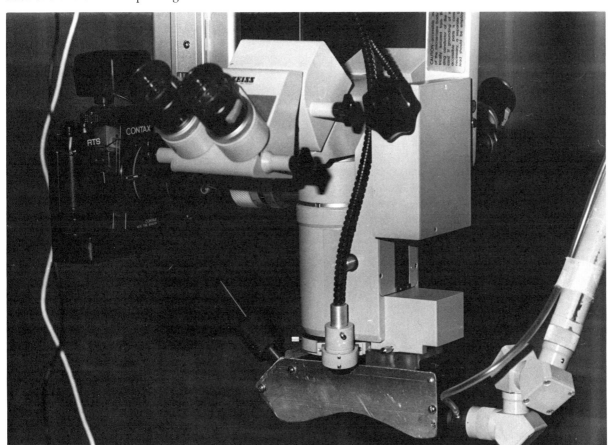

## References

1. Bellina, J. H. Gynecology and the laser. *Contemp. OB/GYN* 4:24, 1974.
2. Bellina, J. H. Reconstructive microsurgery of the fallopian tube with the carbon dioxide laser—procedures and preliminary results. *Reproduction* 5:1, 1981.
3. Bellina, J. H. The Carbon Dioxide Laser and Reconstructive Surgery of the Female Reproductive System. In K. Semm and L. Mettler (eds.), *Human Reproduction.* Amsterdam: Excerpta Medica, 1981. Pp. 481-485.
4. Bellina, J. H., and Seto, Y. J. Pathological and physical investigation into $CO_2$ laser-tissue interaction with specific emphasis on cervical intraepithelial neoplasia. *Lasers Surg. Med.* 47:69, 1980.
5. Christensen, J. Introduction. In I. Kaplan (ed.), *Laser Surgery.* New York: Jerusalem Academic Press, 1976.
6. Einstein, A. Zur quanten theorie der strahlung. *Phys. Zeit.* 68:121, 1917.
7. Fidler, J. P., et al. Comparison of $CO_2$ laser excision of burns with the thermal knives. *Ann. N.Y. Acad. Sci.* 267:254, 1977.
8. Goldman, L., and Wilson, R. G. Treatment of basal cell epithelioma with laser radiation. *J.A.M.A.* 189:773, 1964.
9. Goldman, L. (ed.) *Third Conference on the Laser.* New York: Academy of Science, 1976.
10. Goldman, L., Naprstek, Z., and Johnson, J. Laser surgery of a digital angiosarcoma. *Cancer* 39:1738, 1977.
11. Hall, R. R., Hill, P. W., and Beach, A. D. A carbon dioxide surgical laser. *Ann. R. Coll. Surg. Engl.* 8:181, 1971.
12. Jako, G. J. Laser surgery of the vocal cords: An experimental study with $CO_2$ laser on dogs. *Laryngoscope* 82:2204, 1971.
13. Jako, G. J., et al. Experimental carbon dioxide laser surgery of the vocal cords. *Eye, Ear, Nose and Throat Monthly* 52:171, 1973.
14. Levine, N. S., et al. Clinical evaluation of the carbon dioxide laser for burn wound excision. A comparison of the laser, scalpel, and electrocautery. *J. Trauma* 15:800, 1975.
15. Mihashi, S., and Hirano, M. Surgical Application of $CO_2$ Laser in Otolaryngology. In I. Kaplan and P. W. Ascher (eds.), *Proceedings of the Third International Congress for Laser Surgery* (Graz). Tel-Aviv: Ot-Paz, 1979. Pp. 293-308.
16. Oosterhuis, J. W., Verschueren, R. C., and Oldhoff, J. Experimental surgery of the Cloudman S91 melanoma with $CO_2$ laser. *Acta Chir. Belg.* 74:422, 1975.
17. Patel, C. K. N. Continuous-wave laser action on vibrational rotational transitions of $CO_2$. *Phys. Rev.* 126:1187, 1964.
18. Patel, C. K. N. Vibrational Energy Transfer—an Efficient Means of Selective Excitation of Molecules. In P. L. Kelley, B. Lax, and P. E. Tannenwald (eds.), *Physics of Quantum Electronics.* New York: McGraw-Hill, 1966. Pp. 643-654.
19. Patel, C. K. N. High-power carbon dioxide lasers. *Sci. Am.* 219:22, 1968.
20. Polanyi, T., and Tobias, I. Principles and properties of the laser. Framington Center, Mass.: American Optical Corp. 1970.
21. Polanyi, T. G., Bredemeier, H. C., and Davis, T. W. A $CO_2$ laser for surgical research. *Med. Biol. Eng. Comput.* 8:541, 1970.
22. Schawlow, A. L., and Townes, C. H. Infrared and optical lasers. *Phys. Rev.* 42:1940, 1958.
23. Stellar, S., Cooper, M. D., and Young, J. Recent advances in neurosurgical treatment for the elderly. *J. Am. Geriatr. Soc.* 2:848, 1970.
24. Stellar, S., Polanyi, T. G., and Bredemeier, H. C. Experimental studies of the $CO_2$ laser as neurosurgical instrument. *Med. Biol. Eng. Comput.* 8:549, 1970.
25. Strong, M. S., and Jako, G. J. Laser surgery in the larynx. *Ann. Otolaryngol.* 81:791, 1972.
26. Strong, M. S., et al. Laser surgery in the aerodigestive tract. *Am. J. Surg.* 126:529, 1973.
27. Verschueren, R. C. *The $CO_2$ Laser in Tumor Surgery.* Amsterdam: Van Gorcum, 1976.
28. Wilpizeski, C. R. Otological Applications of Laser. In M. L. Wolbarst (ed.), *Laser Applications in Medicine and Biology*, Vol. 3. New York: Plenum, 1977. P. 289.

# Surgery of the Oviduct

The decade of the 1970s resulted in a dramatic change in surgery of the oviduct. The introduction of magnification and its acceptance since the first edition of this text proved a major advance in achieving the goals of surgical technique advocated by Rock and Mulligan, namely, meticulous hemostasis, atraumatic tissue handling, and accurate tissue reapproximation, all directed toward achieving a high pregnancy rate. This new approach, termed *microsurgery*, actually involved a refinement of recognized principles by a surgeon who simply could "see the tube better." Magnification provided by either the operating microscope or the ocular loupe quickly revealed to the surgeon that techniques previously thought to be meticulous were, in fact, often quite traumatic. These deficiencies were readily corrected, however, as the surgeon learned to work under magnifications of 10 and $20\times$ with suture material barely visible to the naked eye. The advent of microsurgery has given the infertility surgeon an appreciation of the exhilaration felt by Marion Sims a century ago as he watched sperm for the first time under the microscope.

Surgery of the fallopian tube directed toward improving fertility has long challenged the gynecologist. It became clear in a survey conducted by Greenhill in 1937 [84] that the average gynecologist, with minimal training in tubal surgery, had little success with these procedures. At that time, there were only a few centers where infertility surgery was performed in significant volume, and therefore, training in these techniques was available to only a few gynecologists and surgeons.

In the decades that followed, John Rock of Boston provided leadership and an impetus that led gynecologists to approach surgical correction of the blocked oviduct carefully and imaginatively in the laboratory and in the operating room. Centers devoted to evaluation and treatment of female infertility developed in Boston, Philadelphia, and Baltimore and later spread to many medical areas across the United States. In these centers, residents and fellows were able to observe and assist experienced infertility surgeons in the operating room.

Rock became the leading American proponent of tubal surgery in the early 1950s, as he worked to refine existing surgical techniques. Hellman [90], at Johns Hopkins Medical School, published a pioneering study in 1951 using a polyethylene splint in tubal surgery and noted the "impetus for this work was provided by Dr.

John Rock." Experimental data on tubal healing in the monkey published by Castallo in 1950 [26] added support to Hellman's clinical experience with polyethylene. In 1951, Israel [103] supported his clinical experiences with linear salpingostomy with experimental ducts treated in the same manner. During the next decade, many investigators attempted to maintain tubal patency after surgical repair by using fetal membranes or synthetic plastics to protect the opened stoma. The hoodlike device designed by Rock and Mulligan became the prototype of these devices.

During the decade of the 1960s, polyethylene was replaced by a more inert synthetic material, Silastic.* This material was used as a splint for end-to-end tubal anastomoses, for hoods after salpingostomy, and as a ring with limbs in cases of uterotubal implantation [117a]. Early studies published by Swolin [207, 208] and David et al [39] in the late 1960s provided a glimpse of the major change that was to take place during the following decade, namely, the introduction of microsurgery.

During the 1970s, an increased use of various cortisone regimens occurred, the most popular one combining dexamethasone and promethazine. Postoperative hydrotubation, although long advocated by Shirodkar [183], was revived by Grant in a well-documented study [81]. The use of magnification in oviductal surgery, however, was the major change during this decade, and its use rapidly became widespread following a flurry of successes in infertility surgery. Leaders in this field included Winston, Gomel, Diamond, and others.

Social changes occurred in the 1970s that made infertility surgery more important than ever. The increased incidence of pelvic infection and the use of the intrauterine device (IUD) added to the case load of the infertility surgeon, as did the increase in tubal pregnancy, presumably connected with the epidemic of gonorrheal infections. This change was accompanied by a virtual disappearance of babies for adoption.

Increasingly, couples sought treatment for infertility, and surgical correction of tubal pathology was necessary in many patients. Artificial oviducts made from appendix, ileum, bowel, artery, and vein grafts as well as molded plastic were tested and found unsuccessful. Tubal homotransplants were successful for the first time during the 1970s. At least four approaches to tubal transfer were attempted and reported successful. Allotransplants also were tried unsuccessfully, but the complications of immunosuppressive therapy appear to make this approach unacceptable even at the present time.

*Registered trademark of Dow Corning Corporation.

The first successful attempt at in vitro fertilization resulted in baby Louise Brown. Edwards and Steptoe [199], pioneers in the technique, reported four successes, of which two pregnancies produced normal live infants. A similar success was reported by Lopata et al. from Melbourne [126]. The first American center directed toward the study of in vitro fertilization was established by Georgeanna and Howard Jones in Norfolk, Virginia. Other American medical centers are presently pursuing this study, and at this writing numerous live births including twins have been reported.

Also of interest during 1979 was the report of pregnancy following low tubal ovum transfer [122]. Successful in 16 percent of 31 attempts in the monkey, this technique may provide hope for those patients in whom tubal reocclusion occurs following microsurgical salpingostomy.

In spite of these alternatives, microsurgical correction of tubal distortion continues to provide the major hope for pregnancy in the majority of women with oviductal disease. The specialist in female infertility must have both an appreciation of and experience with those surgical procedures designed to improve tubal function. The sections that follow are intended as partial satisfaction of this need.

**Salpingitis and Fertility**

Two changes since the first edition of the *Atlas of Infertility Surgery* have had a profound influence on the development of the field. The first, microsurgery, has permitted the infertility surgeon to see areas of tubal damage at magnifications previously available only to the pathologist. This technique has led to new methods of tubal repair and has resulted in pregnancy successes at almost twice the rate achieved by earlier surgical techniques. The second major change was the marked increase in patients whose tubal damage and infertile status resulted from prior pelvic inflammatory disease (PID) rather than endometriosis. This reflected a sweeping change in American sexual attitudes, as sexual intercourse outside marriage became socially acceptable. An epidemic of venereal disease due to the gonococcus, *Chlamydia, Trichomonas,* and herpes organisms became rampant in the American population under 40 years of age.

An in-depth understanding of the relationship between salpingitis and sterility in American women began to unfold during the 1970s. As the number of patients found to have acute salpingitis continued to rise, it became apparent that as many as 17 percent of these women would be sterile because of postinfection tubal occlusion. The gonococcus was found to account for only about 50 percent of these infections, while anaerobic bacteria, *Chlamydia, Mycoplasma,* and other organisms were responsible for an equal number of cases. The clinical diagnosis of acute salpingitis also became more specific with the use of routine diagnostic laparoscopy in these patients. Finally, this surge in patients requesting tubal repair was heralded by the microsurgeon, who achieved better results than ever when confronted with midtubal disease, but remained thwarted by the hydrosalpinx.

The leadership responsible for relating PID and subsequent sterility to the middle-class female came from the Department of Obstetrics and Gynecology at the University of Lund, Sweden. The initial impetus provided by Sjorvall in the 1950s was carried on by Sunden, Viberg, Jacobsen, Westrom, and others. These investigators anticipated the significance of the surge in acute pelvic infection that occurred in Scandinavia in the 1950s and 1960s and later swept through Europe and the United States. The studies from Lund involving the diagnosis and treatment of acute pelvic infection in unmarried female students and young professional women were carried out during the early 1960s. This homogeneous middle-class white female population was then followed during subsequent years of marriage and attempted pregnancy. This long-term prospective study by Swedish investigators has provided a framework for understanding the relationship between the disease process and subsequent sterility in terms highly relevant to the American gynecologist and infertility surgeon.

An interesting paradox in the American gynecologic literature has been the paucity of information and clinical perspectives relating to the long-term results of acute salpingitis in the middle-class American female. Although the incidence of reported cases of gonorrhea did not begin to rise in the United states until 1965, the ensuing 12 years resulted in a fourfold increase (Fig. 7-1). One million cases of gonorrhea were reported in the United States during 1978, and at least two authors have estimated that this number might be closer to 2 million, which is 1 case of gonorrhea for every 100 Americans [60,133]. Gonococcal salpingitis occurs in approximately 1 in 5 of these female patients but, as discussed later, is responsible for only one-half of all cases of acute PID. Overall, approximately 17 percent of women who have an attack of acute salpingitis will become sterile because of postinfection tubal occlusion [223].

**Figure 7-1.** Incidence of gonorrhea and syphilis in the United States,[a] 1919–1977.[b] (From W. McCormack, Sexually Transmitted Diseases: Incidence and Epidemiologic Considerations. In *Sexually Transmitted Disease.* New York: Science and Medicine, 1979.)

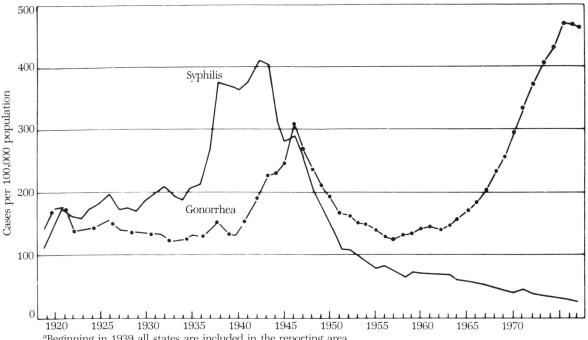

[a]Beginning in 1939 all states are included in the reporting area (military cases included 1919–1940; excluded thereafter).

[b]1919–1940 Fiscal years: Twelve month period ending June 30 of year specified—1919–1940
1941–1977 calendar years.

**Table 7-1.** Laparoscopic diagnosis of acute PID

| Author | No. of patients | Acute PID | | Normal | | Other | |
|---|---|---|---|---|---|---|---|
| Jacobson, 1964 | 218 | 155 | (71%) | 42 | (19%) | 21 | (10%) |
| Jacobson & Westrom, 1969 | 814 | 532 | (65%) | 184 | (23%) | 98 | (12%) |

This rapid rise in the incidence of acute PID has resulted in increasing numbers of patients with tubal adhesions and tubal occlusion. The incidence of endometriosis, the disease process most frequently responsible for tubal and ovarian pathology during the 1960s, lay behind this disease, previously found primarily in females of lower socioeconomic status. The balance clearly changed as the decade of the 1970s advanced, and as this decade closed, the infertility surgeon encountered tubal adhesions and tubal occlusion caused by a previous inflammatory insult far more often then the adhesion and cyst formation associated with endometriosis. This was exemplified by Patton's experience in 257 consecutive infertility laparotomies performed during the years 1977 to 1981. Endometriosis accounted for only 15 percent of the group; 5 percent of these married females underwent reversal of tubal sterilization; and 80 percent were found to have had a previous inflammatory insult involving previous surgery or salpingitis [156].

*Diagnosis*

Diagnostic laparoscopy is the key to an accurate diagnosis of acute salpingitis. In 1959, Sunden [204] reported the first group of patients with acute salpingitis diagnosed by visualization of the pelvis and treated conservatively with antibiotics. Following this initial study, enthusiasm for laparoscopic confirmation of the diagnosis of acute salpingitis developed at the University of Lund, and Jacobson [104] stated: "From 1960 onward, therefore, most of the cases seen in the department were diagnosed or confirmed visually." This gynecologist initially presented 216 patients seen between the years 1960 and 1962 and then expanded the group in a second paper in 1969 with Westrom [105] to include 905 patients with acute salpingitis seen between 1960 and 1967 at Lund. The laparoscopic visualization approach continued during the 1970s, and in 1976, Westrom et al. [224] reported the incidence of IUD usage in 515 patients with acute salpingitis confirmed by laparoscopy seen between the years 1971 and 1975. The diagnostic laparoscopic technique employed and a description of Jacobson's findings were discussed in Chapter 2 in the section on diagnostic laparoscopy. In brief, Jacobson stated: "As minimum criteria for the visual diagnosis of acute salpingitis, three signs had to be present: (1) hyperemia of the tubal surface, (2) edema of the tubal wall, and (3) a sticky exudate on the tubal surface and from the fimbriated end when patent" [104].

In the same paper, Jacobson found that only 71.1 percent (115) of patients suspected of having acute PID by clinical evaluation were actually infected when screened by laparoscopy. Visualization of the pelvis in these patients revealed that 19.3 percent were normal and 10 percent had other pathology that accounted for the symptoms. Only 41 percent of the infected patients in this series had cervical or peritoneal cultures that were positive for gonococcus, and 59 percent were, therefore, classified as nongonococcal. In 1969, Jacobson and Westrom [105] reported the clinical findings in 905 patients studied between the years 1960 and 1967. This included Jacobson's earlier patients and involved 814 patients suspected of having acute PID and 91 patients in whom PID was found unexpectedly after a diagnosis of appendicitis or ectopic pregnancy. In the group of 814 female patients suspected of harboring PID, the diagnosis was confirmed by laparoscopy in only 532 (65 percent); 23 percent had no evidence of pelvic pathology, while 12 percent had other diagnoses. These authors also identified a group of 91 patients in whom acute PID had been found unexpectedly and combined them with the earlier group of 532 patients to form a basic study group of 923 patients. The results of these two studies are summarized in Table 7-1. Jacobson, Westrom, and others [105,222,225] at Lund continue to perform diagnostic laparoscopy on all female patients suspected of acute PID. There has not been the same degree of emphasis on early diagnosis and aggressive treatment of this disease entity in the United States, as demonstrated by the comment by Sweet [206] that 66 to 70 percent of American women with acute PID are treated as outpatients.

The ages of the Swedish female patients found to have acute salpingitis were reported in the studies performed during the 1960s and 1970s (Table 7-2). As might be expected, Jacobson [104] found that most patients were young and unmarried. In this group, 76 percent were under 25 years of age, and "girls aged 15 to 19 years constituted no less than 45.4 percent, and 73.3 percent of the total group were unmarried." Jacobson also observed that "the class labeled as gonococcal salpingitis were on the average younger and more often unmarried than those classified as nongonococcal." These observations regarding age appear similar to those recorded by Westrom 12 years later, and the two studies are compared in Table 7-2. Again, 36 percent of patients were 20 years of age or younger, and 77 percent were 25 years or younger. In addition, 46 percent of those 25 years or younger had never been pregnant. Overall, 52 percent had not been pregnant prior to the episode of acute PID in the series reported by Westrom. These data are similar to reports of the age-specific rates of gonococcal infection in the United States by the Centers for Disease Control (CDC). During the calendar year 1974, females aged 15 to 19 years accounted for 1,342 cases, and the 20 to 24 age group accounted for 1,511 cases (Fig. 7-2).

**Table 7-2.** Age of patients with acute PID

| Age | 1961–1969 415 Patients[a] | 1971–1975 209 Patients[b] |
|---|---|---|
| <15 yrs. | 5.8% | 1.6% |
| 16–20 | 50.4 | 34 |
| 21–25 | 27.2 | 41 |
| 26–30 | 9.4 | 18 |
| 31–35 | 7.2 | 4 |

[a]From L. Westrom, Effect of acute pelvic inflammatory disease on fertility. *Am. J. Obstet. Gynecol.* 121:707, 1975.
[b]From L. Westrom, L. P. Bengtson, and P. A. Mardh, IUD and PID estimations of the risks of acquiring pelvic inflammatory disease in women using intra-uterine contraceptive devices as compared to nonusers. *Lancet* 2:221, 1976.

**Figure 7-2.** Gonorrhea: Age-specific case rates (cases per 100,000 population) by sex in the United States in the calendar year 1974.

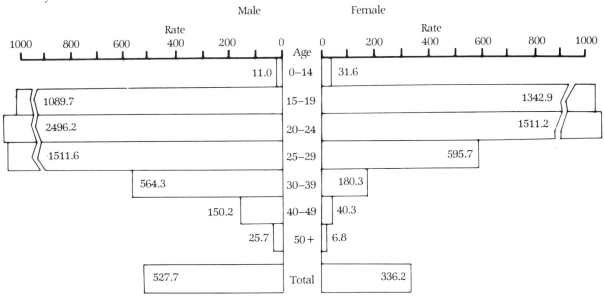

**Table 7-3.** Salpingitis seen at laparoscopy

| | |
|---|---|
| Mild | Tubes reddened, swollen, covered by purulent exudate; "violin string" adhesions or fibrin deposits; tubes open and freely movable |
| Moderate | As above; tubes not freely movable; tubal patency uncertain |
| Severe | Pelvioperitonitis and/or abscess formation; ostia closed |

Source: L. Westrom, Effect of acute pelvic inflammatory disease of fertility. *Am. J. Obstet. Gynecol.* 121:707, 1975.

### Classification of Salpingitis

The infertility surgeon deals with the end result of tubal infection rather than the acute process. This is clearly different from the surgeon's association with endometriosis, where progression of the disease entity is ongoing during treatment for infertility. The patient with tubal occlusion or tuboovarian adhesions resulting from previous acute salpingitis is usually in a stable state. Many patterns of adhesion formation are observed, and they are outlined later in this chapter. Degrees of tubal occlusion are also observed, and an attempt should be made to correlate these findings with the tubal pathology seen at laparoscopy, as well as with the microscopic pathology noted following removal of a tubal segment.

Classification of salpingitis may be considered in terms of the initial observation of acute PID seen at laparoscopy; the surgical classification, reflecting the results of the acute process seen a number of years later under the operating microscope; and the pathologic classification, reflecting tissue changes seen under the pathologist's microscope following tubal removal. Westrom classified acute salpingitis patients at laparoscopy as mild, moderate, or severe (Table 7-3). Westrom correlated these patterns of acute infection with postinfection tubal occlusion found years later and noted that 2.6 percent of patients in the mild category, 13.1 percent of the moderate group, and 28.6 percent of the severe group subsequently demonstrated tubal occlusion.

The aftermath of an acute pelvic inflammatory process is usually encountered a number of years later by the infertility surgeon when attempts are made to improve the functional capability of the involved oviduct. The incidence of a previous inflammatory insult was discussed in Chapter 2. In brief, Patton and Kistner [158] found, in a review of 467 consecutive laparoscopic procedures performed on infertile females, that evidence of prior pelvic infection was present in 48 percent, of whom prior surgery had taken place in 11 percent and endometriosis had occurred in 23 percent. Moreover, 29 percent of these patients appeared normal. As discussed later in this chapter, the residual effect of the disease process may be only a few filmy tubal adhesions or extensive scar formation associated with proximal and distal tubal occlusion and hydrosalpinx formation. The surgical procedures employed to restore tubal function are discussed later in this chapter.

### Pregnancy after Pelvic Inflammatory Disease

The occurrence of sterility in patients following salpingitis dates to early recorded history. During the 1800s and the beginning of the twentieth century, pregnancy was considered very unlikely after bilateral pyosalpinges. A review of Sunden [204] illustrates the point that prior to the use of antibiotic therapy, at most 20 percent of patients conceived following a pelvic infection. After the introduction of antibiotics in the post-World War II era, the pregnancy rates gradually rose, as will be discussed below. Coincident with this improvement in treatment, however, was a marked increase in the number of people with gonorrhea and subsequent salpingitis. Reported cases of gonorrhea in the United States increased from a low point in the 1950–1956 period to a sixfold increase in 1973. In 1977, Sweet [206] estimated that 250,000 to 272,000 women were admitted to hospitals in the United States and two to three times as many were treated with antibiotics in the early 1970s. It was estimated that 750,000 cases of acute PID may have occurred yearly during the 1970s. Despite antibiotics, therefore, increasing numbers of women in the United States have sustained damage to their fallopian tubes following salpingitis. Clearly, this has recently been reflected in the marked increase in the number of women requiring tubal surgery in an attempt to repair damage.

The epidemic of gonorrhea and acute salpingitis noted in American women occurred earlier in the Scandinavian countries. During the years 1945–1954, 944 cases (about 86 per year) of acute salpingitis were treated in Lund, Sweden. Among this group, 59 patients underwent direct visualization of the pelvis by exploratory laparotomy or laparoscopy. All were subsequently treated with hospitalization and antibiotics. A follow-up report in 1959 revealed that 30 of 52 patients (58 percent) had conceived. There were no ectopic pregnancies in this group, and the pregnancy rate was probably higher because patients who were voluntarily sterile were not included. Interest in direct visualization continued at Lund, and during the years 1960–1967, all patients suspected of acute salpingitis underwent diagnostic laparoscopy. The characteristics of this group have been described, and as noted, all underwent hospitalization and antibiotic therapy. In this study, 415 pa-

**Table 7-4.** The relationship of pregnancy and tubal occlusion to the degree of pathology seen at laparoscopy

| Group | Pregnant | Not pregnant, tubal occlusion |
|---|---|---|
| Mild | 76 | 2 (3%) |
| Moderate | 106 | 16 (13%) |
| Severe | 35 | 14 (29%) |

Source: L. Westrom, L. P. Bengtson, and P. A. Mardh, IUD and PID estimations of the risk of acquiring pelvic inflammatory disease in women using intra-uterine contraceptive devices as compared to nonusers. *Lancet* 2:221, 1976.

**Table 7-5.** Pregnancy after repetitive infections

| Infections | Pregnant | Not pregnant* |
|---|---|---|
| Once | 217 | 32 (13%) |
| Twice | 40 | 22 (35%) |
| Three or more | 6 | 18 (75%) |
| Total | 263 | 72 (21%) |

*Involuntary sterility—tubal occlusion; 16 patients not pregnant for other reasons.
Source: L. Westrom, Effect of acute pelvic inflammatory disease on fertility. *Am. J. Obstet. Gynecol.* 121:707, 1975.

tients who had no other abnormality that would affect fertility were studied and reported in the classic paper on this subject in 1975 by Westrom [223]. Overall, 53 percent of patients who had experienced acute PID conceived, including 5 who had undergone tubal surgery. When the group of patients who were voluntarily sterile were estimated, 79 percent of the study group were found to have conceived and 21 percent were found to be involuntarily sterile, presumably because of the prior salpingitis. The ectopic pregnancy rate in this group was 1 in 24 pregnancies, compared with 1 in 147 pregnancies in Westrom's control group.

It is well known that the severity of tubal damage is associated with a decreased pregnancy rate following tubal repair. However, laparoscopic observations at the time of acute salpingitis may also be correlated with the subsequent incidence of fertility. Westrom's classification into mild, moderate, and severe degrees of pelvic infection was discussed earlier. Table 7-4 demonstrates that as the severity of PID increased in girls expe-

riencing their first inflammatory episode, the incidence of subsequent tubal occlusion rose from 2 percent in the mild group to 29 percent in the severe group. Actually, this incidence of tubal occlusion appears low in view of the extensive inflammation present at laparoscopy. These results lend strong support to early specific diagnosis followed by intensive antibiotic therapy. Unfortunately, a comparable study in middle-class girls treated with either outpatient drug therapy or short-term hospitalization, so frequently employed in the United States, is not available. In a similar vein, the occurrence of repetitive infections also was correlated with increasing sterility. Table 7-5 presents Westrom's observation that 13 percent of patients were sterile following a single episode of pelvic inflammatory disease compared with 75 percent following three or more inflammatory episodes.

The results of microsurgical attempts to correct or reverse tubal deformities following salpingitis are discussed later in this chapter. Unfortunately, the Lund gynecologists were not as interested in the surgical aspect of PID as they were in primary diagnosis and therapy. Westrom commented briefly on patients in his series who had undergone conservative infertility surgery, including salpingolysis and salpingostomy. He reported that 88 of 415 patients were sterile, but that only 72 of these patients had tubal occlusion as a result of PID. Of the 72 patients with tubal occlusion, 35 underwent salpingolysis or salpingostomy and did not conceive. Five patients in Westrom's pregnant group achieved pregnancy after tubal surgery. Therefore, one can assume that 40 patients underwent a conservative infertility procedure, and 12.5 percent of these conceived. Unfortunately, the laparoscopic and hysterosalpingographic results observed in this infertile group were not detailed.

All recent long-term studies of pregnancy following prior episodes of acute PID have been published by Swedish gynecologists. A summary of these reports is listed in Table 7-6. Hedberg and Spetz [88] found that only 44 percent of their patients with acute salpingitis had positive gonococcal cultures. These patients were treated with penicillin, while nongonococcal patients, termed *septic salpingitis*, were treated with sulfa drugs in 13 percent of cases and streptomycin in 22 percent.

**Table 7-6.** Pregnancy rates following acute salpingitis

| Author | Study period | No. of patients | Follow-up | Crude pregnancies | Corrected pregnancies | Ectopic |
|---|---|---|---|---|---|---|
| Hedberg & Spetz, 1958 | 1946–1953 | 181 | ≥4 yrs. | 30% | 63 | 1 |
| Sunden, 1959 | 1945–1954 | 52 | 5 | 58 | — | 0 |
| Viberg, 1964 | 1958–1961 | 99 | 2 | 25 | 63 | 0 |
| Falk, 1965 | 1959–1962 | 281 | 2½ | 47 | 82 | 0 |
| Westrom, 1975 | 1960–1967 | 415 | 8 | 53 | 79 | 1:24 |

Remarkably, two-thirds of these patients received no antibiotic therapy. After an interval of at least 4 years, the corrected pregnancy rate in the patients with gonococcal related salpingitis was 67 percent, compared with 60 percent in the nongonococcal salpingitis patients. The overall corrected pregnancy rate in this study was 63 percent. Viberg [222] also compared antibiotic use in 108 patients with acute PID. These patients were randomly assigned to the antibiotic group (A) or the nonantibiotic group (C). Patients in the A group received penicillin and streptomycin, while patients in the C group were maintained at bed rest and did not receive antibiotics. Hospital time for patients in the A group was 26 days compared with an average of 25 days for the C group. There was no statistical difference between these two groups. Overall, 99 patients were followed by Viberg, and almost identical pregnancy rates were found in these two groups. The crude pregnancy rate of 25 percent rose to a corrected 53 percent when those patients who were voluntarily infertile were excluded.

Falk [58] attempted to study the effectiveness of antibiotics and prednisone therapy in the treatment of acute salpingitis. In this study, the A group consisted of 144 patients who received antibiotic and prednisone therapy, and these patients were compared with 139 patients in the C group who received only antibiotic therapy. All patients were hospitalized and placed at bed rest. After an interval of 2½ to 5 years, only two patients could not be located. Comparison revealed no difference in term pregnancy, involuntary sterility, or voluntary childlessness in the two groups. Overall, 47 percent had intrauterine pregnancies. However, this corrected to 82 percent when patients who were voluntarily childless were excluded. The frequency of sterility resulting from prior salpingitis was 19 percent in this series. Of interest, the corrected pregnancy rate in gonococcal-related salpingitis was 85 percent compared with 79 percent in the nongonococcal salpingitis patients.

### Salpingitis and the IUD

An accurate appraisal of the incidence of acute salpingitis and the subsequent degree of tubal damage associated with the use of the IUD is extremely difficult. Certainly the patient who has had a high fever and an elevated white blood cell count and sedimentation rate has experienced an episode of acute pelvic inflammatory disease and may sustain the usual sequelae. As will be discussed later, the presence of an IUD appears to increase the possibility that salpingitis will occur in a patient. The real question, however, is whether an entity

**Table 7-7.** IUD usage rates in patients with acute salpingitis

| Study | IUD users | IUD controls |
|---|---|---|
| Wright & Laemnle, 1968 | 66.2/1000 | 9.6/1000 |
| Noonan & Adams, 1974 | 81% | 47% |
| Targum & Wright, 1974 | 48% | 9% |
| Eschenbach, 1976 | 29% | 13% |
| Westrom et al., 1976 | 24.3% | 9.7% |
| Faulkner & Obey, 1976 | 38% | 11% |

such as "silent salpingitis" exists in a patient who experiences mild uterine cramps and irregular bleeding while using an IUD. Whether this clinical pattern is associated with development of pelvic adhesions, cornual occlusion, or hydrosalpinx formation in certain patients is at present unsettled. Increasingly, the presence of an IUD remains the most apparent clinical cause of these findings in many patients.

Use of the intrauterine device in the United States began in the late 1950s. A review of 22,403 women who used an IUD between 1959 and 1966 was published by Tietze [213] and concluded that "the PID rates among IUD users . . . for the first and second years after insertion do not appear unduly high." This initial optimism concerning IUDs has not been substantiated by recent clinical data from a number of centers, however. Table 7-7, published by Sweet [207] in 1977, dramatically illustrates an apparent association between salpingitis and PID in IUD users. Again, the work of Westrom et al. [224] at Lund appears representative of the middle-class female. During the years 1971–1975, 515 patients with acute salpingitis confirmed by laparoscopy were compared with 741 sexually active, matched controls. In the group of 515 patients found to have acute salpingitis, 24 percent were utilizing the IUD, compared with 9.7 percent of women of equal parity and age in the control group. This contrast was even more striking in the patients 16 to 20 years of age who had never been pregnant. Twenty-three percent of these younger patients found to have acute salpingitis utilized an IUD compared with 2.7 percent of the control group. Overall, 36 percent of the acute salpingitis cases occurred in the 16 to 20 age group, and 76 percent occurred in the 16 to 25 age group. Remarkably, 46 percent of these patients had never been pregnant. Westrom et al. concluded that a trend was observed in which "the younger the women, the greater the difference in IUD use between patients and controls." These authors also concluded that the risk of developing acute PID in a patient utilizing an IUD compared with one using another contraceptive was 3.1:1 for all women and 6.9:1 for women who had never been pregnant, compared with 1.7:1 for those who had previously been pregnant.

## Classifications of Tubal Surgery

In the first edition of the *Atlas*, we proposed the following classification of procedures utilized in tubal surgery:

1. Salpingolysis
2. Salpingoplasty
   a. Fimbriolysis: Separation of partially sealed fimbria
   b. Salpingostomy: Opening of a totally sealed oviduct
3. Uterotubal implantation
4. Midtubal reconstruction

The principles embodied in this classification have been incorporated into a somewhat different classification proposed by an ad hoc committee at the 1977 meeting of the International Fertility Society, in Miami Beach, Florida, under the Chairmanship of Raoul Palmer. This classification of surgical procedures involving the fallopian tube is listed below and is used throughout the chapter:

I. Lysis of adhesions (classified according to the adnexa with least pathology): Salpingolysis and/or ovariolysis
   a. Mild (less than 1 cm of tube or ovary involved in band or strings)
   b. Moderate (partially surrounding tube or ovary)
   c. Severe (encapsulating peritubal and/or periovarian adhesions)
II. Fimbrioplasty
   a. Deagglutination and/or dilation of fimbriae
   b. By incision of peritoneal ring
   c. By incision of tubal wall
III. Salpingoneostomy (salpingostomy)
   a. Terminal
   b. Midampullary (medial)
   c. Isthmic (including linear salpingostomy)
IV. Tubotubal anastomosis
   a. Intramural (tubocornual)
      1. Isthmic
      2. Ampullary
   b. Isthmic
      1. Isthmic
      2. Ampullary
   c. Ampullary
V. Tubouterine implantation
   a. Isthmic
   b. Ampullary
VI. Combinations
   a. Different operations on right and left tubes
   b. Multiple operations on the same tube

The distribution of patients into these groups will vary in different medical centers. Kistner, in Boston, has found a high incidence of endometriosis among patients undergoing infertility surgery and notes that many of these fall into the category salpingolysis and/or ovariolysis. In contrast, Patton, in Charleston, has noted a high proportion of patients in whom prior infection has been the etiologic process responsible for tubal disease. A significant number of these patients have been found to require fimbrioplasty or salpingostomy. Listed below are the types of procedures performed during 257 consecutive microsurgical operations involving disease of the fallopian tube personally performed by this author (G.W.P.).

| PROCEDURE | PERCENTAGE | NO. OF PATIENTS |
|---|---|---|
| Salpingolysis/ovariolysis | 18 | 46 |
| Fimbrioplasty (mixed and pure) | 26 | 67 |
| Salpingostomy (mixed and pure) | 32 | 82 |
| Tubal anastomosis | 19 | 51 |
| Tubal implantation | 5 | 11 |
| Total | | 257 |

## Salpingolysis and Ovariolysis

The surgical approach to removal of adhesions that involve the fallopian tube and ovary has changed dramatically since the first edition of this text. Although the number of patients undergoing only lysis of adhesions to improve fertility has probably not increased, there is no question that the number of surgical procedures performed following prior pelvic infection has increased dramatically, and in almost all these patients, adhesions that require excision are present. Lysis of tubal (salpingolysis) or ovarian (ovariolysis) adhesions, therefore, is performed in almost all procedures involving tubal damage other than those microsurgical operations performed for reversal of prior tubal sterilization.

The microsurgical approach to the repair of tubal disease has produced a significant change in the surgeon's approach to adhesions. The ability to clearly visualize each layer of filmy adhesion under magnification and to remove the entire layer of adhesion by cutting exactly at the reflection of the adhesion and the tubal serosa with a microelectrode, laser, or fine scissors begins to approach the goal of precise incision and absolute hemostasis.

The new classification of infertility surgical techniques discussed earlier describes lysis of adhesions as follows:

I. Lysis of adhesions: Salpingolysis and/or ovariolysis (classified according to the adenexa with the least pathology)
   a. Mild (less than 1 cm of tube or ovary involved in band or strings)
   b. Moderate (adhesions partially surrounding the tube or ovary)
   c. Severe (encapsulating peritubal and/or periovarian adhesions)

This classification clearly separates procedures involving salpingolysis from those involving fimbrioplasty (fimbriolysis). Emphyasis on this separation was made in the first edition of the *Atlas*, and recent clinical studies have supported this distinction [18, 50]. Although the classification into mild, moderate, and severe helps the surgeon define the extent of adhesive disease, the specific location of these adhesions is probably more significant in determining the chance of pregnancy following surgical removal.

Murray [142] has described the "peritoneal factor" in female infertility and suggested a concept that provides a functional approach to the treatment of periovarian and peritubal adhesions. He defined the *tuboovarian hiatus* as the space between the ovary and the tubal infundibulum. This hiatus is the site of the first stage of ovum transport following ovulation. However, it functions normally only if the tubal infundibulum (fimbria) is completely mobile and able to envelop the ovarian site at which follicular rupture and oocyte expulsion have occurred. Normal function of the mesotubarium ovarica (MTO) and fimbria ovarica (discussed later under fimbrioplasty) is essential. This concept also involves normal ovarian motility, presumably to permit contraction of periovarian muscle fibers, as well as normal function of the uteroovarian ligament. The belief that shortening of the uteroovarian ligament and the mesotubarium may occur at ovulation to permit egg pickup has been discussed [138, 148].

*Etiology of Pelvic Adhesions*

Three pathologic processes are the major factors responsible for the development of periovarian and peritubal adhesion formation. These are pelvic inflammation, endometriosis, and surgical trauma. The inflammatory process that produces acute endometriosis and salpingitis also may produce a pelvic peritoneal reaction characterized by erythema, a purulent exudate, fibroblast proliferation, and subsequent adhesion formation between the involved surfaces. The laparoscopic observations of Jackson and Westrom noted earlier described this acute reaction in detail [105]. A result of ascending gonococcal infection in less than half the cases, this process also may follow IUD-associated endometritis as well as post-abortal and posttraumatic endometritis. The texture of these adhesions varies from filmy, almost translucent sheets to dense scar. Fluid-filled vesicles and pocket formation are frequently encountered. The latter is responsible for the confinement of dye as often seen at hysterosalpingography. Surprisingly, tubal and fimbrial architecture may appear normal despite extensive filmy adhesion formation.

Pelvic scarring also may result from the inflammatory insult of a ruptured appendix and the peritoneal irritation that accompanies hemorrhage and surgical manipulation of a ruptured tubal pregnancy. Distortion of the tuboovarian relationship may occur subsequent to the surgical trauma, and adhesion formation may be associated with an ovarian cystectomy, wedge resection, myomectomy, and other surgical procedures designed to improve fertility. Bronson and Wallach [18] recently observed that in 15 of 35 patients undergoing lysis of adhesions for infertility, the etiology of the adhesion was unknown, and it was suggested that "ovarian bleeding associated with follicular rupture at the time of ovulation is more likely to produce significant adhesion formation than previously assumed."

The pathogenesis of tissue repair following a surgical insult to pelvic peritoneum and intraabdominal serosal surfaces has been extensively studied [56,93–95,165,178]. The surgical techniques utilized for removal of adhesions are designed to minimize the postoperative inflammatory reaction that occurs at the site of lysis. Appreciation of the concept of serosal repair aids the gynecologist involved in ovarian cystectomy or faced with removal of an ectopic pregnancy as well as the infertility microsurgeon. Minimal trauma to the surfaces involved is the hallmark of a successful repair.

An initial peritoneal insult destroys the tubal serosal surface (Fig. 7-3). Many authors have discussed the fragile nature of the pelvic peritoneum and, in particular, the serosal epithelium of the fallopian tube [9]. Small-vein permeability is thus increased by a host of permeability factors, including histamine release by mast cells and an accumulation of protein-rich fluid in the involved area. A portion of this exudate may then be removed by fibrinolytic activity, but the remaining portion of this fibrin clot is transformed into collagen by fibroplasia and is organized into scar tissue, termed *adhesions*. Bronson and Wallach [18] have emphasized a group of studies performed during the mid-1960s that contradict the excepted theory of serosal repair and indicate that peritoneum does not heal by ingrowth from the edges, as does skin. "Rather, the true nature of peritoneal repair involves either rapid transformation (within 72 hours) of fibroblasts to form new serosa or the implantation of freely floating mesothelial cells on the raw peritoneal surface" [18]. These authors conclude, therefore, that "large serosal defects would heal as rapidly as small ones." This controversial concept has been championed by Ellis [56], who found that a defect in parietal peritoneum healed without adhesion formation, as opposed to a similar lesion repaired with fine silk sutures in which many adhesions occurred. The suggestion was offered that attempting to cover a denuded surface with peritoneum did not necessarily prevent adhesion formation and might, in fact, increase the formation of adhesions. Bucknam and coworkers [21] discovered that plasminogen activator activity is normally present in the mesothelium and submesothelial blood vessels of peritoneum and that this activity results in the spontaneous lysis of many fibrinous attachments within 72 to 96 hours of development. Bucknam et al. concluded that "reperitonealization to prevent adhesions is an unnecessary and probably harmful practice." Ellis [56] suggested that adhesion formation in these cases was due to a vascular injury produced by the process of reperitonealization. These experimental studies were extended to include ischemic areas produced by crushing or ligating small areas of peritoneum, a process that consistently induced adhesion formation. Ellis also observed in a separate group of animals that a peritoneal graft increased the development of adhesions in that site significantly over a similar ungrafted area, which appeared to heal without adhesions. He theorized that adhesions induced by ischemic tissue represented vascular grafts to the involved surface that eventually becomes fibrotic when the normal blood supply to the area had been reestablished. A recent review of this concept has been published by DiZerega and Hodgia [51].

**Figure 7-3.** Summary of normal tissue repair and adhesion formation after surgical trauma. (From G. S. DiZerega, The Cause and Prevention of Postsurgical Adhesions. In H. J. Osofsky (ed.), *Advances in Clinical Obstetrics and Gynecology.* Baltimore: Williams & Wilkins, 1982. Vol. 1, pp. 277–289. © 1982, the Williams & Wilkins Co., Baltimore.)

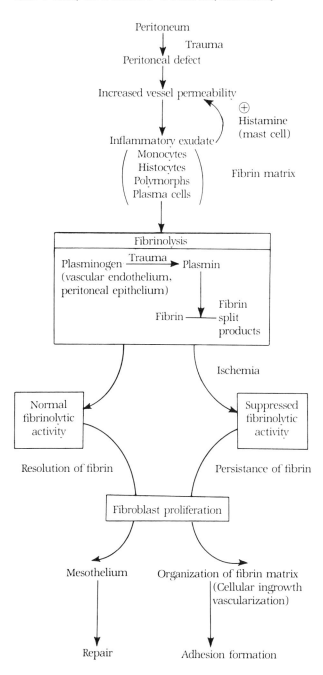

Other factors found to contribute to adhesion formation are drying of the serosa, contact with blood, infection, and foreign-body contamination [162]. Ryan et al. [172] observed that drying alone rarely induced adhesion formation, but that drying of the serosal surfaces and contact with blood produced significant adhesions. Continuous wetting of the involved peritoneal surface during microsurgery with physiologic fluids, including normal saline and Ringer's solution, has become a standard part of the surgical technique. Infection and foreign-body contamination have long been known to induce pelvic adhesion formation. Starch granules have been implicated in adhesion formation following previous surgery [239]. Suture material also may act as a foreign body in the induction of adhesions. The use of silk sutures in the studies of Ellis [56] produced significant postoperative adhesions. Synthetic absorbable suture material, now widely used in microsurgery, appears less reactive and is used in increasingly small gauges. The significance of infection as an etiologic factor in adhesion formation was discussed earlier in association with salpingitis. Prophylactic antibiotic therapy is widely employed following infertility surgery, although the benefit of this treatment is unconfirmed.

Clearly, additional studies of the type performed by Ellis and others [51,93–95,162] are necessary to direct the surgeon's approach to prevention of postoperative adhesions. Of particular significance is the role of electrosurgery in the healing process. This instrumentation, which "simultaneously cuts tissue and seals bleeding vessels" [50, page 291], is designed to "mobilize relatively untraumatized structures in a bloodless, ooze-free field with an intact peritoneum" [50, page 291]. These two quotations from Diamond clearly present the paradox of electrosurgical resection of pelvic adhesions. The question is whether the fine line that results following the use of an electrosurgical electrode and marked hemostasis will result in greater or lesser adhesion formation. Certainly, ischemia at this site will occur and would therefore be expected to contribute to adhesion formation along the line of incision. Utilization of a pure cutting current and bipolar coagulation of small vessels should minimize this insult. The role of the carbon dioxide laser was discussed in Chapter 6. Clearly, it has become essential to obtain a comparison between the degree of tissue damage associated with laser and microelectrode techniques.

Tubal and ovarian distortion caused by endometriosis and the relationship of this process to adhesion formation and infertility are discussed in Chapter 8. Obviously, endometriosis results in diminished conception by altering the oocyte pickup mechanism and tubal motility. However, abnormal follicular rupture and distortion of the posterior cul-de-sac are also possible causes. Correlation of these abnormalities is properly discussed here in this section on salpingolysis. However, procedures that include excision of endometriotic areas involving the ovaries are discussed in Chapter 8.

The surgical and medical regimens described later for the prevention of adhesions are designed to promote minimal tissue trauma and maximal healing of those surfaces which have been injured. Emphasis on meticulous surgical technique as the primary factor responsible for success is more important than ever. The introduction of magnification, improved lighting, and the microelectrosurgical electrode has been a major advance in the surgical approach to the removal of adhesions. Regimens that promote dissolution of the fibrinous exudate, separation of denuded surfaces, and delayed fibroblast proliferation and collagen formation will be discussed.

### Diagnosis of Pelvic Adhesions

Diagnostic procedures used to evaluate abnormal periovarian or peritubal fixation include hysterosalpingography, hysterosalpingography with pneumoperitoneum, and endoscopy (laparoscopy). These are described in Chapters 1 and 2. The role of carbon dioxide insufflation was discussed in the first edition of the *Atlas*. We feel that this technique does not provide significant information regarding adhesions and do not utilize it for this purpose.

Hysterosalpingography may suggest confinement of dye in the tubal infundibulum or lateral pelvis. The fallopian tube may appear stretched along the pelvic side wall, suggesting peritubal adhesions. Many workers use an oil-base dye [40% solution of iodized poppyseed oil (Ethiodiol)] to ensure persistence in the pelvic cavity in order to outline areas of pooling. In the normal pelvis, the dye disperses freely in the cul-de-sac and frequently outlines the loops of the small bowel as ellipses. We recommend a water-soluble dye (Sinografin) to avoid possible granuloma formation and uneven distribution. The dye should be injected under fluoroscopic control, and tubal distortion and pooling should be noted at the time. Oblique views of the pelvis assist in defining the exact area of confinement.

Unless one combines pneumoperitoneography and hysterosalpingography, it is impossible to define ovarian position and thus to evaluate the tuboovarian hiatus or the functional nature of the tubal pick-up mechanism. This combination has not been used by us.

We strongly advocate endoscopy as an integral part of an infertility evaluation (see Chapter 2). Studies reviewed in Chapter 2 compared the diagnostic accuracy of hysterosalpingography and laparoscopy and suggested that these two techniques were complimentary rather than competetive. The reader should recall that the hysterosalpingogram provides information regarding the interior of the fallopian tube and uterus. In comparison, a laparoscopic study visualizes the outside of these structures and the anatomic relationship of tubal fimbria and ovary. Both techniques provide important information regarding tubal anatomy, but laparoscopy is essential for the accurate diagnosis of tubal adhesions.

## Anatomic Forms of Tuboovarian Distortion

As was noted earlier, the processes that lead to formation of peritubal and periovarian adhesions are pelvic inflammation, endometriosis, and surgical trauma. The possibility of a fourth factor in association with bleeding at the time of ovulation has been discussed. These factors produce tuboovarian distortion by a variety of anatomic aberrations. However, three general patterns are most frequently encountered:

1. Fixation of the ovary to the broad ligament
2. Midtubal adhesion to the ovarian surface
3. Fimbrial adhesion to the ovary and broad ligament

Adhesion patterns are reflected in numerous drawings throughout this chapter. In particular, Figures 7-4 and 7-5 demonstrate these common patterns. Midtubal and fimbrial adhesions are depicted in Figure 7-4D and 7-4C. The reader will note fusion of the midtubal segment to the ovarian surface in Figure 7-4D, as well as other tubal and ovarian adhesions associated with the hydrosalpinx in Figure 7-8.

Lastly, it is important to keep in mind the difference between salpingolysis and fimbrioplasty. Although completely separate operative procedures, the two may be confused. In particular, *salpingolysis* refers to the excision of fimbrial-ovarian or fimbrial-peritoneal adhesions. *Fimbrioplasty*, however, refers to the removal of fimbrial-fimbrial adhesions and often involves the repair of a partially closed infundibulum. Fimbrioplasty implies a degree of fimbrial disease, albeit mild, and is in the spectrum of tubal disease that may lead to total occlusion requiring salpingoneostomy. Salpingolysis may involve fimbrial adhesions, but reflects an extrinsic process during which the fimbria have become adherent to another structure. The two processes may occur in the same patient. Commonly encountered tuboovarian adhesons are shown in Figure 7-4.

### Prevention of Adhesions

Since the beginning of this century, a truly enormous amount of work has been carried out on the prevention of adhesions. . . . perhaps in no other aspect of surgery does so much controversy exist.

ELLIS, 1971 [56]

Prevention of postoperative adhesions has been approached from various avenues. Factors that contribute to adhesion formation following surgery are listed below:

1. Vascular injury, ischemia
2. Drying
3. Blood
4. Infection
5. Foreign bodies

**Figure 7-4.** Tubo-ovarian distortion produced by adhesions. **A.** The most commonly encountered adhesion is that which fixes the inferior surface of the ovary to the broad ligament. In the mild form, a filmy adhesion will be seen extending from the ovary to a line along the broad ligament. In a severe case, this same process forms a pocket that almost completely encloses the ovary. Appreciation of this concept permits the surgeon to excise the adhesion at the line of peritoneal reflection and to watch the ovary pop out of this enclosure with minimal damage. Adhesions of this type may occur in association with endometriosis, following ovarian cystectomy, or possibly following rupture of a corpus luteum cyst. A previously ruptured appendix or ectopic pregnancy are also causes. **B.** The combination of ovarian and fimbrial adhesions to the broad ligament is usually associated with previous pelvic infection or prior pelvic surgery. This pattern often involves mild adhesion formation, yet clearly prevents ovum pickup. Surgical excision of these adhesions should be associated with excellent postoperative pregnancy results. **C.** Fimbrial adhesions to the ovarian surface may occur in association with endometriosis, but can be associated with prior ovarian surgery and possibly a ruptured corpus luteum cyst. Removal of this adhesion would be classified as salpingolysis and not fimbrioplasty. **D.** Adhesion formation between the midtubal area and the ovarian surface may occur in two forms. The first, a filmy adhesion, may be elevated with the glass rod and easily resected with a microelectrode. The second, a fusion-type adhesion between the tubal serosa and ovary, is much more difficult to resect and requires the operating microscope. **E.** Other patterns of adhesions are encountered in which the large and small intestine may be found adherent to the tubal, fimbria, or ovarian surfaces. This may be a single band (filmy adhesion) or involve extensive fixation as often found associated with endometriosis.

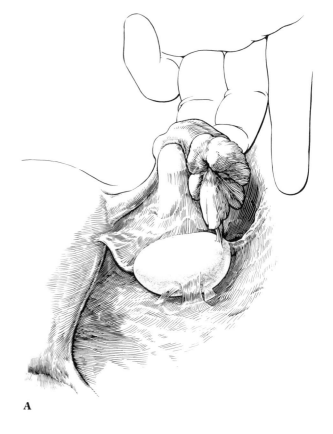

A

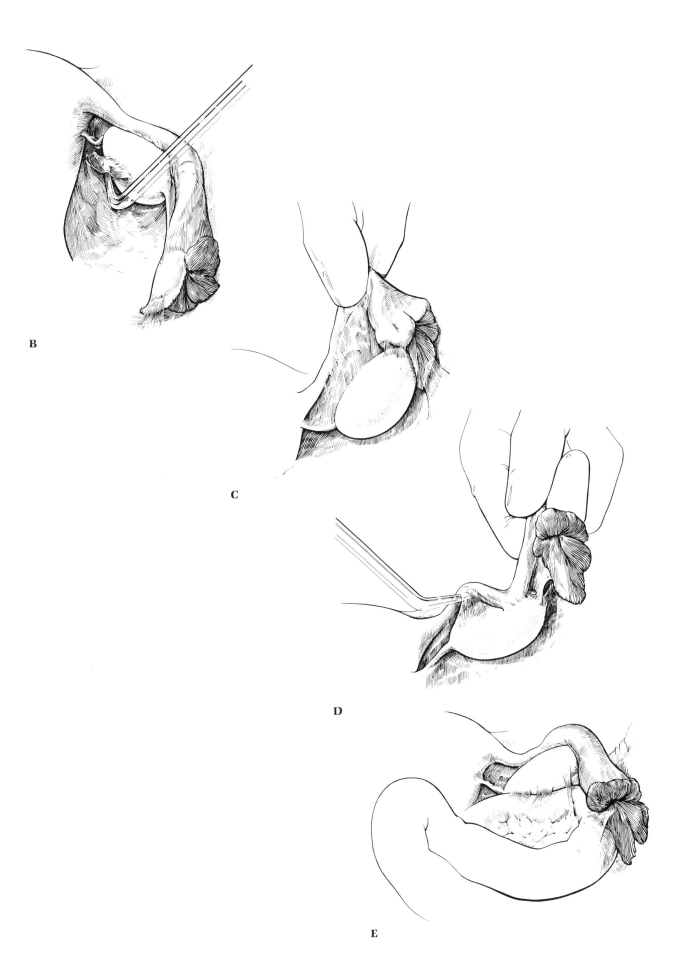

B

C

D

E

227

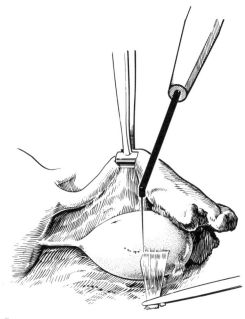

C

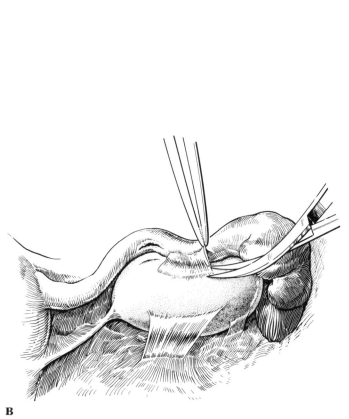

B

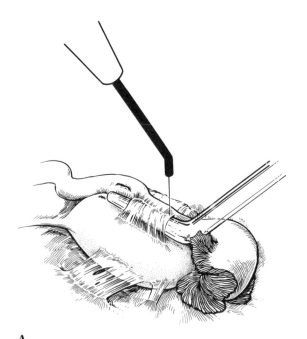

A

228

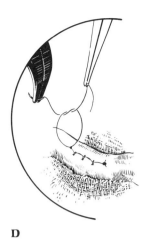

**D**

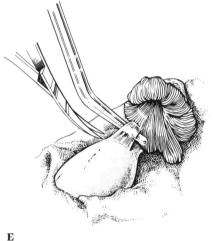

**E**

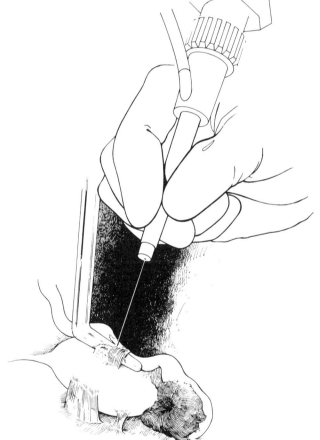

**F**

**Figure 7-5.** Salpingolysis and/or ovariolysis. **A.** The angled
end of a glass rod is slipped beneath the adhesion, exposing
the reflection between adhesion and tubal serosa. Using
magnification, the exact site of attachment to the tubal serosa can be identified and the adhesion cut with a fine microelectrode, virtually without damage to the oviduct. Small
blood vessels can be easily identified and electrocoagulated
when necessary. **B.** Elevation of these filmy tuboovarian
adhesions can be accomplished by gentle traction on the
adhesion with a fine forceps, as well as a glass rod. Wescott
scissors provide a curved blade convenient for excision of the
ovarian attachment of this adhesion. The tubal or peritoneal
reflection is usually cut with a microelectrode, as shown in
Figure 7-5A. **C.** The microelectrode is also a convenient instrument to use during excision of an ovarian adhesion since
small vessels can easily be electrocoagulated to provide an
almost "perfect" ovarian surface. **D.** A small defect on the
tubal serosa should be carefully closed with 8-0 synthetic
absorbable suture under magnification. **E.** Fimbrial adhesions must be handled with extreme care. The author performs this type of excision under the operating microscope.
Fimbrial adhesions to the ovary do not prevent the elevation
of this structure, which is accomplished during the first step
of a microsurgical procedure, and is usually performed
under loupe magnification. Certainly, the normal fimbria
ovarica should not be excised. The glass rod is used to elevate the adhesive band, permitting careful excision from the
ovarian surface. **F.** The hand held laser permits rapid vaporization of fine adhesions. It should be used with a quartz
rod as shown in this drawing. This technique is an alternative to that using the microelectrode (see Fig. 7-5A).

**Table 7-8.** Agents employed for adhesion prophylaxis[a]

| Intended mechanism | Agent |
| --- | --- |
| Inhibit inflammatory reaction and/or fibroplasia | Corticosteroids[b] |
| | Oxyphenbutazone |
| | Antihistamines[b] |
| | Cytotoxic agents |
| Inhibit coagulation | Heparin[b] |
| | Oral anticoagulants |
| | Peptone |
| | Citrates |
| | Hiruden |
| | Oxalates |
| Promote fibrin lysis | Amniotic fluid |
| | Fibrinolysin |
| | Hypertonic glucose |
| | Pepsin |
| | Sodium ricinolate |
| | Streptokinase |
| | Urokinase |
| | Actase |
| | Chymotrypsin |
| | Hyaluronidase |
| | Papain |
| | Protoporphyrin |
| | Streptodornase |
| | Trypsin |
| Mechanical separation | Albumin |
| | Bladder strips |
| | Chyle |
| | Crystalloid solutions[b] |
| | Fat |
| | Gelatin |
| | Lanolin |
| | Mineral oil |
| | Oxidized cellulose |
| | Peritoneum (carp, ox, shark) |
| | Polysiloxanes |
| | Silk and rubber sheets |
| | Vitreus of calf's eye |
| | Agar |
| | Aristol |
| | Camphorated oil |
| | Collodion |
| | Dextran[b] |
| | Fetal membranes |
| | Gum arabic |
| | Metal foils |
| | Olive oil |
| | Paraffin |
| | Pneumoperitoneum |
| | Povidine |
| | Vaseline |

[a]Other modalities include abdominal massage, colibactragen, iron/magnet, bowel stimulants, and diathermy.
[b]Agents presently used.
Source: G. Holtz, Prevention of postoperative adhesions. *J. Reprod. Med.* 24:141, 1980.

Meticulous surgical technique employing accurate hemostasis, fine nonreactive suture material, and constant irrigation was stressed earlier. The issue of whether reperitonealizing a denuded surface is beneficial has not been resolved, although we prefer to cover denuded areas when possible. This controversy also involves the use of peritoneal and omental grafts. The latter have been found to be extremely useful in covering large raw surfaces in patients with severe pelvic endometriosis.

The medical regimens designed to reduce postoperative adhesion formation may be divided into four categories and are listed in Table 7-8. At present, the following adjuncts to surgery of the oviduct are utilized by the authors for the prevention of postoperative adhesions:

1. Irrigating solutions:
   a. Ringer's lactate
   b. Ringer's lactate and heparin
2. Intraoperative 32% dextran 70 (Hyskon)
3. Preoperative and postoperative promethazine and dexamethasone
4. Prophylactic antibiotic therapy

Continuous irrigation of the pelvic organs during infertility surgery, initially proposed by Swolin [207,208], has become an integral part of microsurgical technique. A balanced salt solution, i.e., Ringer's lactate, has been advocated by Blandau [9] and appears to us to produce significantly less fimbrial edema than is encountered when normal saline is used. Addition of dilute heparin to the solution washes away fibrin deposition during the surgical procedure, permitting accurate hemostasis and resulting in a cleaner serosal surface. Anticoagulation with heparin citrate and dicumarol in numerous animal studies has been shown to effectively reduce the incidence of adhesions following intestinal manipulation. However, full systemic anticoagulation is necessary in order for the adhesion-reducing properties to be expressed [56]. The dangers of anticoagulation to patients undergoing surgical procedures are manifest and have led to the abandonment of this therapy. Cohen and Katz [35] reported instilling 2,500 units of heparin with dexamethasone intraoperatively at the time of peritoneal closure in infertility surgery without complication, however. This dosage is significantly lower than that employed by early investigators [16], and the effectiveness of this single small dose is unconfirmed. It is our present practice to add 5,000 units of heparin to 500 ml of Ringer's lactate solution, most of which is utilized as an irrigant during the surgical procedure. In addition, the pelvis is washed with this solution at the completion of surgery.

Dextran solutions of varying molecular weights and concentrations are presently of interest in the attempt to prevent postoperative adhesions. These solutions are slowly absorbed from the peritoneal cavity, and significant amounts of this fluid were present 5 to 10 days after intraperitoneal installation [163]. Dextran also appears to have a siliconizing effect on raw surfaces and to alter fibrin structure, making it more susceptible to plasmin digestion [163]. Low-molecular-weight dextran (dextran 40, Rheomacrodex) was first evaluated for adhesion prophylaxis in 1964 [30]. Reviews of studies with this solution have been reported by Holtz [93] and Pfeffer [162]. The clinical usefulness of this solution was never clearly established, and it did not become a popular postoperative adjunct.

More recently, high-molecular-weight 32% dextran 70 (Hyskon) has been of greater interest. Most studies of this solution have demonstrated its usefulness in preventing postoperative adhesions. Mazuji and Fahhyi [129] found dextran 75 to be effective in decreasing adhesion formation following initial peritoneal injury as well as following lysis of postoperative adhesions. Utian et al. [220] reported both a lower adhesion score and improved fertility when 6% dextran 70 or 32% dextran 70 (Hyskon) in dextrose was instilled intraperitoneally following bilateral tubal resection with subsequent reanastomosis. A similar decrease in adhesions was reported by Neuwrith and Khalaf [143]. More recently, a study performed in monkeys found small quantities of Hyskon highly effective in preventing adhesion formation and in maintaining tubal patency [51]. Holtz [93] has demonstrated that a low volume of 32% dextran 70 placed in the abdomen prior to closure will also reduce adhesion formation following a peritoneal insult. However, this low volume did not decrease adhesion formation following surgical lysis.

Few clinical studies with dextran are presently available. Utian et al. [220] reported the use of 6% dextran 70 in over 300 laparotomies without adverse effect, and Stangel et al. [198] have employed this fluid for intraoperative hydrotubation. Pfeffer [162] has recently reported that of 104 microsurgeons performing oviductal surgery, 45 stated that they utilized intraperitoneal dextran during these operative procedures. At present, no controlled studies evaluating the effectiveness of dextran 70 as an adhesion-reducing agent in humans have been reported.

The two remaining factors, i.e., dissolution of the fibrinous exudate and an attempt to delay fibroblast proliferation and collagen formation have been approached by a medical regimen that employs high doses of promethazine and dexamethasone before, during, and after surgery. First employed experimentally in dogs and later in babies and young children by Replogle et al. [165], this regimen was demonstrated to be associated with improved fertility rates following conservative pelvic operative procedures by a collaborative study involving 240 infertility patients [97]. Although promethazine-dexamethasone has been used by Seitz et al. clinically, their experimental study in the monkey [178] did not demonstrate a significant reduction in adhesion formation when this regimen was compared with intraabdominal saline alone. Extremely careful surgical technique was used in all animals, resulting in 75 percent improvement in both series. A control group was not employed. It is possible that meticulous surgical technique and the small numbers of animals may have blunted the difference in these two treatment regimens.

As described by Replogle et al., the goals of this medical regimen are to reduce the initial inflammatory response, which is characterized by small-blood-vessel dilatation, increased permeability, and exudate formation, by administering an antihistamine, namely, promethazine. Other studies have demonstrated that antihistamines may also delay fibroplasia. However, the inhibitory effects of corticosteroids on this process are well documented, and therefore, a large dose of dexamethasone was employed. Since the inflammatory reaction begins at the time of insult, this therapy was initiated preoperatively.

In the collaborative study by Home et al. [97], all patients were given 20 mg dexamethasone and 25 mg promethazine in separate syringes intramuscularly 2 to 3 hours before surgery. A similar amount of medication was instilled through a rubber catheter into the pelvic cavity prior to final closure of the peritoneum. Beginning 4 hours after surgery, the same dosage regimen was given 12 times at 4-hour intervals. We utilize this regimen on all patients unless acute or subacute pelvic infection is present. A concentrated solution of dexamethasone (Hexadrol) reduces the volume of each injection. Permanent suture material is used to close the fascial layer, and skin sutures are left in place for 10 days. If a suprapubic transverse incision is used, it may be closed with subcuticular 4-0 Dexon.

The use of preoperative and postoperative pseudopregnancy in patients operated on for endometriosis is discussed in Chapter 8. This hormonal therapy is recommended in patients with unresectable endometriosis or extensive involvement of the cul-de-sac.

Broad-spectrum antibiotics are utilized parenterally in all patients with pelvic inflammatory disease. These should be initiated during the procedure. Postoperatively, antibiotics are not given to patients operated on for endometriosis unless specifically indicated.

Postoperative hydrotubation has not been utilized routinely by us in patients undergoing salpingolysis only. Other surgeons have employed this technique in an effort to maintain tubal patency and to secure a high concentration of hydrocortisone and antibiotics in the peritubal area.

*Surgical Techniques of Salpingolysis and Ovariolysis*

The surgical approach to removal of adhesions involving the fallopian tube and/or ovary must incorporate the use of magnification and accessory lighting. As discussed in Chapter 5, difficult-to-reach adhesions involving the inferior surface of the ovary or tubal adhesions extending deep into the cul-de-sac are resected under loupe (2.5 to 4.5×) magnification and fiberoptic lighting provided by a headlamp. Once these adenexal structures can be brought into the plane of the incision and stabilized by packs placed in the pouch of Douglas, the operating microscope is brought into the field and additional tuboovarian and fimbrial-ovarian adhesions are resected. The ability to visualize the entire adhesion in detail permits the surgeon to accurately remove the band, leaving both peritoneal surfaces smooth and free of blood. It is this approach rather than the practice of simply cutting adhesive bands (lysis) without removal that represents the most significant recent change in this surgical technique.

Resection of adhesive bands is performed in most instances with a monopolar microelectrode. Although Swolin [207,208] is given credit for introducing electrosurgery into the field of infertility, Throwbridge [212], in 1929, was apparently the first surgeon to employ this technique during abdominal surgery. His publication, entitled "The Treatment of Abdominal Adhesions by Use of the Electro-Surgical Knife," presented 5 case reports. Throwbridge commented, "In all of my surgical operations during the past 2 years, the electrosurgical knife has displaced the regular scalpel. . . . The adhesions instead of being separated by moist gauze, or being severed by the ordinary knife or scissors are easily separated or cut by the electro-surgical knife leaving a surface sealed over with little or no tendency to adhere to any adjacent structures." This early technique employed the generator designed by Bovie, which delivered a far different current than that presently utilized by the microsurgeon (see Chapter 5).

Sheets of adhesions involving the fallopian tube are gently elevated by the assistant with a nonconducting glass or plastic rod. The surgeon is then able to cut the adhesion exactly at the line of peritoneal reflection with a high-frequency monopolar cutting current. Crushing instruments, i.e., forceps, are never used to grasp the tubal serosa. A tubal clamp designed by Diamond has been found to be useful for this purpose. Hemostasis is accomplished with bipolar coagulation of bleeding sites or with the monopolar needle. Small peritoneal defects are closed with 6-0 and 8-0 synthetic absorbable sutures. Occasionally, a peritoneal or omental patch is employed, particularly in patients with severe pelvic endometriosis (Fig. 7-5D). The admonition of Ellis [56], that tension on a suture line used to cover a denuded area may cause more adhesions than leaving the defect open, is always considered. The microsurgical techniques of salpingolysis and ovariolysis are shown in Figure 7-5.

LASER TECHNIQUE OF SALPINGOLYSIS

Adhesions can be excised by using a carbon dioxide laser beam. Bellina [6] uses power densities ranging from 2,000 to 10,000 W per square centimeter* (spot diameter .55 mm, power 5–24 watts). As shown in Figure 7-5C, each adhesion should be removed from its origin and insertion. The microelectrode has been demonstrated in Fig. 7-5A, however, the carbon dioxide laser used as a hand-held unit or attached to the operating microscope and controlled by a micromanipulator can also be used to cut adhesions (Fig. 7-5F). The dissipation of laser energy is limited, a characteristic that minimizes damage to adjacent tissue, particularly at reasonably high power. Therefore, adhesions arising from serosal surfaces of the bowel can be safely removed with the laser, a procedure not possible with microelectrosurgery. A quartz probe should be used to absorb excess laser energy, as shown in Figure 7-5F. These adhesions separate cleanly when gentle traction is applied.

Bellina [6] believes that all serosal surfaces from which an adhesion has been removed should be relasered with PD 800 to 1,000 W/per square centimeter* (spot diameter .55 mm, power 2–2.5 watts) to reduce postoperative adhesion formation. This procedure has been supported by second-look laparoscopy.

The physical properties of the laser beam permit the surgeon to direct it toward difficult-to-reach adhesions in the abdominal cavity by using a mirror to redirect the beam. Thus the surgeon can operate under such structures as the ovary and the fallopian tube, where adhesions and implants of endometriosis occur. Bellina has pioneered the use of a front-silvered mirror with an integrated light bundle to redirect the laser beam and thus remove adhesions that occur on the inferior and lateral surface on the ovary (see Figs. 8-7 and 8-8). Utilization of energy in this fashion to perform surgery is a unique characteristic of the new laser technology.

*Power density (PD) equals power in watts times 100, divided by the square of the spot diameter (in millimeters).

## Results

The incidence of salpingolysis in a collected series of infertility operations from various medical centers appears in Table 7-9. Variations from 4 to 76 percent were encountered, with an average incidence of 35 percent. The low incidence reported by Crane and Woodruff [37] (4 percent) and Siegler and Konlopoulos [188] (4 percent) was felt to be related to patient selection. In contrast, Garcia [66] reported that 133 of 176 patients (76 percent) required this procedure. However, this series included both fimbriolysis and salpingolysis. At the Boston Hospital for Women (now part of the Brigham and Women's Hospital) [240], salpingolysis was performed in 47 of 114 infertility operations (41 percent) on the residency service. In a collected series from seven hospitals reported by Horne and coworkers [97], salpingolysis alone was performed in 33 of 240 private patients (14 percent), but this operation was combined with other procedures in an additional 158 patients.

Pregnancy occurs in 31 to 63 percent of patients who have undergone macrosurgical salpingolysis, and term pregnancy is reported in 20 to 57 percent of these patients (Table 7-10). Ectopic pregnancy has been reported to occur in 4 to 6 percent of these patients. These reports, however, involve a nonmicrosurgical technique,

**Table 7-9.** Incidence of salpingolysis

| Author | Patients undergoing salpingolysis | Total patients in series | Percent salpingolysis |
|---|---|---|---|
| Arronet et al., 1969 | 46 | 173 | 27 |
| Grant, 1971 | 268 | 592 | 45 |
| Garcia, 1968 | 133 | 176 | 76 |
| Horne et al., 1973 | 33 | 240 | 14 |
| Crane & Woodruff, 1968 | 4 | 96 | 4 |
| Young et al., 1970 | 47 | 114 | 41 |
| Martius, 1959 | 138 | 399 | 35 |
| Siegler, 1969 | 4 | 115 | 3 |
| Hellman (literature survey), 1956 | 931 | 2285 | 41 |
| Moore-White, 1960 | 15 | 69 | 22 |
| Lamb & Moscovitz, 1972 | 46 | 100 | 46 |

**Table 7-10.** Pregnancy following macrosurgical salpinogolysis

| Author | Etiology | No. of patients | Pregnancy | Term pregnancy | Ectopic pregnancy | Comment |
|---|---|---|---|---|---|---|
| Arronet et al., 1969 | | 46 | 21 (46%) | 20 (43%) | 1 (2%) | Postoperative hydrotubation |
| Grant, 1971 | Sepsis | 142 | 63 (44%) | — | 8 (6%) | Preoperative pseudopregnancy in endometriosis |
| | Endometriosis | 126 | 55 (44%) | — | 2 (1.6%) | |
| | Total | 268 | 118 (44%) | | 10 (4%) | |
| Garcia, 1968 | | 133 | 71 (53%) | — | — | |
| Horne et al., 1973 | Inflammatory | 33 | 20 (61%) | 14 (42%) | 2 (6%) | Dexamethasone and promethazine |
| | Endometriosis | 48 | 19 (40%) | 14 (29%) | 1 (2%) | Pseudopregnancy |
| | Total | 81 | 39 (48%) | 28 (35%) | 3 (4%) | |
| Young et al., 1970 | | 47 | 18 (38%) | 15 (32%) | 2 (4%) | Residency service at Boston Hospital for Women (now part of the Brigham and Women's Hospital) |
| Murray, 1962 | | 102 | 32 (31%) | — | — | |
| Martius, 1959 | | 138 | 68 (49%) | 57 (41%) | 7 (5%) | |
| Lamb and Moscovitz, 1972 | | 46 | 17 (37%) | — | — | |
| Spangler et al., 1971 | Endometriosis | 101 | 52 (52%) | 47 (47%) | 0 | |
| Umezaki et al., 1974 | | 24 | 14 (58%) | — | — | |
| Bronson et al., 1977 | | 35 | 23 (63%) | | (4.5%) | |

and only Diamond [50] has reported a large series of patients who have undergone microsurgical salpingolysis.

Siegler and Kouloupoulos [188] found that lysis of adhesions was done in only 6 of 80 (8 percent) microsurgical procedures at Down State Medical Center, Brooklyn, New York. Patton [157] has noted a similar low incidence of pure cases of microsurgical salpingolysis covering 249 microsurgical procedures carried out during the years 1978–1980. It is assumed that the lower incidence of pure salpingolysis procedures noted by Siegler and Kouloupoulous and Patton is related to the use of magnification. Use of the operating microscope has revealed treatable tubal disease in the form of fimbrial adhesions and cornual occlusion that was either not previously recognized or not previously treated.

Diamond included only "those patients whose infertility was primarily due to adhesions and to adnexal fixation resulting from previous pelvic surgery" [50]. Patients with endometriosis and additional tubal disease were excluded from the survey. Diamond was able to increase total pregnancy from 34.1 to 61.4 percent while lowering the ectopic pregnancy rate from 11 to 1 percent. The uterine pregnancy rate therefore rose from 30 to 61 percent when a microsurgical approach was utilized by that author.

A study by Bronson and Wallach [18] that reported the results of nonmicrosurgical salpingolysis performed in 35 patients is often quoted. All patients were operated on by the same surgeon using "delicate surgical technique." Pregnancy occurred in 63 percent of these 35 patients, and only one pregnancy was ectopic (4.5 percent). Comparison of this study with results obtained by Diamond is not possible, because the indications for surgery in the two groups were quite different. Endometriosis occurred in 11 of 35 of the patients reported by Bronson and Wallach [18], and in 16 of 35 of the patients, the etiology of adhesion formation could not be determined. In contrast, all of Diamond's patients were felt to have tubal and ovarian adhesions caused by previous pelvic surgery performed for benign disease. Patients with endometriosis were not included in Diamond's report.

Kistner [117] reviewed his experience with endometriosis over 20 years and his data are presented in Chapter 8. Infertile patients with moderate or severe endometriosis, including ovarian endometriosis, underwent surgical excision. Approximately 33 percent of 338 patients were found at surgery to have tuboovarian, uteroovarian, or sigmoidovarian adhesions. Pregnancy occurred in 76 percent of 232 patients with endometriosis who did not have additional adhesions compared with 38 percent of those patients in whom adhesion formation complicated pelvic endometriosis.

## Fimbrioplasty and Salpingoneostomy (Salpingostomy)

Schroeder [175] is credited with one of the first attempts at salpingoplasty when he opened and repaired an infected fallopian tube of a 21-year-old female in 1884. Unfortunately, her postoperative fertility status was not reported. Skutsch, in 1889, appears to have been the first to use the term *salpingostomy* in its present context [191]. In 1903, Martin [128] reported 24 cases of tubal resection but only one pregnancy, a spontaneous abortion. Polk [164] and Burrage [24], and later Solomons [194], were also pioneers in this area of conservative surgery of the oviduct.

One of the first drawings of a salpingoplastic procedure was a linear salpingostomy reported by Gouillioud [79] in 1900. Ferguson, in 1903 [61], depicted a procedure that closely approximated the cuff technique popularized by Holden and Sovak [92].

### Definitions

Distortion of the fimbriated end of the fallopian tube may occur as partial or complete closure. In the first edition of the *Atlas*, the surgical procedures used for repair of these two conditions were considered under the term *salpingoplasty*. Repair of partial fimbrial occlusion was defined as *fimbriolysis*, and repair of total occlusion was termed *salpingostomy*. This classification is briefly outlined:

I. Salpingoplasty
   A. Fimbriolysis: Separation of partially sealed fimbria, leaving almost normal fimbria
   B. Salpingostomy: Technique for opening the distal portion of a completely sealed oviduct, including a hydrosalpinx

The essential factor in this classification was the combination of these two surgical procedures into a single category of fimbrial surgery, since both the etiologic disease processes and the surgical approach to these two patterns of fimbrial occlusion were felt to be similar.

In an attempt to standardize the classification of infertility surgical techniques, a somewhat different nomenclature (presented in detail at the beginning of this chapter) was agreed upon by an ad hoc committee at the 1977 meeting of the International Fertility Society. In regard to fimbrial surgery, the following categories were given:

II. Fimbrioplasty
   A. Deagglutination and/or dilation of fimbriae
   B. By incision of peritoneal ring
   C. By incision of tubal wall
III. Salpingoneostomy (salpingostomy)
   A. Terminal
   B. Midampullary (medial)
   C. Isthmus (including linear salpingostomy)

This new classification has been adopted in this text. Correlation has been made between the terms *fimbrioplasty* (previously fimbriolysis) and *salpingoneostomy* (salpingostomy), and the intended surgical procedures within the context permitted by drawings.

Although the distinction between these terms may appear clear, a recent review demonstrates a possible discrepancy in this view. The review by Siegler [187] defines salpingoneostomy as follows: "This operation is performed for distal obstruction in which no identifiable fimbria are seen or recovered." Fimbrioplasty is described as follows: "Often the radiologic and gross appearance of these club-shaped tubes is not distinguishable from the hydrosalpinx requiring salpingostomy." It appears that this reviewer considered fimbrioplasty to be the repair of a totally occluded distal oviduct in which recognizable fimbriae were recovered. In contrast, salpingoneostomy referred to a somewhat different surgical procedure, also on a totally occluded oviduct, in which no fimbriae were found. Neither Rock [167] nor the authors feel this was the intention of the new nomenclature.

In the discussion that follows, *fimbrioplasty* will refer to a surgical procedure performed for partial occlusion of the fimbria. This may occur in mild degree as agglutination of two or three folds, or it may appear as an infolding of the fimbria surrounded by a band, giving the appearance of almost total occlusion. It is our opinion that the infolding of the fimbria seen in these oviducts represents a mild degree of the disease process which in a severe form leads to complete closure and hydrosalpinx formation. If any opening exists in the distal tube, we would classify the restorative procedure as a fimbrioplasty. In contrast, *salpingoneostomy* (salpingostomy) refers to the repair of a totally occluded distal tube. In some cases, almost normal appearing fimbriae will exude from this new opening. However, in others, a bare, denuded surface will confront the surgeon. These degrees of fimbrial pathology found at salpingostomy have been classified and correlated with postoperative pregnancy rates later in this section.

*Etiology of Fimbrial Obstruction*

Fimbrial obstruction is most often a result of bacterial salpingitis or endometriosis. This blockage is but one of the sequelae of these disease processes, which may also be responsible for pelvic adhesions and cornual obstruction. Surgical trauma is an infrequent cause, although a ruptured appendix or ectopic pregnancy can be an etiologic factor. Fimbrial adhesions to ovarian endometriosis may also cause occlusion of the distal oviduct. Differentiation of the disease process involved in pelvic infection (intrinsic mucosal damage) and endometriosis (extrinsic damage) is important for proper surgical correction and evaluation of prognosis.

Occlusion of the distal oviduct may be only a loose agglutination of fimbrial strands, or it may be complete closure in which a mere dimple remains to identify the prior opening. Complete closure may result in fluid accumulation and distension of the ampullary portion, usually termed a *hydrosalpinx* or *sactosalpinx*. Unfortunately, the exact etiology of saccular distension of the tube is not clear. Novak et al. [145] believe this follows a pyosalpinx and is always the result of an infectious process. Others believe that any type of fimbrial obstruction may lead to hydrosalpinx formation.

Recent studies of human tubal fluid under normal conditions and in a hydrosalpinx have been reported. Moghissi [136], in 1970, studied the protein composition of tubal fluid from four normal women undergoing surgery for tubal ligation. He observed that the total protein concentration in tubal fluid was 3.26 gm/100 ml, which is only half as much protein as is present in serum. However, the electrophoretic patterns of the two fluids were similar. Immunoelectrophoretic studies revealed 15 different proteins in tubal fluid, with increased concentration of haptoglobin and cerruloplasm. Levels of IgA and IgG were comparable with those in serum, but IgM was found in only trace amounts in tubal fluid. David et al. found that sodium and chloride concentrations differed little from serum levels, but potassium levels were about twice the serum levels. In this study, total protein concentrations were only about 1.0 gm/100 ml [41].

Assays of similar components of hydrosalpinx fluid were reported by David and associates in 1969 [40]. These values revealed little difference from those found in normal tubal fluid. David et al. noted that the pH of hydrosalpinx fluid varied from 7.28 to 7.70. Results of protein electrophoresis of this fluid closely approximated normal serum values, with some reduction in the alpha$_1$-, alpha$_2$-, and gammaglobulin fractions. These latter results are comparable with the electrophoretic pattern of normal tubal fluid reported by Moghissi. The data of David and associates [40,41] on tubal fluid composition did not make it possible to differentiate between epithelial secretion and transudation through the wall from vascular channels as sources of this fluid. In view of the marked reduction in secretory cells in these fallopian tubes, "transudation and/or lack of reabsorption through the wall" was felt to be the major factor in fluid accumulation.

It is apparent that hydrosalpinx formation occurs after complete fimbrial occlusion, usually as a result of a prior episode of acute salpingitis. The relationship between PID and sterility was discussed earlier in this chapter. Unfortunately, the studies of fluid physiology associated with hydrosalpinx formation have not correlated these data with the state of the fimbriae at the time of investigation, nor have these data been useful thus far in predicting the potential regenerative capacity of the fimbriae. Evidence discussed later supports the belief that it is this regenerative capacity that determines subsequent pregnancy.

*Fimbrioplasty*

A review of the literature reveals remarkably little data relating to the surgical repair of partially sealed fimbriae. Discussed in the first edition of the *Atlas* as *fimbriolysis*, fimbrioplasty involves first the separation of agglutinated fimbriae, which are fimbriae that have adhered to each other by a firm scar. Second, fimbrioplasty refers to the opening of a partially occluded oviduct, which in our opinion appears to be a step prior to complete occlusion. This process involves an infolding of a fimbria that is encircled by a fibrous band. At times, this will appear as a constricting ring compressing a "tuft" of fimbria. However, the pathologic process of reaction to intrinsic tubal infection appears similar in both instances. A ruptured appendix or previous surgery may be responsible for fimbrial agglutination and tubal adhesions, but they do not lead to the process of gradual fimbrial infolding. Endometriosis is responsible for tubal adhesions to the ovary and broad ligaments, but these rarely lead to fimbrial agglutination. In most instances, the surgical procedure for resection of endometriosis will be classified under *salpingolysis*.

The number of patients whose infertile status appears to be caused by partial fimbrial closure and who subsequently undergo tubal surgery varies in different medical centers. This number is influenced by the indications used to select the patients for restorative tubal surgery, the classification scheme used to define these operations, and the pattern of referral in various communities. The change in selecting patients for infertility surgery is reflected in the practice at Johns Hopkins Medical University, where prior to 1974, "it was the general practice in the department not to operate on such patients . . . with patent tubes and peritubal adhesions . . . on the theory that if the tubes were really open, surgery could not improve the situation" [218]. Between 1965 and 1972, this concept changed, and 24 patients underwent salpingolysis, representing almost one-third of all infertility surgery cases during that interval. The

pregnancy rate in these patients was 58 percent, thus raising the overall pregnancy rate during 1965–1972 to 39.4 percent compared with 23.2 percent for the years 1940–1965, when only 4 of 82 patients underwent salpingolysis. The Johns Hopkins study also demonstrates the confusion associated with previous classification schemes. The authors used the term *fimbrioplasty* to refer to a surgical procedure performed for totally occluded oviducts, i.e., salpingoneostomy in the present terminology. The authors did not include a separate category for those surgical procedures involving repair of partial fimbrial occlusion, probably including these patients in the category *salpingolysis and/or ovariolysis* [218]. Certainly Garcia's early data appear to place these patients in the group termed *salpingolysis* [66]. In contrast, Palmer [152], the chairman of the ad hoc committee that outlined the present classification, used the term *codonolysis* to refer to a surgical technique "which is gentle separation of agglutinated fimbria." We emphasized in the first edition that surgical procedures involving partially agglutinated or partially sealed fimbriae should be included in a separate category, i.e., fimbriolysis. These patients should not be included in the salpingostomy group, nor in the group of patients who undergo lysis of adhesions, because the prognosis for pregnancy in each of these groups is quite different.

Finally, it would appear that the practice of referral in each community influences the selection of these surgical procedures. Kistner in Boston has noted a high proportion of endometriosis in patients undergoing infertility surgery. This has also been noted by Shapiro in Madison, Wisconsin [179]. Patton in Charleston has noted that a large portion of his surgical patients in a private middle-class practice have undergone a previous inflammatory insult. In this regard, Patton has noted that during 1978–1979, approximately 60 percent of 145 patients undergoing infertility surgery had fimbrial disease, presumably related to a previous inflammatory insult, since in none of these patients was endometriosis observed. In one-half of these 80 patients, partial fimbrial occlusion was encountered, such that in these patients, fimbrioplasty and salpingostomy were performed in almost equal numbers. The pregnancy rate in the two groups is significantly different and will be discussed later. These cases did not include those patients in whom endometriosis was responsible for adhesion formation. Most patients with endometriosis undergo salpingolysis and/or ovariolysis. However, when a fimbrioplasty is performed in a patient, a proper appreciation of prognosis is obtained by separating endometriosis and nonendometriosis patients. A point of confusion occurs when fimbrial adhesions occur to a site of ovarian endometriosis. In general, we have classified these patients as salpingolysis, not as fimbrioplasty, since endometriosis rarely involves the fimbriae primarily.

*Surgical Technique of Fimbrioplasty*

A. Deagglutination and/or dilation of fimbriae
B. Incision of peritoneal ring
C. Incision of tubal wall

The microsurgical technique of fimbrioplasty is similar to that employed during salpingoneostomy with minor variations. Magnification is essential and may be accomplished by the use of a loupe (4.5×) and fiberoptic headlamp or the operating microscope. We have found the operating microscope to be essential during salpingostomy, and we also employ it during almost all cases of partial fimbrial occlusion. Since it is our practice to begin an infertility operation with excision of adhesions present in almost all patients to some degree, and since this procedure is performed with the aid of an ocular loupe and headlamp, inspection of the fimbriae under loupe magnification is frequently performed. At this point the surgeon must determine whether the degree of magnification is adequate for fimbrioplasty. In most cases it will not be adequate, and one must be able to switch quickly to the operating microscope. As was discussed in Chapter 5, the ability to change easily from the loupe and headlamp to the microscope requires extensive preoperative operating room organization. Our microsurgical technique of fimbrioplasty was outlined earlier [155].

USEFUL INSTRUMENTS

1. Operating microscope: The OpMi-7ph or OpMi-6s ph is used for most cases of advanced partial occlusion. The ocular loupe (4.5×) and fiberoptic headlamp are also useful for mild degrees of agglutination.

2. Microelectrode: The fine monopolar microelectrode is employed to cut fimbrial adhesions. Bipolar current is used for coagulating small bleeding vessels.

3. Special operating room table, i.e., Kifa, that permits the surgeon to sit comfortably.

4. Glass or Teflon rods: An essential tool.

5. Fine angled scissors: Also useful.

6. Heparin-Ringer's lactate irrigating solution: 5000 units heparin diluted in 500 ml Ringer's lactate.

DEAGGLUTINATION AND/OR DILATION

We no longer use the dilation technique of fimbrioplasty described earlier [5a], because under magnification it is possible to see the exact site of fimbrial agglutination. Large, coiled fimbrial vessels will be seen in each fimbrial strand and easily avoided. In the accompanying drawings, the glass rod is used to identify and elevate a site of fimbrial adhesion. This adhesion is usually firm and requires surgical separation with either a microelectrode or scissors. Small bleeding sites are coagulated with bipolar current. The technique of fimbrial deagglutination is shown in Figure 7-6 A and B.

INCISION OF PERITONEAL RING AND/OR TUBAL WALL

The most commonly encountered condition requiring microsurgical fimbrioplasty appears as a ring of scar tissue that has compressed a tuft of fimbria. The fimbrial elements appear to have been enfolded inward by this process, which constricts the distal opening in various degrees. The mild form may represent the condition referred to as *tubal phimosis*, while in the severe form the tube appears very similar to a hydrosalpinx until a small opening is located, usually by a small fragment of fimbria. This technique is shown in Figure 7-6 C through F.

**Figure 7-6.** Fimbrioplasty. Technique of deagglutination and dilatation: **A.** The glass rod is used to identify and to elevate a site of fimbrial adhesion (agglutination). This adhesion will usually be firm and require surgical separation by a microelectrode. The avascular line of agglutination can be seen under magnification and cut with the microelectrode. It is essential to use a nonconducting probe (i.e., a glass rod) with electrosurgical cutting current to avoid damage to surrounding tissue. Small bleeding sites are coagulated with bipolar current. **B.** A second approach to the removal of fine fimbrial adhesions uses a small probe (i.e., a Winston probe) to elevate the filmy adhesion, which is then cut with a small angled iris scissor under high magnification. A microelectrode should not be used in combination with a metal conducting probe. Incision of peritoneal ring and/or tubal wall: **C.** The most commonly encountered condition requiring fimbrioplasty appears as a partial enfolding of the fimbria resulting in a constricting ring as this scar tissue compresses a tuft of fimbria. The area of the fimbria ovarica has been completely covered. Tubal patency is easily demonstrated by hysterosalpingography and at the time of surgery. **D.** Under magnification provided by the operating microscope, the avascular lines of scar formation can be easily visualized and cut. Elevation of this area with the glass rod and incision with a microelectrode has been demonstrated. Scissors may also be employed for this purpose. The fimbria will be seen to "pop out" following this line of incision and will appear almost normal. **E.** The area of the fimbria ovarica should be carefully studied under magnification before an incision is made. Pressure with a glass rod or a metal probe will usually identify the area of agglutination and permit incision with a total release of this important fimbrial element.

**F.** The outcome of microsurgical fimbrioplasty results in an almost normal appearing fimbrial structure. The fimbria ovarica and mesotubarium ovarica have been completely preserved. One or two sutures of 8-0 synthetic absorbable suture or a small atraumatic needle may be employed to cover denuded serosal surfaces with fimbrial folds.

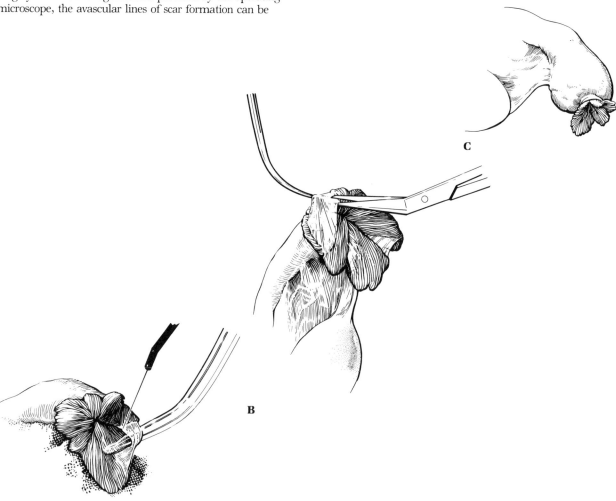

C

B

A

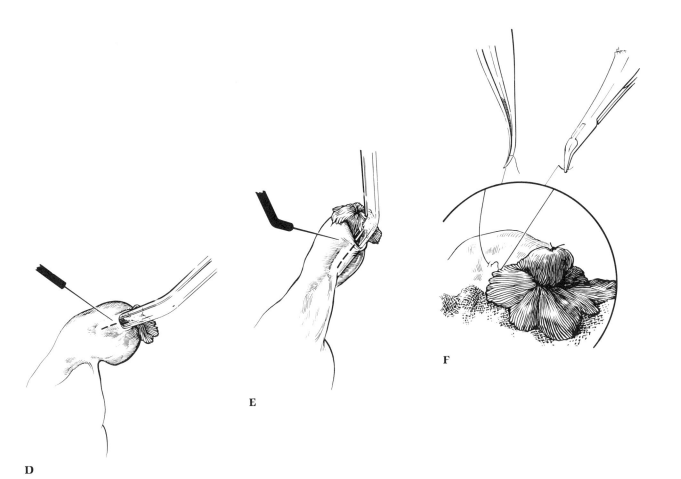

D

E

F

**Table 7-11.** Pregnancy following fimbrioplasty

| Surgeon | No. of patients | Percent uterine | Percent ectopic | Percent total | Technique |
|---|---|---|---|---|---|
| Palmer, 1960 | 10 | 40 | 20 | 50 | Macrosurgical |
| Swolin, 1967 | 20 | 20 | 0 | 20 | Microsurgical |
| Siegler, 1979 | | | | | |
|     Macrosurgical | 11 | 18 | 50 | 36 | |
|     Microsurgical* | 9 | 56 | 17 | 67 | |
| Patton, 1982* | 40 | 63 | 5 | 68 | Microsurgical |

*Microsurgical fimbrioplasty.

**Table 7-12.** Pregnancy following microsurgical fimbrioplasty*

| Group | No. of patients | Uterine pregnancies | Ectopic | Total |
|---|---|---|---|---|
| Pure | 35 | 60% (21) | 3% (1) | 63% (22) |
| Mixed | 5 | 80% (4) | 20% (1) | 100% (5) |
|     Total | 40 | 63% | 5% | 68% |

*Numbers of patients are listed in parentheses.
Source: G. W. Patton, Pregnancy outcome following microsurgical fimbrioplasty. *Fertil. Steril.* 37:150, 1982.

### Results of Fimbrioplasty

As was noted earlier, there are few clinical studies of infertility operations that fit clearly into this classification. Palmer, in 1960, performed "gentle separation of agglutinated fimbria" [152] in 10 patients, of whom 5 became pregnant (1 with an ectopic pregnancy). In addition, 41 patients underwent a terminal salpingostomy in Palmer's series, and postoperative pregnancy occurred in only 20 percent. In Swolin's now classic report of microsurgical salpingostomy, first published in 1967, in addition to 33 patients who underwent a salpingostomy procedure, 10 patients underwent salpingolysis. Only 2 of these 10 patients who presumably had a fimbrioplasty procedure had a subsequent pregnancy [207,208]. A detailed report of pregnancy in the salpingostomy group is presented later in this chapter. Siegler and Konlopoulous have reported 11 patients who underwent macrosurgical fimbrioplasty and 9 who had fimbrioplasty by a microsurgical approach [188]. In the macrosurgical group, 4 patients conceived, but 2 of these had a tubal pregnancy. In contrast, 6 of 9 patients conceived after microsurgical fimbrioplasty, and only 1 of the 6 pregnancies was ectopic. The uterine pregnancy rate in this small group of patients was, therefore, 56 percent (Table 7-11).

Patton [155] has recently reported the results of microsurgical fimbrioplasty in 40 patients operated on during the years 1978–1979. These patients accounted for almost one-half the patients with fimbrial disease and for 29 percent of the 140 patients operated on for infertility during these 2 years. Remarkably, 74 percent of the 23 patients who underwent microsurgical fimbrioplasty during 1978 conceived. There was only 1 ectopic pregnancy associated with a pure fimbrioplasty procedure. Five of 40 patients underwent fimbrioplasty on one tube and salpingostomy on the other. All 5 conceived after surgery, and only 1 of these 5 pregnancies was ectopic. In the group of 40 patients, pregnancy occurred in 65 percent, and ectopic pregnancy occurred in 4.5 percent of pregnancies or in 2.5 percent of all surgical cases (Table 7-12).

A high proportion of postoperative pregnancies following microsurgical fimbrioplasty occurred during the first postoperative year, in contrast to a delayed pattern found by Rock et al. [167], Gomel [76], and Swolin [210] following salpingostomy. Patton [155] noted that 46 percent of those patients achieving a pregnancy following microsurgical fimbrioplasty did so within 3 months of surgery and 81 percent did so within the first year. However, 26 percent of patients attempting a pregnancy during the second postoperative year were successful (Table 7-13).

**Table 7-13.** Interval between microsurgical fimbioplasty and pregnancy

| Months | Pregnancies | Cumulative pregnancy rate (%) | Percent total pregnancies | Chance of pregnancy | |
|---|---|---|---|---|---|
| | | | | Fraction | Percent |
| 1–3 | 12 | 30 | 44 | 12/40 | 30 |
| 4–6 | 3 | 38 | 11 | 3/28 | 11 |
| 7–12 | 6 | 53 | 22 | 6/25 | 24 |
| 13–24 | 6 | 68 | 22 | 6/19 | 32 |

Source: G. W. Patton, Pregnancy outcome following microsurgical fimbrioplasty. *Fertil. Steril.* 37:150, 1982.

It would appear that microsurgical fimbrioplasty results in a high incidence of postoperative pregnancy because of degree of fimbrial damage is slight. The data presented by Patton [155] may be compared to that of Rock et al. [167], in which patients who underwent salpingostomy for total tubal occlusion were classified according to the extent of tubal damage. In this retrospective study from Johns Hopkins Hospital, Rock et al. noted that in a group of patients in whom recognizable fimbriae were encountered during the operative procedure leading to a diagnosis of mild tubal damage, pregnancy occurred in 67 percent, and only 1 of 13 patients had an ectopic pregnancy. In contrast, 30 patients in whom the extent of distal tubal damage was classified as moderate had a postoperative intrauterine pregnancy rate of 17 percent, and 4 of 9 pregnancies were ectopic.

Thus when excellent fimbriae are encountered following surgical repair by salpingostomy, as reported by Rock et al. [167], or following microsurgical fimbrioplasty, as noted by Patton [155], excellent pregnancy results with a low rate of ectopic pregnancy can be expected. The treatment of different degrees of fimbrial damage occurring in the same patient has not been established. The unanswered question relates to the management of patients in whom total fimbrial occlusion is found in one tube and partial occlusion in the opposite tube. The lower pregnancy rate and higher ectopic occurrence following repair of totally occluded oviducts would suggest the possible removal of the totally occluded tube when partial occlusion is encountered in the opposite oviduct. All 5 patients in the mixed fimbrioplasty-salpingostomy group reported earlier [155] conceived postoperatively, and only 1 of the five pregnancies was ectopic. The single ectopic pregnancy occurred in a tube that had undergone a microsurgical salpingostomy procedure. It is significant that the fimbriae of the totally occluded oviducts in this series reported by Patton were graded as moderate or excellent in all 5 patients [155]. The classification proposed by Rock et al. [167] should assist in delineating the prognosis for pregnancy in patients with total fimbrial occlusion. Certainly, in those patients whose distal oviduct meets the criteria of Rock et al. for moderate or severe disease, the tube should be removed if the contralateral fimbriae are almost normal. It appears, however, that the combination of partial and complete fimbrial occlusion usually reflects a mild inflammatory insult, and it is therefore unusual to find severe disease in the presence of a contralateral oviduct that is partially occluded.

## Salpingoneostomy (Salpingostomy)

Perhaps no other problem in the surgical treatment of the infertile patient arouses more controversy and has more emotional impact than does treatment of a terminal hydrosalpinx. It is generally agreed that the failure to achieve pregnancy after opening a cystically dilated tube and creating a new stoma rests on prior deterioration of tubal structures and the inability of the surgical corrected tube to recover normal physiologic mechanisms. This failure may involve many aspects of tubal physiology and biochemistry, including the following:

1. Failure of adequate regeneration of mucosal elements
2. Failure of regenerated secretory elements to function normally, i.e., abnormal tubal fluid
3. Failure of distorted and stretched muscle fibers to return to normal, resulting in abnormal tubal peristalsis
4. Failure of obstructed lymphatic or vascular channels to recanalize, possibly contributing to abnormal tubal secretion or abnormal intraoviductal oxygen tension surrounding the incubating egg, sperm, or blastula

The surgeon must attempt to establish an accurate prognosis in a specific patient with a hydrosalpinx. Preoperative evaluation would be of utmost value in selecting patients in whom salpingostomy would be useful. However, at present proper classification can be made only during surgery. We have presented a classification scheme that provides useful prognostic information. At the Boston Hospital for Women (now part of the Brigham and Women's Hospital), as well as at other centers, pregnancy outcome has been correlated with the presence or absence of rugal patterns on preoperative hysterosalpingography [167,240]. Pregnancy occurred in 70.3 percent of 37 patients with moderate to excellent rugal patterns and in 42.1 percent of 19 patients with poor rugae. In contrast, only 7.4 percent of 41 patients with no demonstrable rugae conceived postoperatively. In summary, if the patients at the Boston Hospital for Women were classified according to the presence or absence of rugae on the hysterosalpingogram, pregnancy occurred in 65 and 7.4 percent, respectively.

Shirodkar [183] has classified oviductal hydrosalpinx formation into two groups on the basis of digital size: grade 1, fallopian tube dilatation ranging from the size of the little finger to that of the thumb; and grade 2, fallopian tube dilatation greater than the size of the thumb.

The best pregnancy results occurred in reconstruction of grade 1 hydrosalpinges. Shirodkar noted that the result of salpingostomy depended on the condition of the fimbriae, tubal muscularis, and ciliated epithelium. He noted that grade 1 was the preferred size because of the likelihood of preserving these three anatomic structures in the smaller hydrosalpinx. Determination of prognosis remained difficult, however, since only the state of the fimbriae could be adequately judged at the time of surgery. When the fimbriae were of normal length and

**Table 7-14.** Classification of the extent of tubal disease with distal fimbrial obstruction

| Extent of disease | Findings |
|---|---|
| Mild | Absent or small hydrosalpinx ≤ 15 mm diameter |
| | Inverted fimbria easily recognized when patency achieved |
| | No significant peritubal or periovarian adhesions |
| | Preoperative hysterogram reveals a rugal pattern |
| Moderate | Hydrosalpinx 15–30 mm diameter |
| | Fragments of fimbria not readily identified |
| | Periovarian and/or peritubular adhesions without fixation, minimal cul-de-sac adhesions |
| | Absence of a rugal pattern on preoperative hysterogram |
| Severe | Large hydrosalpinx ≥30 mm diameter |
| | No fimbria |
| | Dense pelvic or adnexal adhesions with fixation of the ovary and tube to either the broad ligament, pelvic sidewall, omentum, and/or bowel |
| | Obliteration of the cul-de-sac |
| | Frozen pelvis (adhesion formation so dense that limits of organs are difficult to define) |

Source: Rock et al. Factors influencing the success of salpingostomy techniques for distal fimbrial obstruction. *Obstet. Gynecol.* 52:591, 1978.

character, salpingostomy resulted in 100 percent patency and 50 percent pregnancy rates. Fimbriae that appeared as "well-marked elevations around the stoma" resulted in a pregnancy rate of 20 percent. Salpingostomy in the absence of fimbriae resulted in a pregnancy rate of only 0 to 5 percent. Unfortunately, the condition of the muscularis can be judged only after the release of fluid, and the condition of ciliated and secretory epithelial elements can be evaluated only by biopsy, a procedure that could result in considerable bleeding. In addition, it would be expected that both epithelial elements would require some time to recover a degree of normal function.

Rock et al. [167] have suggested a classification of the extent of tubal disease in patients with total fimbrial occlusion that includes four factors relevant to condition of the fimbriae and tubal mucosa. There are included in the following list:

1. Size of hydrosalpinx
2. Condition of the fimbriae; evaluated at surgery
3. Associated peritubal and periovarian adhesions
4. Rugal pattern determined during hysterosalpingography

These factors have been utilized to classify total fimbrial occlusion into the three categories of mild, moderate, and severe disease. A detailed classification is presented in Table 7-14.

It is significant that patients with incomplete distal fimbrial obstruction and isolated tubal adhesions requiring "fimbriolysis" were excluded from the study by Rock et al. These authors also stated that "the presence or absence of fimbriae was not used to differentiate between salpingoneostomy and fimbrioplasty, as reported by Siegler." The details of the patients classified by Rock et al. will be discussed later. However, in brief, pregnancy occurred in 87 percent of the 15 patients classified in the mild category and in only 5 percent of 42 patients in whom the extent of tubal damage was classified as severe at the time of surgery.

In summary, our approach to a hydrosalpinx is to attempt distal reconstruction if adhesions are slight or moderate and if rugal markings have been noted on the preoperative hysterogram. If mobilization of the occluded tube is extremely difficult, and if rugal markings have not been seen preoperatively, further corrective surgery is usually hopeless. Garcia [68] has stated that the size of a hydrosalpinx does not influence his decision concerning repair. We agree with this opinion, but if the mucosa of the newly opened tube is smooth and there are no recognizable fimbriae, pregnancy is not anticipated. We agree with Shirodkar [183] that the presence of fimbriae is essential for success, and we look forward to the increased use of the classification suggested by Rock et al. (Table 7-14) as an intraoperative guide to the prognosis of postoperative pregnancy.

*Use of Prosthetic Devices*

Interest in tubal surgery, and particularly salpingoplasty, was revived following World War II with the introduction of imaginatively designed prosthetic devices used to maintain tubal patency following a corrective procedure. Although the hoodlike device designed by Rock and Mulligan became the prototype of these devices, these surgeons were not the first to employ this concept. Gepfert [71], in 1939, reported the use of cow allantoic membrane to cover the ostium of reconstructed fimbriae in the monkey. The material was absorbable and postoperative adhesions were minimal. In 1943, Gepfert [72] reported the use of allantoic membrane in 28 infertile patients. Patency was maintained at 6 months in 18 of 21 patients, but only 2 pregnancies occurred during that interval. Six months, however, is too short an interval for adequate evaluation of postoperative fertility. In 1954, Ten-Berge and Lok [211] reported the use of human chorioamniotic membrane to protect the ostium after salpingostomy in 6 patients. No pregnancies occurred subsequently.

**Table 7-15.** Results of salpingoneostomy with application of a hood

| Surgeon | No. of patients | Percent tubal patency | Percent pregnant | Percent living child | Percent tubal pregnancies | Comment |
|---|---|---|---|---|---|---|
| Mulligan et al., 1953 | 21 | 66 | 24 | — | — | |
| Rock et al., 1954 | | | | | | |
|   No splint | 41 | 43 | 17 | — | — | Early hood |
|   Polyethylene hood | 18 | 62.5 | 28 | — | — | |
| Mulligan, 1966 | | | | | | |
|   1949–1954 | 21 | 64 | 14 | 10 | — | Polyethylene hood |
|   1955–1959 | 45 | 87 | 36 | 21 | — | Silastic hood |
| Garcia, 1968 | 25 | 76 | 40 | 28 | 8 | Silastic hood |
| Buxton and Mastroianni, 1962 | | | | | | |
|   No splint | 31 | 46 | 12 | 7 | 6 | All had bilateral tubal |
|   Hood | 9 | — | 33 | 22 | 11 | obstruction |
| Young et al., 1970 | | | | | | |
|   No splint | 24 | — | 37.5 | 25 | 8 | Hoods placed on only |
|   Hoods | 18 | — | 16.7 | 16.7 | 0 | severely diseased tubes |
| Crane and Woodruff, 1969 | 17 | — | 17 | 6 | 6 | |
| Lamb and Moscovitz, 1972 | | | | | | |
|   Polyethylene splint | 23 | — | 17 | 8 | 8 | Bilateral operations for |
|   Hood | 12 | — | 25 | — | — | hydrosalpinx |
| Comminos, 1979 | | | | | | |
|   No hood | 15 | 27 | 20[a] | 20 | 20[a] | |
|   Hoods | 15 | 53 | 33[b] | 33 | 13[b] | Scurasil device of Cognat |

[a]A total of 5 pregnancies occurred in 3 patients. One of 5 pregnancies was ectopic.
[b]A total of 8 pregnancies occurred in 5 patients. One of 8 pregnancies was ectopic.

In 1950, Castallo [26] published a study of tubal regeneration in monkeys in which he resected a 2-cm section of midtube and observed mucosal regeneration over splints of various materials. The polyethylene used in one monkey produced the best results. In 1951, Hellman [90] published the first report in which polyethylene tubing was utilized to maintain tubal patency in 8 patients. Seven of the 8 maintained tubal patency, but only 1 pregnancy was reported in a rather short follow-up interval.

It was in this environment that a flurry of reports appeared in 1953 and 1954 describing the use of additional devices to cover a newly created tubal ostium. Barsky and Blinick [5] reported using autogenous cartilage fashioned into a ringlike shape to maintain patency of the ostia in 2 patients. Six months later, both tubes were obstructed. A polyethylene ring was designed by Kahn [113] for permanent retention after salpingoplasty, and recently, Roland [170] advocated placement of a polyethylene-coated "wire spiral" device to maintain fimbrial patency. In 1953, Mulligan and associates [141] reported using a polyethylene hood that was, in fact, little more than a saclike device to cover the repaired ostium. Recently, Silastic has replaced polyethylene as a less reactive material. In 1954, Rock and associates [169] reported pregnancy in 5 of 18 (28 percent) patients in whom a polyethylene hood had been used and compared this group with 7 of 41 (17 percent)

pregnancies in patients in whom hoods had not been used. A summary of reported results with the hood is shown in Table 7-15.

The Silastic hood prosthesis* was designed by William J. Mulligan, M.D. It was utilized to cover and protect a newly created fimbrial ostium following salpingostomy. Mulligan [139] and Garcia [68] used this prosthesis when total fimbrial occlusion and hydrosalpinx formation necessitated the procedure described previously as salpingostomy. The hood was placed over this opening to protect raw surfaces of endosalpinx from agglutination and adhesion formation. Approximately 4 months later the prosthesis was removed at a second laparotomy.

The Silastic fimbrial prosthesis (Mulligan design) is essentially nonreactive to body tissue and fluids over prolonged periods of use. It is nonadherent to tissue and thus permits quick, easy removal with minimal trauma. Furthermore, it will not calcify or degenerate on long-term implantation. This prosthesis may be autoclaved without change in physical properties and has an indefinite shelf life. It is supplied individually in sterile packs and is available in two sizes: small (35.0 mm long by 22.4 mm maximum diameter) and large (50.8 mm

*Marketed by Dow Corning Corporation, Medical Products Division, Midland, Michigan.

long by 28.6 mm maximum diameter). It is recommended that both sizes be at the surgeon's disposal during the operative procedure. Due to the cost of the prosthesis and the difficulty of resterilization, the surgeon should be familiar with these sizes prior to making a choice, and he or she should attempt to "guess right" as frequently as possible. The prosthesis should be handled as little as possible because talc and lint tend to adhere to the surface. Garcia has designed an adaptor that eliminates touching the prosthesis during the operative procedure.

Approximately 4 months postoperatively, a second laparotomy is recommended for removal of the hood prosthesis. Adhesions present at that time should be lysed. The fimbriae usually appear erythematous at the time, and postoperative hydrotubation is suggested following the second laparotomy. In addition, dexamethasone and promethazine should be given to diminish adhesion formation further.

Two surgeons [4,31] have reported utilizing the laparoscope or culdoscope to remove the hood. This may be difficult because of omental adhesions and the need to cut the Mersilene sutures. In addition, the advantage of removing other adhesions would be lost by this approach.

A modified hood device, the Scurasil salpingoplasty device designed by Cognat [33], was introduced in 1971. This Silastic prosthesis contained a pliable cone-shaped hood designed to cover the newly created tubal ostium and prevent adhesion formation in this area. A nylon cord attachment was passed out through the anterior uterine wall, and removal of the entire prosthesis was possible by traction on this cord, thus avoiding a second laparotomy. A report by Comminos in 1977 [36] compared the use of this device during salpingostomy in 30 patients. The device was used in 15 patients, and 15 other patients underwent only salpingostomy. Pregnancy occurred in 33 percent (5 patients) of patients in whom a device was used, and in 20 percent (3 patients) in whom it was not employed.

At present, we do not use a prosthetic device during salpingoneostomy. We feel that increased use of the microsurgical approach provides the best avenue for improved pregnancy results and are working to perfect the technique. Hoods of the Mulligan design are still employed by other surgeons, including Garcia. The technique of hood placement was presented in detail in the first edition of the *Atlas*. The Scurasil salpingoplasty device is no longer marketed.

### Postoperative Hydrotubation

Although intraoperative tubal lavage and postoperative hydrotubation were employed by Green-Armytage [83] and Chalier [27], in 1960, Shirodkar [183] described the regimen of repetitive lavage. He advocated keeping the stoma open following salpingoplasty "by injecting sterile normal saline through the cervix with a Rubin or screw cannula. . . . Postoperative hydrotubation is done once in 24 hours for 4 days and then every 4 days for a fortnight." As noted previously, he achieved 100 percent patency and 50 percent pregnancy results in grade 1 patients, but in cases where the fimbriae were "poorly preserved," pregnancy occurred in only 10 to 20 percent.

This early postoperative hydrotubation was utilized infrequently by other surgeons until Grant [81] reported a study in which early hydrotubation clearly improved the conception rate. In one group of 103 patients, salpingoplasty was performed without adjuvant therapy; 16 percent of these patients conceived, 3 percent had tubal pregnancies, and 70 percent of the tubes were patent postoperatively. In Grant's second group, "hydrotubation was done every 3 days after the operation for 2 weeks and then less often." Forty-one percent of these patients conceived, and no tubal pregnancies occurred. This level of pregnancy success has been unequaled by any other surgeon attempting salpingostomy, including the microsurgeons. Hydrocortisone and chymotrypsin were utilized by Grant for lavage. Both appeared to give the same incidence of pregnancy, and currently Grant advocates using hydrocortisone for 2 weeks and then changing to chymotrypsin. The dose of hydrocortisone was 25 mg dissolved in 10 ml sterile saline, and the dose of chymotrypsin was 5 mg (or 5,300 Armour units or 25 chymotrypsin hemoglobin units) dissolved in 10 ml sterile saline. Grant noted that chymotrypsin apparently "depolymerizes the macromolecules of fibrin that tend to become trapped in a fine mesh of young connective tissue and capillaries." He observed that 75 percent of those patients who achieved a pregnancy did so in less than 6 months. Again this has not been the observation of others in this field, since pregnancy following salpingostomy is often delayed, frequently occurring at intervals of greater than 6 months.

In a third group of 61 patients who did not become pregnant during the year following surgery, Grant performed late hydrotubation. Thirteen percent of the group conceived following this treatment. Other surgeons have modified Grant's approach. Arronet and coworkers [2] reported using "transfundal tubal washings" with 10 ml normal saline, 1 vial of Elase,* and a few drops of indigo carmine at the completion of surgery in 74 patients. Hydrotubation with hydrocorti-

---

*One vial as a lyophilized powder contains 25 units of fibrinolysin and 15,000 units of deoxyribonuclease with 0.1 mg thimerosal. Manufactured by Parke-Davis.

**Table 7-16.** Results of salpingoneostomy using postoperative hydrotubation

| Surgeon | No. of patients | Percent tubal patency | Percent pregnant | Percent term pregnancies | Percent tubal pregnancies | Comment |
|---|---|---|---|---|---|---|
| Shirodkar, 1966 | Not reported | | | | | |
|   Good fimbriae | | 100 | 50 | — | — | Early hydrotubation |
|   Poor fimbriae | | — | 10–20 | — | — | on day 1 |
| Arronet et al., 1969 | | | | | | |
|   Salpingostomy | 11 | 40 | 30 | — | 0 | Lavage at surgery |
|   Salpingostomy and lysis | 74 | 57 | 24 | — | 3 | Hydrotubation on day 8 |
| Grant, 1971 | | | | | | |
|   Early hydrotubation | 53 | 66 | 41 | 35 | 0 | |
|   Late hydrotubation | 61 | 62 | 13 | 3 | 3 | |
|   Surgery only | 103 | 68 | 16 | 12 | 3 | |
| Swolin, 1967 | 33 | | 27 | | | Hydrotubation on day 8 |
| Jessen, 1972 | 25 | | 36 | | | $CO_2$ insufflation on day 7 |

sone was then initiated on about the eighth postoperative day and repeated once a month for 2 to 6 months. Pregnancy occurred in 30 percent of patients undergoing salpingostomy only and in 24 percent of patients who also required salpingolysis.

Swolin [210] reported the results of microsurgical salpingostomy in 33 patients, of whom 15 became pregnant (46 percent). At the conclusion of surgery, 2,000 mg hydrocortisone solution was lavaged into the pelvis, and dexamethasone was given for 20 days. Hydrotubation was performed on the ninth postoperative day and again just prior to ovulation during the next two menstrual cycles. Table 7-16 summarizes the results these workers obtained. Gomel [76] has apparently also utilized early hydrotubation following microsurgical salpingoneostomy.

A report by Jarvinen and associates [107] described postoperative hydrotubation in patients undergoing conservative surgery for tubal pregnancy. A Foley catheter was inserted into the uterine fundus, and hydrotubation was performed daily postoperatively. Twenty-six pregnancies (22 intrauterine and 4 ectopic) occurred in 43 patients so treated. Six of 10 patients having only one tube conceived, and 5 of these delivered normally.

When utilizing postoperative hydrotubation following microsurgical salpingoneostomy, we prefer the regimen advocated by Grant [8]. Hydrotubation should be started on the first postoperative day and continued on alternate days for 3 to 4 injections. The solution [25 mg hydrocortisone sodium succinate (Solu-Cortef) diluted in 10 ml normal saline] is injected gently and slowly. We have not used chymotrypsin.

The purpose of early hydrotubation is to remove the coagulum that forms following surgical manipulation of the fimbriae. Early clearing by this technique is important to prevent coalescence of the mucosa. The use of

dilute heparin as an irrigating solution during surgery also fulfills this role. Garcia [68] has noted the possibility of introducing infection with hydrotubation. However, the incidence is low in most series and infrequent in our experience. The optimum time to perform hydrotubation is in the early proliferative phase of the cycle, and surgery should be scheduled accordingly. Postoperative hydrotubation is not included as a routine part of a microsurgical salpingostomy procedure.

*Surgical Approach*

Innumerable surgical techniques have been used since 1890 to open the obstructed distal oviduct. Many of these were performed in the absence of fimbriae, and in some cases, the distal tube was excised prior to reconstruction of a new stoma. Numerous series of disappointing pregnancy results accumulated during the first half of the twentieth century and gradually led to the realization that the presence of fimbriae was essential and that the simplest operation was frequently the most successful. The concept of Holden and Sovak [92] that "tubal patency was the indicator" of successful tubal surgery has also been replaced by the criterion of live babies obtained by a corrective procedure.

Significant changes have occurred in this area of tubal surgery since the first edition of the *Atlas*. The use of prosthetic devices, very popular during the 1960s and 1970s, has given way to a microsurgical approach. Improved visualization provided by loupes and the operating microscope have permitted the surgeon to examine the fimbriae closely at the time of surgery. An improved understanding of fimbrial anatomy has permitted better reconstruction of the fimbrial opening. An awareness of the vascular pattern of the fimbriae, published by Diamond [49,50], permits the surgeon to avoid injury to

**Figure 7-7.** The distribution of spiral-shaped corkscrew arterioles in the tubal fimbria has been demonstrated by Diamond. Microsurgical procedures involving fimbrial repair must avoid damage to these vessels. (From E. Diamond, Lysis of postoperative pelvic adhesions in infertility. *Fertil. Steril.* 31:288, 1979.)

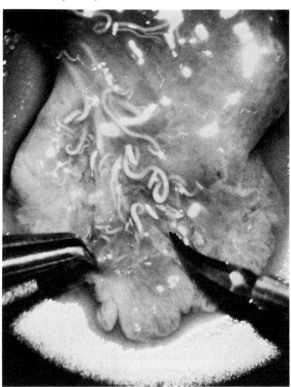

these coiled vessels (Fig. 7-7). As will be noted later, the microsurgical approach to the repair of fimbrial occlusion is in its infancy. Although microsurgical fimbrioplasty has produced excellent pregnancy results, microsurgical salpingoneostomy has not.

The classification proposed earlier defines salpingoneostomy as follows.

III. Salpingoneostomy (salpingostomy)
    A. Terminal
    B. Midampullary (medial)
    C. Isthmic (including linear salpingostomy)

The surgical procedure described later in this chapter is a terminal salpingoneostomy (salpingostomy). Midampullary salpingostomy results in few pregnancies. Recent evidence suggests that an ampullary salpingostomy performed for reversal of prior sterilization by fimbriectomy may result in pregnancy [146]. One of us (G.W.P.) has visualized the spontaneous occurrence of such an opening in the distal ampulla following a failed fimbriectomy in which a term pregnancy occurred. Tubal length appeared significant in this instance, associated with a residual tube of 8 cm, producing an ostium that easily hung over the ovarian surface. Isthmic salpingostomy is no longer performed.

CUFF EVERSION TECHNIQUE

Distal excision of a hydrosalpinx accompanied by cuff eversion was a popular technique in the hands of Skutsch [191], Polk [164], and later Bonney [11], Solomons [193], Moore-White [137], and Holden and Sovak [92]. Holden and Sovak published a detailed account of this technique in 1932 and were responsible for its popularity in America during the 1940s and 1950s. Ingersoll noted in 1949 [102] that "in 18 salpingostomies . . . a procedure of amputating the end of the hydrosalpinx and then suturing the mucosa to the serosa was employed. . . . None of the patients became pregnant, although in 33 percent tubal patency was proved." Shirodkar, in 1966 [183], summarized the present surgical thinking when he noted that "cuff salpingostomy . . . is in my hands a very unsound procedure."

LATERAL SALPINGOSTOMY

Lateral salpingostomy, described in 1899 by Skutsch and in 1903 by Ferguson [61,191], has become a procedure of historical interest only. In this technique, a linear opening is made along the medial aspect of the dilated ampulla adjacent to the ovary. Moore-White utilized this technique occasionally when both tube and ovary were involved in adhesions. The obvious purpose of this procedure was to provide an ostium for severely compromised fimbriae. However, Shirodkar succinctly appraised the procedure by stating that "making a lateral opening . . . in the dilated portion of the fallopian tube has not been successful in my hands."

## TOTAL LINEAR SALPINGOSTOMY

Another salpingostomy technique seldom employed is that of total linear salpingostomy. An incision is made along the entire length of the oviduct from fimbriae to cornu, with no attempt at closure. Although first reported by Bourne [13] in 1923, the technique was popularized by Israel [103], when he recommended its use in "instances of unexpectedly encountered acute suppurative salpingitis." Over a period of 15 years (1935–1949), he performed this operation on 8 patients. Seven of these women were thought to have gonococcal salpingitis and the eighth had pelvic tuberculosis. Four of the 7 patients in the former group subsequently conceived. In spite of these observations, Israel commented that "total linear salpingostomy is neither recommended as a treatment for occluded fallopian tubes nor as the therapy of choice in preoperatively recognized acute suppurative salpingitis."

Increased utilization of endoscopy in patients with suspected acute salpingitis should facilitate the nonoperative approach to this disease. It is possible that the surgical approach may be of value in the conservative treatment of distal tubal pregnancy, as will be discussed later in this chapter.

## MICROSURGICAL SALPINGOSTOMY

The present technique of microsurgical salpingostomy was first suggested by Swolin [207,208] and is a refinement of the technique described in the first edition of the *Atlas*. We stated, "Identification of the sealed ostea is aided by distending the ampullary portion of the tube with dye. A small indentation or thinning of the tube is noted as the most distal point of closure." Without magnification, it was not possible to accurately delineate the lines of fimbrial agglutination that met at this central point. Early use of the ocular loupe and now the operating microscope permit the surgeon to cut accurately along these vascular lines of agglutination and avoid the excessive bleeding frequently encountered when one erroneously cuts across the center of a fimbrial fold. The technique described in this text is a modification of the microsurgical approach suggested by Swolin in which the operating microscope, microelectrode, and glass rod are commonly employed tools.

## ESSENTIAL INSTRUMENTS

1. Operating microscope: We use either the Zeiss OPMI-7PH or OPMI-6S microscope. An experienced assistant is invaluable. Loupes do not provide adequate magnification in most cases.
2. Special operating room table, i.e., Kifa, that permits the surgeon to sit comfortably.
3. Microelectrode: This standard tool is used to cut avascular lines of fimbrial adhesions.
4. Bipolar forceps: Used for coagulating small vessels.
5. Dilute heparin solution: Used for irrigation.
6. Angled Wescott scissors and angled Iris scissors.
7. Glass or Teflon rods.
8. Suture: 8-0 Vicryl or Dexon with fine atraumatic needle.
9. Smooth microforceps.

The technique of microsurgical salpingoneostomy is presented in Figure 7-8 A through E.

## LASER APPROACH TO SALPINGOSTOMY

The carbon dioxide laser has been used in place of the microelectrode during microsurgical salpingostomy [6]. When one is using the laser technique, the occluded oviduct should first be placed on saline soaked telfa. Adhesions are excised either with the hand-held or with the micromanipulated laser at power densities of 2,000 to 10,000 W per square centimeter* (power 5–24 watts, spot diameter .55 mm). The tubal ostea is then identified under the operating microscope as shown in Figure 7-8B. The central dimple is identified and opened with the laser beam using a power density of 5,000 W per square centimeter (12 watts, spot diameter .5 mm) for .5 second [6]. A glass rod is then inserted into the osteum and the avascular lines of agglutination cut with radial incisions to power densities of 5,000 to 8,000 W per square centimeter* (power 12–20 watts, spot diameter .5 mm; Fig. 7-8F). This power-density range creates precise lines of tissue separation with minimal thermal injury, although the zone of thermal necrosis is usually sufficient to seal microcapillaries and prevent bleeding.

---

*Power density (PD) equals power in watts times 100, divided by the square of the spot diameter (in millimeters).

Arterioles greater than 1 mm in diameter require high frequency bipolar electrocoagulation. Irrigation with normal saline or Hartman's solution is performed at this time to remove loose debris and carbonated matter.

A unique aspect of the carbon dioxide laser technique during salpingostomy is the ability to irradiate the serosal surfaces adjacent to the radial incision at power densities 100 to 300 W per square centimeter (power .25–.8 watts, spot diameter .5 mm). This serosal heating causes linear protein contraction and eversion of the tubal mucosa. In fact, the tubal mucosa can be seen to roll back and assume an almost normal appearance during this procedure. Bellina [6] has found that three or four sutures of 8-0 polyglactin 910 are necessary to hold the mucosal elements in normal proximity during healing in spite of the laser effect as shown in Figure 7-8 E.

RESULTS

A better understanding of the factors that determine the postoperative pregnancy rates following fimbrial surgery has developed since the first edition of the *Atlas*. As was discussed earlier, the concept that fimbrial disease should be rigidly separated on the basis of partial and complete distal tubal occlusion has been advanced and is now established in the new classification proposed by Palmer. Early studies by Young et al. [240] that identified the significance of ampullary rugal markings have been confirmed. The significance of hydrosalpinx size and the presence of tubal and ovarian adhesions has been acknowledged. Finally, the quality of the fimbriae noted at the time of surgery has become an important prognostic indicator. These four parameters of tubal

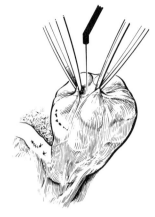

C

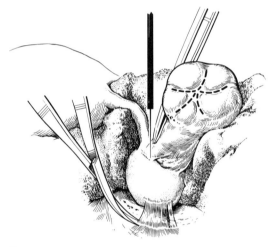

B

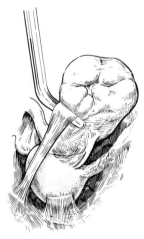

A

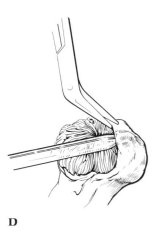

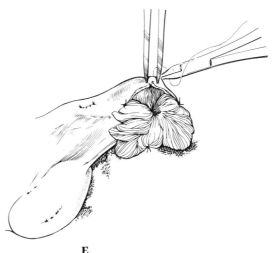

**D**

**E**

**Figure 7-8.** Surgical technique of salpingoneostomy.
**A.** Close inspection of the site of distal occlusion. The lines of agglutination are visible under high magnification and the center of these folds is the site at which the initial incision should be made. Distention of the ampullary portion of the tube with dilute indigo carmen serves to accentuate these lines. Elevation with a glass rod, as demonstrated in this drawing, permits atraumatic handling of the tube. Note the tubal and ovarian adhesions. **B.** Excision of adhesions must be carried out prior to performing salpingoneostomy. Use of the microelectrode and the curved iris scissors (Wescott) are demonstrated. The author employs the ocular loupes and headlamp during resection of difficult-to-reach ovarian–broad-ligament adhesions. In contrast, the tubal-ovarian adhesions shown here should be resected under microscope control. These two adhesions are also of a different character. In A and B, the ovarian–broad-ligament adhesion appears as a filmy sheet fixed only at the ovarian and broad ligament sites. In contrast, the tubal-ovarian adhesion being resected with the microelectrode in this drawing is almost a fusion of the two serosal surfaces. Under high magnification it is possible to cut between these surfaces, but often a small defect occurs. The "fusion" type adhesion is the more problematic. Sites of subsequent incision in the distal tube have been drawn in dotted lines to emphasize the concept of cutting between the fimbrial folds. **C.** The initial incision in the closed ostea is made with the microelectrode employing a pure cutting current in a field magnified by the operating microscope. Fine smooth forceps are useful to delineate the proper line of incision. Eversion of the mucosal folds permits the surgeon to visualize the avascular area of scar formation. Optimal technique is associated with minimal bleeding. Constant irrigation with dilute heparin solution is employed during this step. **D.** A glass rod is a useful tool to expose the line of fimbrial agglutination. An angled iris scissor is also very useful to cut along this line. **E.** Suturing is kept to a minimum. An average of three sutures (8-0 synthetic absorbable material or 9-0 nylon) are employed to maintain the fimbrial opening. Note the reconstruction of the fimbria ovarica and normal-appearing mesotubarium ovarica. Suture technique is demonstrated in which the forceps are held sideways and the needle passed through this space. This is in contrast to grasping the tissue and squeezing as is usually done. **F.** The laser beam, controlled by the micromanipulator and visualized under the operating microscope, may also be used to open the tubal ostea. Power density of $1 \times 10^5$ w/cm$^2$ for 0.5 second is employed. Lines of agglutination are cut and the fimbrial edges sutured to the tubal serosa, as shown in Figure 7-8E.

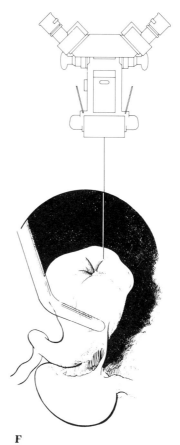

**F**

disease have been combined in the classification presented earlier (see Table 7-14):

1. Size of hydrosalpinx
2. Condition of fimbriae
3. Tubal and ovarian adhesions
4. Rugal pattern on hysterosalpingography

The earlier confusion involving the classification of fimbrial disease and identification of specific types of tubal operations appears to have been clarified. The new nomenclature advocated by R. Palmer in 1977 has been used in this text and has been employed by both Siegler and Gomel in other writings [78,185]. The surgical technique of salpingostomy first advocated by Swolin in 1967 and termed *microsurgical salpingostomy* has been standardized. The use of magnification, the microelectrode, and the glass rod to open a totally occluded duct in a manner that preserves the fimbriae was outlined earlier in this chapter. Proof that microsurgical salpingostomy produces more uterine pregnancies than earlier salpingostomy techniques is still lacking. A perspective on this question will be developed by reviewing the three nonmicrosurgical studies that provided the best pregnancy results following terminal salpingostomy and comparing these with the microsurgical results of Swolin and Gomel.

Garcia [68] employed "Mulligan hoods" during a terminal salpingostomy when hydrosalpinx formation was encountered. In 25 patients operated on by this surgeon, pregnancy occurred in 36 percent, of which 28 percent (7 of 25) were uterine and 24 percent (2 of 9) were ectopic. This study typifies a pattern involving uterine and tubal pregnancies that will be encountered in other salpingostomy studies. Overall, pregnancy occurred in slightly more than one-third of Garcia's patients who underwent salpingostomy. Of the patients who conceived, ectopic pregnancy accounted for over one-fourth the pregnancies.

Grant [81] reported the results of 156 personal cases of terminal salpingostomy. Early hydrotubation was performed in 53 patients in this series. Comparison of the two groups of patients, salpingostomy alone and salpingostomy plus hydrotubation, revealed exciting results. In 103 patients who underwent only salpingostomy, pregnancy occurred in 17 percent, and a uterine pregnancy occurred in 14 percent of patients. These data are similar to those of many other studies [2,167, 184]. In 53 patients who also underwent early hydrotubation following salpingostomy, pregnancy occurred in 42 percent without an ectopic pregnancy, a result that has never been equaled. In other studies, including those of Gomel, the combination of early hydrotubation and microsurgical salpingostomy have produced a high pregnancy rate. However, a significant number of these pregnancies had been ectopic.

Horne et al. [97], utilizing a preoperative and postoperative regimen of dexamethasone and promethazine (Phenergan), reported the pregnancy results in a series of 254 patients operated on by four surgeons. In this group, 29 patients had a pure terminal salpingostomy. Overall, 38 percent of these patients conceived postoperatively. There were 9 (31 percent) intrauterine pregnancies and 2 (2 of 11, or 28 percent) ectopic pregnancies.

These three nonmicrosurgical approaches to salpingostomy are summarized in Table 7-17. These studies should be compared against the background of many other reports of terminal salpingostomy in which pregnancy occurred far less often [152,171]. These studies were presented in the first edition of the *Atlas* and are summarized in Table 7-18. A recent retrospective review of terminal salpingostomy at Johns Hopkins University School of Medicine has been reported by Rock et al. [167]. The study included the years 1935 to 1976 and involved 87 patients. Overall, pregnancy occurred in 28 percent of these patients; 22 percent of the patients had a uterine pregnancy and 21 percent had ectopic pregnancies. These results are similar to those reported by other authors [66,81] and appear to constitute the usual pregnancy outcome following nonmicrosurgical salpingostomy.

In contrast to these earlier studies are two recent reports of microsurgical salpingostomy. The study of Swolin [207,208] (1967) reported 33 patients who underwent microsurgical salpingostomy. By the time of his initial report, nine pregnancies occurred (27 percent), for a uterine pregnancy rate of 18 percent and an ectopic pregnancy rate of 33 percent (3 of 9). The same patients were reviewed by Swolin [210] 7 years later (1974), by which time pregnancy had occurred in 14 patients (46 percent). However, the ectopic pregnancy rate had increased to 40 percent (6 of 15), while the uterine pregnancy rate increased slightly to 27 percent (9 of 25). In 1978, Gomel [76] reported pregnancy results following microsurgical salpingostomy in 50 patients. After a follow-up interval greater than 1 year, he reported that pregnancy had occurred in 16 patients (32 percent). Uterine pregnancy occurred in 25 percent of these patients (12), and 25 percent (4 of 16) of the pregnancies were ectopic. Siegler [188] also achieved pregnancy in 35 percent of 23 patients who underwent microsurgical salpingostomy. Uterine pregnancy occurred in 22 percent of these patients, and 38 percent of the pregnancies were ectopic. The results of microsurgical salpingoneostomy are summarized in Table 7-19.

The reports of microsurgical salpingostomy have been combined into a single group comprising 106 patients and are summarized in Table 7-20. In this same table, for comparison, are the results of the three non-microsurgical series presented in Table 7-17 and the patients reviewed by Rock et al. in whom nonmicrosurgical salpingostomy was employed.

**Table 7-17.** Pregnancy following nonmicrosurgical salpingostomy

| Surgeon | No. of patients | Percent pregnant | Percent uterine | Ectopic Percent total | Ectopic Percent pregnancy | Technique |
|---|---|---|---|---|---|---|
| Garcia, 1972 | 25 | 36 | 28 | 8 | 22 | Hoods |
| Grant, 1971* | 53 | 42 | 42 | 0 | 0 | Hydrotubation |
| Horne et al., 1973 | 29 | 38 | 31 | 7 | 18 | Dex./Phen. |
| Total | 107 | 39 | 36 | 4 | 10 | |

*Results significantly different from other two series.

**Table 7-18.** Summary of results of all techniques of nonmicrosurgical salpingostomy

| Technique | Percent patency | Percent pregnant | Percent living child | Percent tubal pregnancies |
|---|---|---|---|---|
| Cuff method | 33–71 | 0–39 | 0–27 | 0–12 |
| Hood method | 62.5–87 | 14–40 | 6–28 | 0–11 |
| Postoperative hydrotubation | 40–100 | 24–50 | 35 | 0–3 |
| Postoperative cortisone | 49–100 | 18–52 | 37 | 2–7.4 |

**Table 7-19.** Pregnancy following microsurgical salpingoneostomy

| Surgeon | No. of patients | Percent pregnant | Percent uterine | Ectopic Percent total | Ectopic Percent pregnant |
|---|---|---|---|---|---|
| Swolin, 1967 | 33 | 27 | 18 | 9 | 33 |
| Swolin, 1975 | 33 | 46 | 27 | 18 | 40 |
| Gomel, 1978 | 50[a] | 32[b] | 24 | 10 | 31 |
| Siegler, 1978 | 23 | 35 | 22 | 13 | 38 |

[a]The 9 patients lost to follow-up have been included as failures.
[b]One patient who had both an ectopic and an intrauterine pregnancy has been included in each group.

**Table 7-20.** Pregnancy following microsurgical and nonmicrosurgical salpingostomy

| Group | No. of patients | Percent pregnant | Percent uterine | Ectopic Percent total | Ectopic Percent pregnant |
|---|---|---|---|---|---|
| Microsurgical (Table 7-20) | 106 | 37 | 25 | 13 | 36 |
| Nonmicrosurgical* (Table 7-18) | 107 | 38 [42] | 34 | 4 | 10 |
| Rock et al., 1978 | 87 | 28 | 22 | 6 | 21 |

*Group weighted by 53 patients reported by Grant (1971).

7. Surgery of the Oviduct

**Table 7-21.** Pregnancy associated with extent of fimbrial disease

| Group | No. of patients | Percent pregnant | Percent uterine | Ectopic | |
| | | | | Percent total | Percent pregnant |
|---|---|---|---|---|---|
| Fimbrioplasty: | | | | | |
| Patton, 1982 | 40 | 68 | 63 | 5 | 8 |
| Salpingoneostomy: | | | | | |
| Rock et al., 1978: | | | | | |
| Mild | 15 | 87 | 80 | 6 | 8 |
| Moderate | 30 | 30 | 17 | 13 | 44 |
| Severe | 42 | 5 | 5 | 0 | 0 |

A review of the data presented above indicates similar pregnancy results in the series reported by Garcia [66], Horne et al. [97], and Rock et al. [167]. Uterine pregnancy occurred in 28, 31, and 22 percent of these respective groups, while ectopic pregnancy occurred in 22, 18, and 21 percent of the pregnancies. The exception to this pattern are the results of Grant's series, in which early hydrotubation was performed. Pregnancy occurred in 42 percent of these patients, without an ectopic pregnancy. A further unusual feature of Grant's series was the preponderance of pregnancies that occurred less than 6 months postoperatively, since most authors have reported that pregnancy is often delayed following terminal salpingostomy, occurring as late as 36 to 40 months postoperatively [76,167]. Microsurgical salpingostomy reported by Swolin [210], Gomel [76], and Siegler [188] resulted in uterine pregnancy in 27, 24, and 22 percent of cases, while ectopic pregnancy occurred in 40, 31, and 35 percent of pregnancies. The overall pregnancy rate of 46 percent reported by Swolin [210] was the highest for any reported series of salpingostomy patients.

It would appear that the pregnancy results following terminal salpingostomy have not improved with the use of microsurgical technique. We do not feel that this is the case, however, since the extent of fimbrial disease was not defined by the earlier surgeons. Patton [155] has shown that microsurgical fimbrioplasty in partial fimbrial occlusion usually associated with normal fimbriae results in excellent pregnancy yields with a low number of ectopic pregnancies. Rock et al. [167] carried this point further by demonstrating that when mild fimbrial disease was encountered following repair of a totally occluded distal oviduct, pregnancy occurred in 87 percent (13 of 15) of patients, and only 8 percent (1 of 13) of the pregnancies were ectopic. In contrast, among 72 patients whose tubal damage was classified as moderate or severe at the time of surgery, pregnancy occurred in only 14 percent, and 34 percent (4 of 11) of these pregnancies were tubal. Gomel [73] commented on this point in a recent text with the statement: "The authors [Swolin and Gomel] have attributed the higher incidence of ectopic pregnancy to the greater severity of pathology as well as to the very high postoperative patency rate (over 90 percent). In both these microsurgical series, minimal patient selection was employed. . . . The procedure itself may lead to ectopic implantations by creating patency in a severely damaged oviduct. Conventional surgery is contrasted in its success or failure, leaving few of the severely repaired tubes patent."

It has become apparent that the incidence rates of uterine and of ectopic pregnancy following salpingoneostomy are related to the extent of fimbrial and mucosal damage encountered at the time of surgery. As expected, the surgical repair of partial tubal occlusion involving mild fimbrial disease is associated with a high uterine pregnancy rate and a low incidence of ectopic pregnancy [155]. Total fimbrial occlusion associated with the preservation of fimbrial structures and normal mucosa is also associated with a high pregnancy rate and low ectopic rate following corrective surgery. However, as the extent of tubal disease increases, surgical repair results in a decreased incidence of pregnancy and in an increasing percentage of ectopic pregnancies (Table 7-21).

The classification of the extent of tubal disease proposed by Rock et al. [167] combines the concepts of Young et al. [240], Shirodkar [184], and others [185] to provide a means of arriving at a prognosis for postoperative pregnancy. In the study by Rock et al. it was highly significant that 48 percent of patients were classified in the severe category and that pregnancy occurred in only 5 percent of these women. In contrast, 53 percent of those patients whose tubal disease was classified as mild or moderate conceived postoperatively, and tubal pregnancy occurred in 21 percent of the pregnancies. Evaluation of further reports of patients who undergo salpingoneostomy must include this type of classification in order to ascertain the value of the surgical technique employed. Since both Swolin [210] and Gomel [73] stated that severe tubal disease was encountered in many patients, one must await results of a series of patients undergoing microsurgical salpingostomy whose tubal disease has been divided into the categories designated by Rock et al. [167].

## Tubal and Uterine
## Anastomosis Procedures

The most dramatic change in surgery involving the fallopian tube since the first edition of this text has occurred in the area of tubal anastomoses. The statement made in the first edition that "experience with end-to-end anastomosis of the oviduct has been less common than other tuboplastic procedures" has changed. In fact, now it may be said that tubal and uterine anastomoses have become one of the most commonly employed surgical techniques involving the fallopian tube. The increasing numbers of patients requesting reversal of prior tubal sterilization provide a constant demand for tubal reanastomosis and permit reconstruction of essentially normal fallopian tubes. Recent advances in this microsurgical technique also include correction of isthmic and cornual occlusion caused by pathologic processes including prior infection and salpingitis isthmica nodosa (SIN).

The introduction of microsurgical technique into infertility surgery was popularized by the demand for reversal of tubal sterilization and the dramatic successes reported by Gomel [76], Winston [233], and Diamond [48]. Following Swolin's introduction of magnification and microelectrosurgery for lysis of adhesions and salpingostomy in 1967, Clyman [32] reported a 45 percent pregnancy rate in 27 patients utilizing the operating microscope for tubal reanastomosis. David, Brackett, and Garcia [39] had reported experimental results of uteroisthmic anastomosis in the rabbit, but Garcia [67] did not report his clinical experience with microsurgical tubal reanastomosis until 1972, at which time pregnancy had occurred in 50 percent of his patients.

Subsequently, four surgeons working independently reported their results during the early and middle 1970s. In 1975 Winston [232] established a microsurgical technique for tubal anastomosis in which, following excision and reanastomosis of the fallopian tube, 23 of 25 rabbits conceived and delivered normal litters, a success rate of 92 percent. Although reports of clinical successes following microsurgical reanastomoses were presented at the Fourth Annual Meeting of the American Association of Gynecologic Laparoscopists in Atlanta (November 1975) and at the 32nd Annual Meeting of the American Fertility Society (April 1976), these studies were not published until 1977. In January of 1977, Gomel [76] reported that following reversal of tubal sterilization by microsurgery in 16 patients, "72.7 percent of those attempting a pregnancy and having more than 6 month follow-up have had uterine pregnancies." In the following month, Winston [233] reported that 12 of 16 (76 percent) of his patients had conceived following microsurgical uterotubal anastomosis and that 5 of 8 patients (63 percent) "who had anastomosis after diathermy had normal uterine pregnancies." One ectopic pregnancy occurred in Winston's group. In July of the same year, the Australian group of Owen and Picket-Heaps [150] reported experimental work in the rabbit as well as results of 10 patients who had microsurgical tubal reanastomoses. They reported pregnancy in 6 of 10 patients. Six of 7 patients who had Pomeroy tubal ligation conceived following reanastomoses. However, none of 3 patients who had tubal diathermy conceived following tubal repair. In November of 1977, Diamond [48] reported a 75 percent pregnancy rate in 16 patients undergoing microsurgical reversal of a previous tubal sterilization. There were no ectopic pregnancies in this group, although one molar pregnancy was reported.

By the conclusion of 1977 it was evident that utilization of microsurgical technique improved the results of tubal reanastomoses following previous tubal sterilization. The improvement in uteroampullary anastomoses following previous tubal diathermy suggested that this surgical approach would also help those patients with cornual and isthmic occlusion caused by salpingitis isthmica nodosum, endometriosis, or abortion. It was clear that a new era had arrived in infertility surgery.

### Types of Tubal Anastomoses

Five types of tubal anastomoses are possible and have been diagramed later in this chapter. These are as follows:

1. Ampullary-ampullary
2. Ampullary-isthmic
3. Isthmic-isthmic
4. Uteroampullary
5. Uteroisthmic

The disease processes that lead to reconstruction by one of these forms of tubal anastomosis will be discussed at length. Of equal significance for the microsurgeon, however, is an understanding of the tubal architecture in the ampullary, isthmic, and cornual tubal segments. Successful tubal and uterine anastomoses require an ability to work comfortably with these three anatomically different structures. Details of the anatomic characteristics of these three structures have been included in the discussion that follows.

### Anatomic Considerations

The structural differences of the parts of the fallopian tube, including the interstitial segment, the isthmus, and the ampulla, must be appreciated in order to perform a successful tubal anastomosis between two of these segments. An appreciation of the anatomy of each segment is also of value during investigations of tubal pathology by hysterosalpingography and laparoscopy. The infertility surgeons may now appreciate the entire spectrum of normal and pathologic tubal anatomy as they move from a gross (laparoscopic) view of the fallopian tube to a view magnified 20 to 30 times by the operating microscope.

The gross anatomy of the fallopian tube is outlined in Figure 7-9, and the four anatomic divisions are identified. Inclusion of the infundibulum is of significance in view of the markedly large diameter and more numerous mucosal folds in this area. The interconnecting blood supply through the uterine and ovarian arteries has been included because an appreciation of the pattern of vascular arcades that exists in the mesosalpinx is extremely important during an anastomosis procedure.

INTERSTITIAL SEGMENT

The portion of the fallopian tube contained within the wall of the uterus is termed the *intramural* or *interstitial segment*. Prior to the introduction of microtubal surgery, the gynecologic surgeon had little cause to consider the anatomy of this area, since the surgical treatment of interstitial or cornual occlusion was widely accepted to be the complete excision of the area by the technique of uterotubal implantation. Despite this surgical approach, many investigators proceeded with anatomic studies of the area during the first half of this century in search of the uterotubal sphincter. A report by Peel [159] reviewed the studies that supported and opposed the presence of a sphincter and concluded that available evidence opposed the presence of a sphincter at the uterotubal junction. As early as 1891, however, Williams [230] described the anatomic configuration of the cornu that is accepted today. A photomicrograph from this early publication (Fig. 7-10) demonstrates a cross-sectional area of the cornu showing four primary folds of mucous membrane and three layers of muscle forming the wall. Williams stated, "Sections at the cornu uteri show a starlike lumen which is formed by a few folds of the mucous membrane, usually four in number, although the number may vary from three to six. . . . We may designate these folds as primary folds." The gynecologic microsurgeon had rediscovered these primary mucosal folds in the search for normal interstitial and isthmic anatomy during uteroisthmic anastomosis following resection of a segment of oviduct distorted by salpingitis isthmica nodosum or a cornual polyp.

An interesting diagram of the architectural pattern of the interstitial portion of the fallopian tube was published by Lisa et al. [125] in 1954. The transition from tubal to endometrial epithelium was noted to occur approximately one-third the distance of the myometrium. The transition between the inner longitudinal muscle and the outer circular muscle is also significant.

**Figure 7-9.** Anatomical divisions of the fallopian tube. (From R. W. Kistner, *Gynecology: Principles and Practice* (3rd ed.). Chicago: Year Book, 1979.)

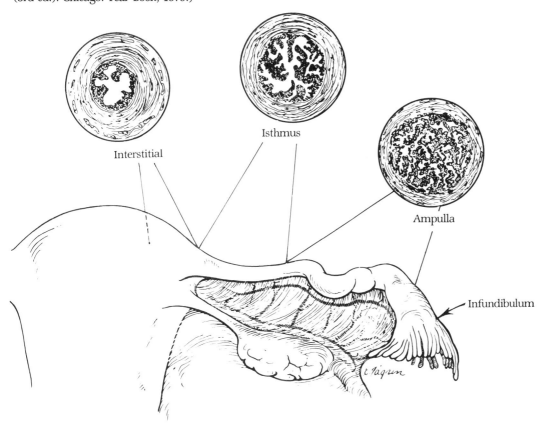

Interstitial

Isthmus

Ampulla

Infundibulum

**Figure 7-10.** Cross-sections of tube at cornu and isthmus. (From J. W. Williams, Contribution to the normal and pathological histology of the fallopian tubes. *Am. J. Med. Sci.* 102:377, 1891.) **A.** Cross section of tube at cornu uteri, showing the four primary folds of the mucous membrane and the three layers of muscle forming the tube wall. **B.** Cross section of the same tube at isthmus, one inch from the section shown in A, showing a more complicated arrangement of the mucous membrane and the disappearance of the inner longitudinal muscular layer.

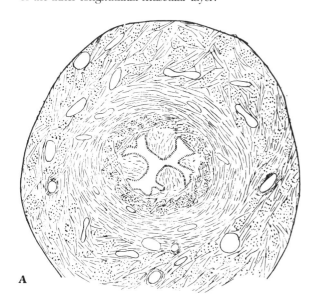

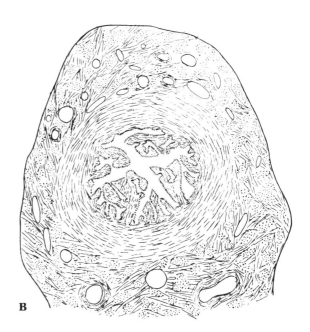

A

B

Variations in the course of the interstitial segment as it travels through the uterine wall are also of interest. Sweeney [205] dissected 100 interstitial segments and observed that "the length in the fresh state was 1.5 and 3.5 cm. Twenty-five specimens had short courses and in these the length of the tubal segment was 1.0 to 1.5 cm. In the remaining 69, however, the course was tortuous with many variations which appeared to fit three general patterns: (1) a course making almost a 90 degree turn halfway through the myometrium (short, stocky tube 1.0 to 1.5 cm), (2) 2 to 4 general convolutions (tubes 1.5 to 3.0 cm long), (3) a course diagonally down through the myometrium with 2 to 4 convolutions and kinks and emerging from the uterine wall at a lower level than with other variants (2.0 to 3.5 cm)" (Fig. 7-11).

**Figure 7-11.** Variations in course of interstitial segment. (From W. J. Sweeny, The interstitial portion of the uterine tube–Its gross anatomy, course, and length. *Obstet. Gynecol.* 19:3, 1962. Reprinted with permission from the American College of Obstetricians and Gynecologists.) **A.** A dissection of the interstitial portion of a tube demonstrating a curved course through the myometrium. *A* marks the endometrial cavity, and *B*, the serosal surface of the uterus. Note that as the tube approaches the endometrial cavity the diameter increases. **B.** A dissection of the interstitial portion of a tube demonstrating a straight course. *A* marks the endometrial cavity; *B*, the serosal border of the uterus. Note that even though this tube courses directly through the myometrium, there are several small gentle curves present. **C.** A dissection of the interstitial portion of a tube demonstrating a second variation of a tortuous course; a straight course through the myometrium, with 2 to 4 gentle convolutions. *A* marks the endometrial cavity; *B*, the serosal border of the uterus. Note that as the tube approaches the endometrial cavity, the diameter increases and the tube projects slightly into the cavity.

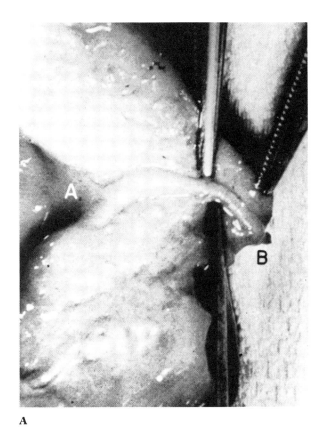

**A**

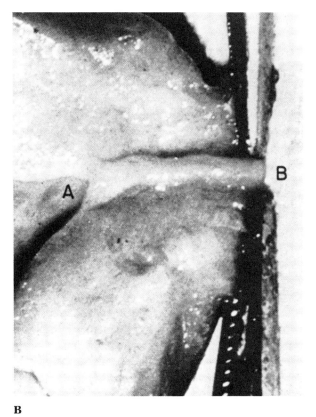

**B**

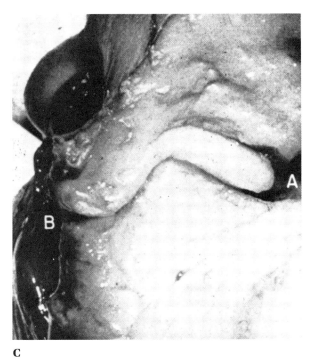

**C**

Finally, the microsurgeon must study the x-ray picture of the interstitial segment and relate this to the thickness of the uterine wall. Hysterosalpingographic studies fail to outline the exterior of the uterus unless pneumoperitoneum is performed, a technique rarely used today. Therefore, it is impossible to be certain of the length of the intramural segment prior to surgery. Geist and Goldringer [70] studied the intramural segment by x-ray and concluded that the diameter varied from 0.5 to 1.0 mm and length varied from 1.5 to 5.0 cm. Of interest was the observation of cornual polyps during this study.

ISTHMUS

The anatomy of the isthmic segment is similar to that of the cornual area, namely, a thick-walled muscular tubal segment with a narrow lumen characterized by four or five mucosal folds (see Fig. 7-10). The average length of the isthmus is 2 to 3 cm, and the lumen diameter is reported to be 0.1 to 1 mm [238]. Woodruff and Pauerstein [238] have also noted that the midisthmic segment often has the smallest lumen, which is estimated to be 0.4 mm. The primary mucosal folds described by Williams [230] run almost the entire length of the isthmus, dividing into secondary folds at the ampullary-isthmic junction. A thick layer of circular muscle is present in this segment and is the layer approximated during surgical anastomosis.

AMPULLA AND INFUNDIBULUM

This thin-walled tubal segment is usually 5 to 8 cm in length and extends from the ampullary-isthmic junction to the infundibulum (see Fig. 7-9). The lumen of the ampullary segment is densely packed with primary and secondary mucosal folds. The diameter of the lumen is estimated to be approximately 1 to 2 mm at the ampullary-isthmic junction, enlarging to a diameter of 1 to 1.5 cm at the infundibulum.* It is often difficult to pass a fine suture through the muscularis layer of the ampullary and infundibulum segments without also including the mucous membrane.

---

*The number of secondary folds increases dramatically as one approaches the fimbriae, and the muscular wall appears to become thinner.

## Factors that Lead to Tubal and Uterine Anastomoses

The clinical indications that lead to tubal anastomosis include prior tubal sterilization and a group of pathologic entities that includes salpingoisthmica nodosa and endometriosis, which usually cause cornual or isthmic occlusion, but occasionally are responsible for a mid-tubal block. An outline of these entities follows:

1. Reversal of prior tubal sterilization
   a. Pomeroy-type procedures, including falope ring and clip
   b. Electrosurgical excision or coagulation, "diathermy"
2. Pathologic processes
   a. Salpingoitis-isthmica nodosa
   b. Postabortal infection
   c. Salpingitis, IUD
   d. Cornual polyps
   e. Endometriosis
   f. Partial salpingectomy for ectopic pregnancy
   g. Others

## Reversal of Tubal Sterilization

End-to-end anastomosis of the midportion of the fallopian tube is most often performed following prior tubal ligation.

ATLAS OF INFERTILITY SURGERY, 1975

This statement from the first edition of this text remains correct. However, the introduction of microsurgery and the increased demand for reversal have resulted in broader application of this area of tubal surgery. As will be discussed later, the term *midportion* is no longer adequate, since there are three types of midtubal anastomosis procedures. Therefore, one must define the exact type of anastomosis being performed, i.e., ampullary-isthmic. In addition, since 1975, the use of magnification has resulted in the introduction of two new surgical uterotubal anastomosis procedures that have markedly affected the surgical approach to reconstruction of the previously ligated oviduct.

The most dramatic change in the overall surgical approach to reversal of tubal sterilization has been the replacement of uterotubal implantation by one of the uterotubal forms of anastomosis made possible by the operating microscope. The premicrosurgical approach of Williams [228] is summarized in the statement that "it seems, therefore, that these sterilized patients are ideal cases for uterotubal implantation." In his published series of patients [229] who were undergoing reversal of prior tubal sterilization, 10 of 16 patients underwent uterotubal implantation. In fact, prior to the introduction of magnification, uterotubal implantation was thought to offer a better prognosis for pregnancy than end-to-end anastomosis. This is not surprising, since tubal lumen diameters of 0.1 to 1.5 mm present in the intramural and tubal isthmic segments cannot be manipulated successfully without magnification. This concept changed, however, with the advent of microsurgical tubal anastomosis, and at present, uterotubal implantation is rarely performed during reversal of tubal sterilization.

Tubal sterilization became increasingly popular as a method of female contraception during the 1970s. Hulka [99] stated in 1977 that over 1 million men and women rely on surgical sterilization. This author estimated that 674,000 female sterilizations were performed in the United States in 1975. At that time, 60 percent were performed postpartum (usually a Pomeroy-type procedure) and 40 percent at a later interval. Of 217,000 interval sterilizations in the United States during 1975, only 6 percent did not involve electrosurgical coagulation, 16 percent were by a bipolar technique, and 68 percent were performed by a form of monopolar coagulation. A survey by the AAGL in 1975 found that most physicians who performed laparoscopic sterilization utilized a coagulation and division technique.

Use of the Falope ring (introduced by Yoon) and, to a lesser degree, the spring-loaded Hulka clip increased markedly after 1977, and at present, monopolar electrocoagulation is rarely used for tubal sterilization. Bipolar tubal coagulation, championed by Kleppinger [120], continues in use. Fear of electrosurgical burns has led most surgeons to adopt nonelectrical techniques, with an increased use of minilaparotomy by those surgeons who are not comfortable performing laparoscopy. By 1979 it was estimated that 10 million individuals had been sterilized in the United States, and 53 percent were female [166].

The reasons for requesting reversal of sterilization were reviewed by Gomel [78]. This author (G.W.P.) found that change in marital status accounted for 63 percent of these requests. Crib death accounted for 17 percent, and the desire to have more children accounted for 10 percent. Certainly the present divorce rate, which is nearing 50 percent in the United States, will remain the major indication for microsurgical reversal of a tubal ligation procedure.

*Anatomic Forms of Tubal Ligation*
The surgeon should be familiar with the types of tubal ligation in use during the past decade and the resulting forms of tubal injury. These surgical techniques have been reviewed by Hafez and Evans [86]. However, a brief summary is presented in Figure 7-12.

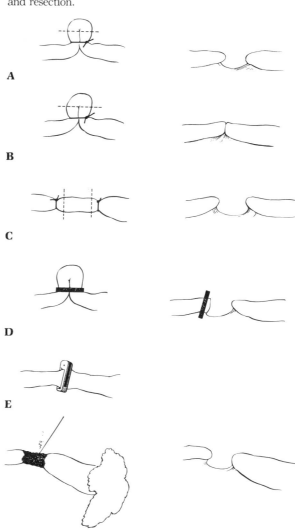

**Figure 7-12.** Type of tubal sterilization procedures and subsequent tubal anatomy. **A.** Pomeroy procedure. **B.** Madliner modification of Pomeroy procedure using permanent suture material. **C.** Midtubal resection. **D.** Falope ring technique. **E.** Clip technique (Hulka). **F.** Electrocoagulation and resection.

As was noted earlier, the most frequently used technique of tubal sterilization removes a portion of the fallopian tube that usually includes the ampullary-isthmic junction. These procedures involve the Pomeroy technique, or a modification, as well as a Madliner procedure, the Falope ring technique, and the minilaparotomy. As was noted, all remove a segment of the midportion of the fallopian tube that usually includes the ampullary-isthmic junction, but can also include only a portion of the midampullary or midisthmic tubal segments (Fig. 7-12).

The Falope ring technique produces a type of tubal injury similar to the Pomeroy technique, with the exception that a shorter segment of tube is involved. In addition, the tubal isthmic is easier to pull inside the ring applicator, thus producing pure isthmic occlusion far more often than found following a Pomeroy ligation. The mildest tubal injury appears to be the 0.3-mm area of tubal damage associated with application of the Hulka clip. This technique of tubal occlusion has been studied in the female pig and human by Hulka and others [235]. The injury usually occurs in the midisthmic segment and has been found readily reversible in both the animal and human models. It is significant that neither the clip nor the Falope ring should be placed on an ampullary segment of the fallopian tube, since the wider lumen of this segment is difficult to occlude and the failure rate increases dramatically when this is done.

Of greater concern to the infertility surgeon will be the decision as to whether reversal of a previously coagulated tubal segment is possible. The major difficulty is the ability to ascertain the length of the residual ampullary tubal segment without visualizing the pelvis. It is in this area that the hysterosalpingography and laparoscopy are necessary preoperative adjuncts. The extent of the fallopian tube injury will vary from a small midtubal defect to almost complete tubal destruction. Surgical techniques of electrocoagulation vary and include the following:

1. Three-burn technique: Coagulation and cutting, one-puncture technique
2. Coagulation only: Single or double puncture
3. Coagulation and resection of a segment: Two-puncture technique
4. Bipolar coagulation: One- or two-puncture technique

One would assume that the coagulation resection technique would lead to the greatest injury. However, in our experience, this has not been the case. We had the opportunity to perform a reversal procedure in two patients on whom we had personally performed tubal coagulation and resection by an electrosurgical approach utilizing the two-puncture laparoscopic technique. In each of these patients, the ampullary segment measured at least 6 cm, and uteroampullary or uteroisthmic anastomoses were possible. In contrast, coagulation only has been reported to lead to extensive injury, presumably because the surgeon attempts to destroy as much of the tube as possible rather than to simply produce coagulation and transection.

FIMBRIECTOMY

Of continuing controversy is the possibility of reversing a prior fimbriectomy-type ligation. Previously thought to be impossible, pregnancies have recently been reported following distal ampullary salpingostomy in these patients by Novy [146]. The length of ampulla or infundibulum necessary for success in these patients is as yet not established. Winston and Margara, however, have reported no successes in 6 such patients [235].

SUMMARY

The Pomeroy tubal sterilization technique or a modification thereof that includes excision of a midtubal segment is commonly performed at the time of cesarean section or immediately postpartum. It is also the procedure occasionally used at the time of minilaparotomy and during vaginal tubal ligation, although fimbriectomy is more commonly employed during the latter procedure. Ligation with the Falope ring also simulates this procedure, although, of course, the Silastic ring is permanent. The area of the ampullary-isthmis junction (AIJ) is frequently removed during this type of ligation, although occasionally a midampullary or midisthmic segment has been excised. The least destructive sterilization procedure at present would appear to be the Hulka clip technique. Placement of the clip on a midisthmic segment permits subsequent isthmic-isthmic reanastomosis, the most successful type of reanastomosis procedure. Laparoscopic tubal coagulation and/or resection (diathermy) was the most popular interval sterilization procedure employed in the United States during the years 1970–1975, and bipolar coagulation is still practiced. This form of electrosurgical tubal resection was for a number of years virtually impossible to reconstruct successfully. The low pregnancy rate reported by Wheeless [227] following uterotubal implantation in 10 of these patients discouraged further attempts at repair until Winston reported in 1977 that 5 of 8 diathermy patients conceived following microsurgical uteroampullary reanastomosis. At present, microsurgical technique permits the repair of this type of tubal defect with excellent success in patients whose tubal remnant measures 4 cm or greater.

*Pathologic Processes Treated by*
*Tubal and Uterine Anastomoses*

An ever-expanding group of pathologic entities resulting in segmental tubal occlusion is now reparable by resection and tubal reanastomosis. A significant change in the surgical approach to salpingitis isthmica nodosa has taken place since the first edition of the *Atlas*. Championed by Winston and Gomel, this change is based on the observation that the site of tubal occlusion associated with salpingitis isthmica nodosum is usually limited to the proximal isthmus and outer one-third of the intramural portion of the fallopian tube and rarely involves the entire intramural segment. It has become possible, therefore, to excise the occluded segment under magnification provided by the operating microscope and to perform uteroisthmic anastomosis rather than uterotubal implantation, as recommended earlier [118]. In fact, uteroisthmic and isthmic-isthmic anastomoses have replaced uterotubal implantation in the treatment of most cases of cornual and isthmic occlusions.

Occlusion of a cornual segment by a polyp was recently found to be an additional cause of cornual occlusion. As discussed earlier by Sweeney and others, including Geist [70], this entity has been found to be the cause of cornual occlusion in instances in which an inflammatory process is not present.

Midtubal occlusion may occasionally be caused by a pathologic entity other than tubal sterilization. Perhaps the most common factor at present is a midtubal defect produced by excision of the site of an unruptured tubal pregnancy. Conservation of the fallopian tube during the treatment of an ectopic pregnancy has been advocated [118], and reanastomosis of this tubal segment does not appear to increase the incidence of subsequent tubal pregnancies in that oviduct. Although it is occasionally possible to perform reanastomosis at the time of excision of a tubal pregnancy, many surgeons are not prepared to perform a microsurgical anastomosis at this point and should not attempt to do so. There is no evidence to show, however, that an unsuccessful anastomosis at the time of tubal pregnancy leads to a more difficult reanastomosis at a later interval, and in fact, a shorter segment of the fallopian tube is removed during an attempted anastomosis than when the tubal segments are individually ligated.

## Reflections on Tubal Function

The increasing skill of the microsurgeon has introduced dramatic changes in the gynecologist's perception of fallopian tube function. The following reflections were made possible by the ability of the operating surgeon to successfully transect and anastomose the animal (rabbit) oviduct. Winston [232] introduced the present technique of microsurgical anastomosis of the rabbit oviduct with a remarkable 93 percent postoperative pregnancy success rate in 1975. Similar successes have been reported by Eddy et al. [54] and Owen and Pickett-Heaps [150] following transection and reanastomosis of the rabbit fallopian tube. This ability to successfully reunite a transected segment of the fallopian tube has permitted the experimental surgeon to study the effects of removal of segments of the oviduct on subsequent pregnancies, as well as to study the effect that reversing a small segment of isthmic or ampullary tube would have on subsequent pregnancy rates. In the sections that follow, interesting animal and human results of tubal anastomoses have been discussed as they apply to the function of the uterotubal junction, the tubal isthmus, the ampullary-isthmic junction, and the ampullary segments.

INTERSTITIAL SEGMENT AND UTEROTUBAL JUNCTION (UTJ)

The first experimental study that utilized a microsurgical technique to perform reanastomosis of the rabbit fallopian tube was reported by David, Brackett, and Garcia in 1969 [39]. These surgeons, at the University of Pennsylvania Hospital, resected the UTJ (a 1.5-cm segment of isthmus and uterine cornu) in 25 rabbits, after which they performed uteroisthmic anastomosis over a polyethylene stent aided by a Zeiss operating microscope. Postoperatively, 48 percent (11 of 15) of the rabbits conceived in the reattached tube. However, a comparison of corpora lutea and implantation sites revealed a decreased 41 percent incidence of implantation in the operated tube compared with a 96 percent correlation in the unoperated side. David et al. concluded that "sperm migration, fertilization and ovum transport can occur in the absence of the UTJ," but these authors also stated that removal of the UTJ appeared to decrease the ability of the oviduct to retain ova until they were ready to implant. It will be pointed out later that a major defect in the study by David et al. was the use of polyethylene stents left in situ for a prolonged interval following microsurgical uterotubal anastomosis [39]. Recent studies in the human and in the rabbit demonstrate markedly lower pregnancy rates when stents are used for prolonged intervals, and certainly a repeat study involving resection of the UTJ in rabbits without the use of stents would be of great value. This type of anastomosis has become a standard part of the armamentarium of the gynecologic microsurgeon and has, in many instances, replaced the more destructive procedure of uterotubal implantation.

ISTHMUS

Transection of the isthmic segment followed by microsurgical anastomosis has been widely studied in the rabbit, pig, and human. Winston [232] and Eddy et al. [54] reported excellent pregnancy results following transection of the rabbit isthmus (93 and 100 percent). Removal of a small segment of isthmus lowers the pregnancy rate only slightly, as demonstrated in the studies of Winston [232], as well as those involving reversal of clip ligation in the pig and human [100]. In fact, Winston reported that pregnancy occurred in 8 of 8 patients undergoing clip reversal. As was noted earlier, isthmic-isthmic reanastomosis may achieve the highest pregnancy success rate. Both Winston and Gomel have studied the effect on pregnancy of removing increasing segments of isthmus: "Fewer animals became pregnant when greater lengths of isthmus were removed, the trend leveling off after 50 percent or more had been resected. . . . More than this did not reduce absolute fertility and about one half of the animals conceived when 90 to 100 percent of the isthmus was resected" [232]. The study by McComb and Gomel [132] noted almost no decrease in pregnancy when 20 percent of the total oviduct was resected (about two-thirds of the isthmic segment). However, when 40 percent was removed (the entire isthmus), pregnancy fell to one-third. Removal of more than 60 percent of the fallopian tube, i.e., all the isthmic segment and about one-half the ampulla, reduced the pregnancy rate to 0. The ability to achieve a pregnancy in the absence of the isthmus has clearly been demonstrated by the successful pregnancies reported in the female following uteroampullary anastomosis employed to repair electrosurgical destruction of the entire isthmus. One might also recall that many cases of uterotubal implantation were actually ampullary implantation, and that pregnancy occurred in 20 to 40 percent of these patients.

The functional role of the tubal isthmus was further studied by Eddy et al. [54] in a study in which reversal of a segment of isthmus was performed. A segment approximately 1 cm in length was cut, the vascular pedicle maintained while the segment was reversed, and the ends reattached by microsurgical anastomosis. Although Kuo and Lim [123] performed a similar experiment in 1928 without successful pregnancy, Eddy et al. [55] noted that "reversal of 1-cm segments of the rabbit oviductal isthmus did not interfere with normal pregnancy." These studies, including reversal of both the proximal and distal isthmic segments, led to the conclusion that "in the isthmus, with its sparse ciliation and prominent mesosalpinx, segmental reversal imparts a weak adovarian ciliary bias easily overcome by the contractile activity of the isthmus" [53]. In fact, it appeared that the muscular activity of the isthmus reverted to its original function following reversal and did not lead to a substantial decrease in pregnancy.

AMPULLARY-ISTHMIS JUNCTION

The junction of tubal isthmus and ampullary segments has been thought to represent a type of sphincter that acts to delay ovum transport through the ampulla and as such to be essential for a normal pregnancy [238]. It was startling, therefore, when early microsurgical studies demonstrated that ampullary-isthmic reanastomosis resulted in excellent pregnancy results; i.e., Owen and Pickett-Heaps [150] found that 6 of 7 such patients conceived following ampullary-isthmic reanastomosis. Pomeroy-type tubal sterilization procedures frequently remove a tubal segment that includes the ampullary-isthmic junction, and reanastomosis is successful in over 50 percent of these patients. Eddy et al. [54] removed the ampullary-isthmic junction from rabbit tubes and found no change in normal fertility following microsurgical reanastomosis of isthmic and ampullary segments. It should be noted that microsurgical reconstruction of the human ampullary-isthmic junction is not anatomically perfect, since postoperative pregnancy rates are approximately 55 to 64 percent, a lower success rate than that obtained with other types of reanastomosis (see Table 7-27).

AMPULLA

A paradox has occurred in the area of the ampullary-ampullary reanastomosis, since prior to the use of microsurgical technique, this type of anastomosis produced a pregnancy more often than did other types of tubal reanastomosis. However, recent microsurgical studies indicate a reversal in this trend and, in fact, have noted that the lowest postoperative pregnancy rate often follows ampullary-ampullary reanastomosis (see page 278). Although it is a relatively simple matter to reoppose the ends of two ampullary segments, two possible defects may occur: (1) malpositioning of the rugal mucosal folds, which then interfere with ovum transport through the ampulla, and (2) shortening of the ampullary segment, thereby preventing an adequate delay in ovum transport. Winston [232] resected various lengths of ampulla in 46 rabbits and found that "the number of pregnancies fell in linear fashion to 0 when 70 percent had been removed." Merely transecting the ampulla did not appear to alter fertility in the rabbits, however. Eddy (1980) reported that double transection of proximal, middle, and distal ampullae in the rabbit followed by microsurgical anastomosis did not significantly alter fertility. These studies appear to eliminate the first objection, which suggested that rugal (mucosal) folds might not be properly aligned following reanastomosis. It would appear, therefore, that the most significant factor determining pregnancy following ampullary-ampullary reanastomosis is the amount of ampulla that has been resected.

Reversal of ampullary segments has been reported by two groups of experimentors. Eddy et al. [53] performed reversal of middle, proximal, and distal ampullary segments without achieving a viable pregnancy. This was consistent with the concept that ciliary activity is primarily responsible for ovum transport in this tubal segment. McComb and Gomel [131], however, also performed segmental reversal of ampullary segments and found that pregnancy occurred in one such animal following a delay of 70 to 90 days. These authors surmised that ciliary movement had become reoriented during this prolonged interval.

## Techniques of Tubal and Uterine Anastomosis

Five types of tubal anastomoses are possible, and all five must become "second nature" to the microsurgeon. In the discussion that follows, two of the procedures have been outlined in detail. The general principles of a two-layer closure, including tissue handling, tubal lavage, and incision of the tubal lumen, are applicable to the other types of anastomoses. The first, ampullary-isthmic anastomosis, is representative of tubotubal anastomoses and is probably the most commonly performed anastomosis utilized in reversal of prior tubal sterilization. Abbreviated sketches of the techniques of isthmic-isthmic and ampullary-ampullary anastomoses have been included.

The second anastomosis diagramed in detail is a uteroisthmic anastomosis most commonly performed for tubal occlusion due to intrinsic cornual pathology rather than prior sterilization. The second type of uterotubal anastomosis, ampullary-uterine, is diagramed in brief, but it uses the principles demonstrated during uteroisthmic anastomosis. The types of tubal anastomoses are as follows:

1. Tubotubal anastomoses
   a. Isthmic-ampullary*
   b. Isthmic-isthmic
   c. Ampullary-ampullary
2. Tubouterine anastomoses
   a. Uteroisthmic*
   b. Uteroampullary

*Techniques diagramed in detail.

## HIGHLIGHTS OF MICROSURGICAL ANASTOMOSIS TECHNIQUE

The basic microsurgical technique described in detail at the beginning of this chapter is employed during a tubal or uterine anastomosis. Specific highlights that apply to tubotubal or tuboovarian anastomoses are discussed below:

1. *Suture material.* The sutures employed during microsurgical anastomosis are either 8-0 synthetic absorbable suture (Vicryl or Dexon) or 9-0 nylon. We utilized 8-0 polyglactic 910 (Vicryl) on a cutting needle (GS-9) during our early anastomosis techniques, but then found 9-0 nylon easier to handle and a more comfortable suture. The stock needle selection provided with 9-0 nylon was also superior at that time, since a taper needle was not available with Vicryl or Dexon (see Chapter 5 for this discussion). Addition of a small-diameter taper needle to 8-0 synthetic absorbable suture material now appears to make this the preferable suture. We now use 8-0 Dexon or 8-0 coated Vicryl on a 130-$\mu$ or 145-$\mu$ taper needle in almost all cases. Pregnancy rates have not differed with the use of these two sutures. Polyglactin 910 (Vicryl) suture has been used by Gomel [77] and nylon by Winston [232] and Diamond [48]. Two additional sutures are 6-0 coated polyglactin 910 (Vicryl), which is very useful for opposing the mesosalpinx, and 10-0 nylon, which is used occasionally for isthmic-cornual anastomoses. The needle used with 10-0 suture is a taper point of 50- to 70-$\mu$m wire diameter.

2. *Stents.* Although the use of polyethylene stents has clearly been abandoned, 2-0 nylon thread is occasionally useful during uteroisthmic anastomosis because of its small size, stiffness, and dark color. It is usually removed immediately following anastomosis so that lavage can then be performed. Passage of a 2-0 nylon suture through the isthmus is occasionally not possible, and we have utilized a technique in which the nylon is threaded through the intramural segment and coiled within the uterine cavity for removal 48 to 72 hours postoperatively.

*3. Placement of sutures during closure of first layer.* A controversy exists regarding placement of the first layer of sutures during tubal reanastomosis. The issue is whether the suture should pass into the tubal lumen or whether care should be taken to exclude the tubal mucosa with this suture, thereby placing it through only the muscularis layer (Fig. 7-13).

In early clinical microsurgical studies, Winston [233] and Gomel [74] stated that the suture utilized in the first layer of a tubal reanastomosis should not pass into the tubal lumen for fear of establishing an inflammatory reaction at that site and thereby contributing to partial obstruction. Diamond [48], however, used 9-0 and 10-0 nylon passed through the lumen with excellent pregnancy results. The debate regarding placement of sutures during midtubal anastomosis still exists. It has become apparent, however, that placement of the sutures used in the first layer depends partially on the site of anastomosis and partially on the difficulty encountered achieving an accurate tubal approximation.

Seki et al. [176] have published the only experimental study that compared these two suturing techniques in microsurgical anastomosis of the rabbit oviduct. These investigators asked the following question: "When the suture penetrates the endosalpinx, are the results of tubal anastomosis different from results obtained when the mucosa is carefully excluded?" In eight rabbits, 10-0 monofilament nylon sutures were passed through serosa and through myosalpinx and mucosa, and in two rabbits, a similar anastomosis was performed excluding the mucosa. It should be noted that this team of researchers has published numerous studies of tubal reanastomosis in which the mucosa was excluded with excellent pregnancy results. Three of the rabbits were then mated and all three conceived. Fourteen of 16 oviducts were patent at the time of sacrifice. One oviduct demonstrated partial occlusion, and the other was totally occluded. Examination of the anastomotic site revealed disturbance of the mucosal folds "showing some discontinuity," and these "were bunched slightly to the center. Similar changes are observed in tubes that have been sutured to include the mucosa and in those in which the mucosa had been carefully excluded." Interestingly, the surface of the intralumenal suture became completely covered by 9 weeks, at which time most of the intralumenal sutures were completely epithelialized. These cells were, however, "very large and misshapened in comparison with normal epithelium cells" [176]. In summary, "The results with through-and-through sutures were not different from those in another group of animals . . . in which the sutures were placed to avoid the mucosa" [176]. These authors concluded that "there seems to be no practical advantage to placing the sutures to exclude the endosalpinx."

It is our opinion that during closure of the muscularis layers, the suture should not pass into the tubal lumen.

**Figure 7-13.** Placement of the first suture during tubal anastomosis. **A.** Suture passed through muscularis layer carefully avoiding the tubal mucosa. **B.** The suture has included the muscularis and mucosa layers.

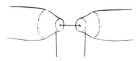

**A**

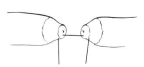

**B**

However, placement of this suture depends in part on the tubal anatomy, and the first tenet of a successful anastomosis should be accuracy of anatomic approximation of the two tubal lumina. Although, in general, during ampullary-ampullary anastomosis, the first layer of suture is placed in the muscularis, at times the surgeon will be more comfortable placing the first suture through the muscularis layer into the tubal lumen. The folds of tubal mucosa make accurate identification of the lumen somewhat difficult, and the thin muscularis layer may preclude restriction of the suture to this layer. This point also applies to an ampullary-isthmic anastomosis. The usual placement of sutures during ampullary-isthmic anastomosis permits the approximation of the muscularis layer in most cases. However, on occasion the suture may enter the ampullary lumen. Uteroampullary anastomoses present a totally different technical problem, involving placement of the suture at the cornual end. The surgeon will find it technically difficult to approximate ampullary and cornual tubal segments, since the cornual opening is a stiff muscular type of tissue. It is therefore much easier to place the initial suture outside the cornual opening and to overlap this cornual nipple with the tubal ampulla.

4. *Microelectrode*. Both monopolar and bipolar electrodes are useful during tubal reanastomosis. The monopolar microelectrode is useful during dissection of the occluded remnant, although incision of the mucosal surfaces directly involved in the anastomosis is performed nonelectrically. Bipolar coagulation of small vessels is also useful, although again, care is taken not to coagulate extensively near the inner surface of the anastomotic site. The injection of dilute Pitressin in this area eliminates much of the bleeding from the cut surfaces and is used routinely.

5. *Instruments*. A fine-tip needle holder without lock and fine, smooth-tip forceps are utilized. A fine-tooth forceps is necessary during uterine anastomosis procedures involving the cornual area. A special sharp scissors is used to cut the isthmic segment, and a Winston probe is always useful.

6. *Other adjuncts*. Dilute Pitressin—1 ampule mixed in 100 ml (a 1:20 dilution) and used with a 3-cc syringe and a No. 30 needle. Irrigation solutions—lactated Ringer's (plain) 1000 ml; dilute heparin solution, 5000 units heparin (5 cc) in 500 ml lactated Ringer's solution.

TECHNIQUE OF TUBAL LAVAGE (HYDROTUBATION)

A prerequisite during surgical repair of the oviduct is the ability to ascertain tubal patency at various times during a procedure. Although preliminary x-ray and laparoscopic studies have indicated the status of the oviduct, the surgeon should have the ability to verify these findings during surgery.

As discussed earlier, we have used the term *tubal lavage* to refer to the passage of dye from the uterine cavity outward through the oviducts. The terms *transfundal hydrotubation* and *chromopertubation* have been used synonymously. The popular technique of transfundal injection through a cannula placed into the uterine fundus while occluding the cervix with a Buxton or Shirodkar clamp is now infrequently used. Rather, a HUI (Harris uterine insufflator) catheter can be placed into the uterine cavity prior to surgery and dye injected when necessary. We have utilized this technique in over 200 patients without evidence of complication. In 5 to 10 percent of patients, a problem with the flow of dye may require use of the Buxton clamp technique. A recent development has been reverse hydrotubation through the fimbrial end of the oviduct in order to establish patency of a distal isthmic segment. An angled Stangle type perfusion cannula is utilized for this purpose. The techniques of tubal lavage are presented in Figure 7-14.

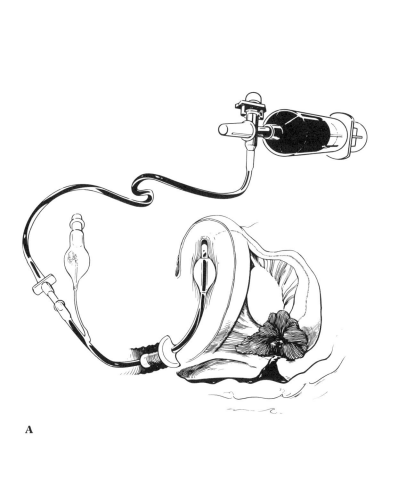

A

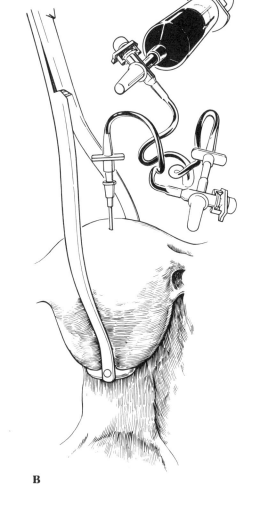

B

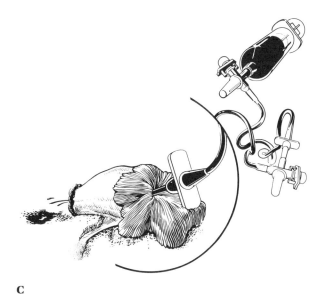

C

**Figure 7-14.** Techniques of tubal lavage (hydrotubation): **A.** A Harris intrauterine device (HUI transcervical canula) is presently utilized in place of the transuterine needle and Buxton clamp technique shown above. This technique does not require a uterine puncture and it eliminates the cumbersome uterine clamp from the incision. The catheter is placed in the uterine cavity at the beginning of surgery. A K-50 extension tubing is then carried into the sterile field and a 20 cc syringe containing blue dye attached. Injection of dye is then possible when indicated. The Buxton clamp and needle technique should, however, be held in reserve should the catheter be displaced during a surgical procedure. **B.** The Buxton clamp can be utilized to occlude the lower uterine segment. A 20 gauge Jelco-type catheter is placed through the uterine fundus into the endometrial cavity. K-50 and K-52 plastic extension tubing is then attached to the 20 cc syringe containing indigo carmen or methylene blue dye. This technique has been in wide use since its description by Buxton in 1964. It was described at length in the first edition of the *Atlas.* **C.** It is important to ascertain patency of the ampullary and isthmic segment during a tubal anastomosis procedure. Blue dye should, therefore, be injected into the fimbriated end by placing the tip of the K-50 extension tubing or an angled perfusion canula, shown in Fig. 5-47, into the fimbriated opening. Although an ampullary segment can easily be proved, this will not be possible when a small isthmic segment remains attached. This type of reverse hydrotubation is therefore of great value. An angled perfusion canula, which attaches to the K-50 tubing, is an added convenience.

Figures 7-15, 7-16, and 7-17 demonstrate the three techniques of tubotubal anastomosis. Most often performed following Pomeroy or Falope ring-type ligation procedures, isthmic-ampullary anastomosis will occasionally be required following partial salpingectomy due to midtubal ectopic pregnancy and, less frequently, midtubal occlusion caused by implants of endometriosis. A second technique of isthmic-isthmic anastomosis is usually employed during repair of a clip-type tubal sterilization procedure. The third technique of ampullary-ampullary anastomosis also follows a prior sterilization procedure, usually a Pomeroy-type performed in the midampulla.

**Figure 7-15.** Isthmic-ampullary anastomosis. **A.** The site of occlusion, including the ampullary-isthmic junction, is identified under the operating microscope. This segment is elevated with fine forceps and excised with a fine monopolar electrode, taking care not to cut into the normal mesosalpinx. Note the use of a glass rod to gently stabilize the distal tubal segment. Injection of dye through the transcervical canula assists in identifying the distal isthmic segment. **B.** Sharp straight or angled scissors are used to cut the isthmic segment cleanly. Fine toothed forceps may be used on the tissue segment being excised, but should not be used to hold tubal serosa whenever possible. **C.** Demonstration of distal (isthmic) patency by transcervical lavage is extremely important at this time. The surgeon must also examine the isthmic mucosa under high magnification to ascertain the normal four-fold pattern. Use of the fingers to gently hold the tube is emphasized in this drawing. It is the surgeon's usual policy to prepare both isthmic segments prior to anastomosis. This is particularly valuable when there is difficulty in ascertaining tubal patency and repetitive injections of dye are necessary. Should one anastomosis have been completed, a repetitive injection of dye might lead to

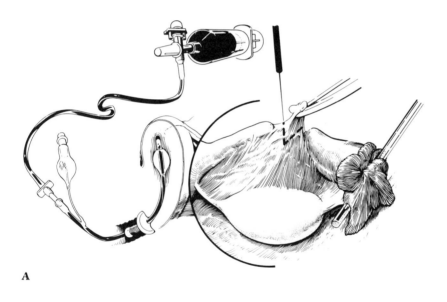

A

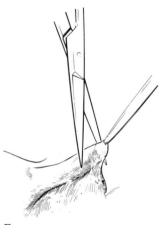

B

infiltration and damage of this anastomosis. **D.** The technique of opening the ampullary segment is extremely important. Creation of a small opening that matches the isthmic lumen size greatly facilitates anastomosis. It is, therefore, important to make a small opening rather than to simply cut across the ampullary lumen. This is accomplished by using fine forceps to hold a small segment of lumen which can then be cut with the curved Wescott scissors. The right-hand part of the figure shows a second approach in which a Winston probe has been used to distend a part of the ampullary segment permitting excision of a small distal segment. In both cases, the outer serosal layer should be gently trimmed so that it falls back from the inner muscularis, identified as a white layer. **E.** Again, demonstration of patency of the ampullary segment is very important. If a probe has been placed through this segment, lavage is not necessary. However, during isthmic-isthmic and isthmic-uterine anastomoses, this technique of reverse pertubation or reverse chromopertubation is extremely important. The small plastic tip of the K-50 extension tubing fits nicely into the fimbrial opening and can be held in place to achieve a tight fit during injection of dye. A right-angled perfusion cannula (shown earlier) is also useful for this purpose.

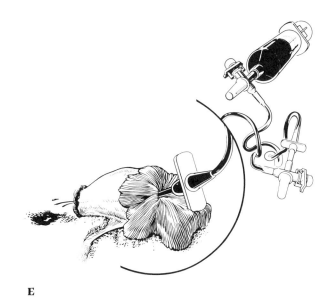

E

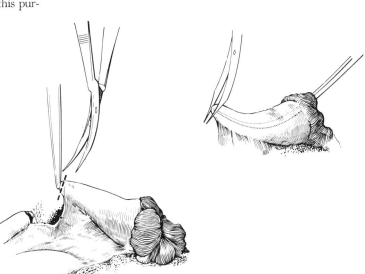

D

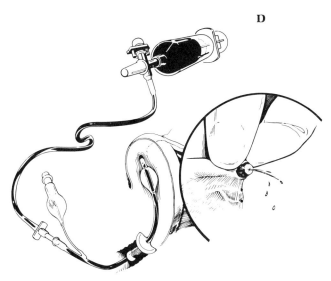

C

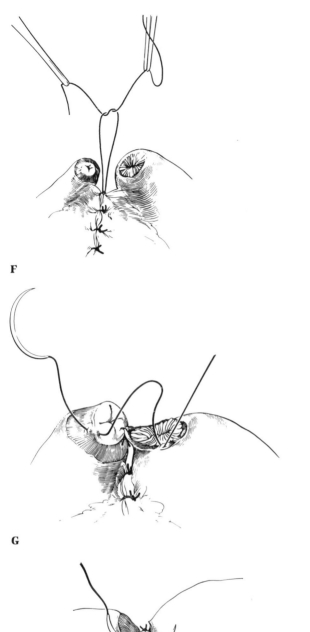

**F**

**Figure 7-15 (continued)**
**F.** Approximation of the tubal ends prior to anastomosis removes tension from the line of anastomosis. This is
accomplished by placement of a 6-0 Dexon Vicryl or PDS
(polydioxanone) suture in the mesosalpinx right below the
tubal serosa. In usual practice, the suture closest to the fallopian tube is placed first. **G.** The first layer of the anastomosis is performed with 8-0 synthetic absorbable suture
(Vicryl or dexon) or 9-0 nylon. A taper needle, diameter 130 to
145 μm, should be used at this time. Placement of the suture
through the muscularis layers has been shown although this
is not always possible, particularly in the ampullary segment. The most difficult suture on the inferior edge of the
lumen (6 o'clock) must be placed first, followed by placement of lateral sutures, and finally the 12 o'clock suture.
Placing the overhand tie squarely will maintain the suture
tension and permit placement of the second row without
spillage or separation of these ends of the oviduct. **H.** The
serosal (second) layer is closed with interrupted sutures of
8-0 synthetic absorbable Dexon or Vicryl. Again, a fine taper
needle is used. Accurate approximation is very important
during this closure, and again, the most difficult suture (6
o'clock) is placed first. **I.** Demonstration of patency by transcervical lavage is performed following closure of the first
layer and then again upon completion of the anastomosis.
Small degrees of leakage at the anastomotic site are generally overlooked. Infiltration of dye into the distal segment is
sometimes observed.

**G**

**H**

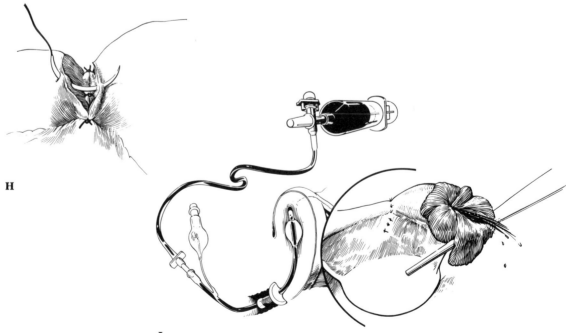

**I**

**Figure 7-16.** Isthmic-isthmic anastomosis. Reanastomosis of two isthmic segments is technically satisfactory for the microsurgeon and produces excellent pregnancy results. Two muscular lumina of nearly equal size appear to fall together with ease following placement of the initial 6-0 synthetic absorbable suture in the mesosalpinx. Tubal patency should be determined by injection of dye through the transcervical canula and again through the fimbriated end, using an angled perfusion canula. This is particularly important during isthmic-isthmic anastomosis since passage of a probe across this small lumen is often difficult. The first layer of the anastomosis employs 8-0 synthetic absorbable suture on a small taper needle or 9-0 nylon passed through the tubal-muscularis layer. Again, the most difficult 6 o'clock suture is placed first. The suture should include only the muscularis. A nylon stent is unnecessary at this time, since it is possible to visualize the lumen under the high magnification provided by the operating microscope during the entire first layer closure. Approximately 10 to 12 power magnification may be used during placement of this suture, and lower 2 to 3 power utilized during tying and cutting of the suture. After completing this layer, injecting dye through the transcervical canula (HUI) verifies patency of this anastomosis. Closure of the second layer is performed with interrupted 8-0 synthetic absorbable suture.

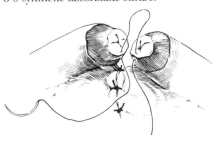

**Figure 7-17.** Ampullary-ampullary anastomosis. This anastomotic technique should not be taken casually even though it presents a significantly smaller technical challenge to the microsurgeon; postoperative pregnancy results are often relatively low following this type of anastomosis. The approach to opening the occluded ampullary segments has been shown in Figure 7-15D. Patency of the proximal segment should be demonstrated by transcervical lavage as demonstrated earlier. Figure 7-17 demonstrates the first layer of the ampullary-ampullary anastomosis in which an attempt is made to oppose only muscularis layers. Occasionally, this is not possible, and passage of the needle into the tubal lumen is necessary. Eight-0 synthetic absorbable suture is employed for this anastomosis. Closure of the serosal layer should be performed carefully with interrupted 8-0 synthetic absorbable suture in order to avoid distortion of the tubal lumen. After completion of the anastomosis, patency is again demonstrated by lavage as shown in Figure 7-15I.

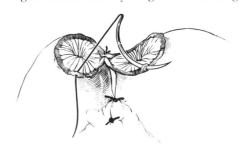

Figure 7-18 demonstrates the technique of uteroisthmic anastomosis in detail. This procedure is most often performed for the treatment of tubal pathology that has caused cornual or isthmic occlusion and includes SIN, prior infection, endometriosis, and prior abortion. The first three processes require excision of a 1- to 2-cm tubal segment in order to remove the disease process. Anastomosis of normal segments is then possible. A second technique of uteroampullary anastomosis is usually performed for reversal of a sterilization procedure that involved electrosurgical coagulation (diathermy) of a midtubal segment (Fig. 7-19).

**Figure 7-18.** Utero-isthmic anastomosis. **A.** Following injection of dilute pistressin, incision of the isthmic segment is made at a distance of 1 cm from the uterine cornu with sharp straight or angled scissors. The dotted line in this drawing defines the subsequent incision of the mesosalpinx close to the tubal wall. The monopolar electrode is used to make this incision and extreme care is taken to avoid transecting the ascending branch of the uterine cavity artery or major vessels in the mesosalpinx. **B.** Again, following injection of dilute pitressin, sharp incision of the intramural tubal segment is made with a specially designed knife blade. The outer serosal layer may be incised with the fine electrode. Fine-toothed forceps are necessary at this point to hold the muscular tubal segment while cutting in order to provide traction. Observe the normal appearance of the cut end of the isthmic segment. **C.** Documentation of normal architecture of the intramural segment is necessary and the normal intramural mucosa will be revealed under high

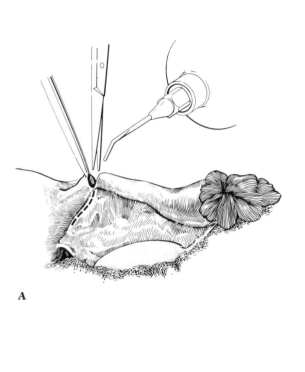

A

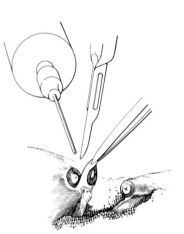

B

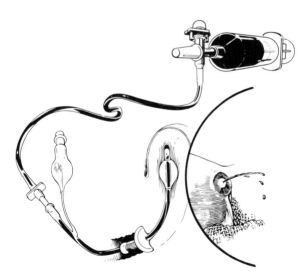

C

power magnification. Lavage through the transcervical canula should produce a stream of fluid that will shoot out of the tubal lumen with great force. **D.** When necessary, to ensure accurate approximation of the tubal lumen, a 2-0 nylon stent is threaded through the intramural segment into the uterine cavity. The coiled nylon should be placed inside the uterine cavity for removal 24 to 48 hours later. In these cases, only 2 to 3 cm of the nylon is threaded directly into the distal isthmic segment. When possible, the nylon is threaded through the entire oviduct and removed through the fimbriated end immediately following anastomosis. **E.** The mesosalpinx has been approximated with 6-0 synthetic absorbable suture (Dexon or Vicryl). The first layer of the anastomosis is performed with 8-0 synthetic absorbable suture or 9-0 nylon. The 6 o'clock suture has been placed first, as always, and is located outside the tubal lumen. The nylon stent is shown in this drawing. Fixation of the anastomotic site provided by careful packing permits the surgeon to move easily from low to high power during close inspection; the narrow depth of field at high magnification requires a virtual absence of tubal motion. **F.** The second layer of this anastomosis usually employs 8-0 synthetic absorbable suture to oppose the tubal and uterine serosa. As with ampullary-ampullary anastomosis, care must be taken not to distort the first layer when difficulty is encountered because of a large serosal defect. Occasionally, 6-0 synthetic absorbable suture is utilized at this point to ensure strength in this layer. **G.** Finally, tubal patency is confirmed by transcervical or transfundal lavage. As noted earlier, lavage had been performed following closure of the first layer since correction of a defect is easier at that time. This drawing demonstrates use of the Buxton clamp to perform hydrotubation through a transfundal canula. Although this small opening is a potential site of adhesion formation, facilitating with this technique is necessary when the transcervical canula becomes occluded or falls out of the uterus during a microsurgical procedure, preventing reinsertion.

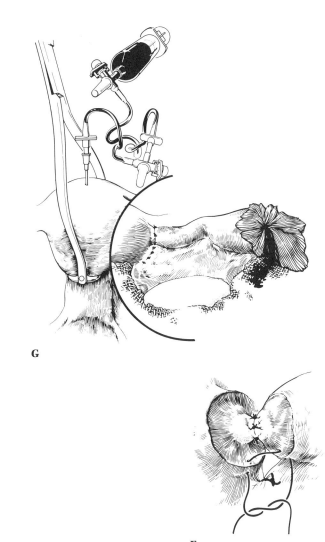

G

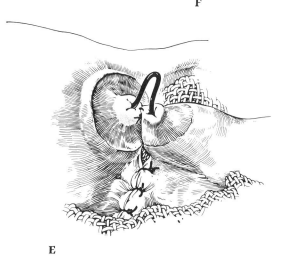

F

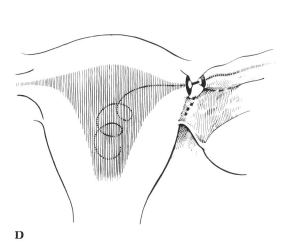

D

E

**Figure 7-19.** Utero-ampullary anastomosis. **A.** The usual tubal defect associated with prior tubal electrocoagulation in which the entire isthmic segment has been destroyed is outlined. A small isthmic stump may be present at the uterus. The residual ampullary segment should measure at least 4 cm. **B.** The cornual and ampullary segments are injected with diluate pitressin and carefully opened. Great care is taken not to produce an overly large ampullary opening. Anastomosis of the thin walled ampullary segment to the thick walled intramural (cornual) tubal segment is accomplished by suturing the muscularis layer of ampulla over the cornual opening. A suture of 8-0 synthetic absorbable suture or 9-0 nylon is placed in the muscularis layer adjacent to the cornual opening in such a fashion that the ampullary segment covers the rigid cornual segment. A 2-0 nylon stent may be used during the first layer of anastomosis and then removed through the fimbrial end. Lavage at this time confirms patency and a second layer of 8-0 synthetic absorbable suture (Vicryl or Dexon) is placed circumferentially about the anastomosis opposing the serosal edges.

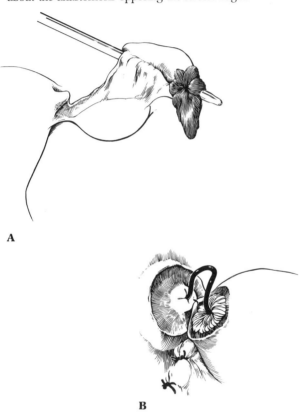

**A**

**B**

ROLE OF THE CARBON DIOXIDE LASER DURING TUBAL ANASTOMOSIS PROCEDURES

The carbon dioxide laser has been used in place of the microelectrode during preparation of an occluded tubal segment for tubal reanastomosis. This technique permits the surgeon to selectively cut individual layers of the tubal wall. The tubal serosa can be vaporized with the power density ranging from 800 to 1,000 W per square centimeter (power 2–2.5 watts, spot diameter .5 mm) [6]. The underlined muscularis layer can then be incised without damaging the mucosal layer by using a power density of 5,000 W per square centimeter (power 12 watts, spot diameter .5 mm). Incision of the mucosa is then performed sharply, using scissors or the knife as shown earlier.

Bellina [6] prefers reanastomosis with 8-0 polyglactin 910 suture and does not employ a technique called *laser welding*. At present there have been no studies to demonstrate the usefulness of attempting to weld the tubal ends together with the laser beam.

*Results of Tubal and Uterine Anastomosis*
It is firmly established that the use of magnification during an anastomosis procedure for reversal of tubal sterilization significantly increases the chance of a subsequent uterine pregnancy and decreases the number of postoperative ectopic (tubal) pregnancies. It appears that the two most significant factors that influence subsequent pregnancy are the specific type of anastomosis procedure and the length of the residual oviduct. It also has become apparent that a form of uterotubal anastomosis can be utilized in the treatment of cornual occlusion with higher pregnancy results than have been attained following uterotubal implantation.

A review of the nonmicrosurgical studies of sterilization reversal by tubal reanastomosis is presented in Table 7-22. The large series reviewed in the first edition of the *Atlas* has been included. However, unfortunately, the tubal pregnancy rate was not reported by many of these surgeons. In all studies included in Table 7-22 patients underwent an anastomosis procedure and postoperatively pregnancy occurred in 129 (39%) of the entire group. The number of tubal pregnancies was recorded in only 163 of these patients, and in this group, there were 71 pregnancies (44%). However, in 16 of 71 patients (23%), the pregnancies were ectopic. The largest series in this nonmicrosurgical group of 163 patients was reported by McCormick et al. [134,135]. These surgeons attained the highest pregnancy rate (64%) reported following use of a nonmicrosurgical technique for reversal of tubal sterilization by selecting only the better of the two tubes for repair. Unfortunately, 8 of 34 (24%) of the pregnancies reported by McCormick et al. were ectopic, lowering the uterine pregnancy rate in his patients to 43 percent. A high ectopic pregnancy rate also was reported by Hodari et

**Table 7-22.** Pregnancy following reanastomosis for reversal of tubal sterilization, nonmicrosurgical reanastomosis technique

| Study | No. of patients | Percent uterine pregnancy | Ectopic | Percent total | Comments |
|---|---|---|---|---|---|
| Kistner & Patton, 1975 | 159 | N/A | N/A | 33 | Lit. review |
| Siegler, 1975 | 46 | 37 | 1 | 39 | Lit. review |
| Siegler, 1975 | 17 | 24 | 1 | 29 | Reversal cases |
| McCormick, 1976 | 13 | 62 | 1 | 69 | Repaired better tube |
| McCormick, 1979 | 53 | 49 | 8 | 64 | Ectopic 8 of 34 (24%) |
| Hodari, 1977 | 14 | 29 | 3 | 50 | Ectopic 3 of 7 (43%) |
| Wheeless, 1977 | 10 | 10 | 0 | 10 | Uterine implant for "diathermy" |
| Diamond, 1977 | 12 | N/A | N/A | 42 | |
| Patton, 1977 | 10 | 40 | 2 | 60 | Personal cases prior to 1977 |
| Total | 334 | 55/163 | 16/71 | 129/334 | |
| Percentage | | 34% | 23%[a] | 39[b] | |

[a]Ectopic pregnancies in series were 16 of 163 (10%).
[b]Total pregnancies in series were 71 of 163 (44%).

**Table 7-23.** Pregnancy following reanastomosis for reversal of tubal sterilization: microsurgical reanastomosis technique

| Study | No. of patients | Percent uterine | Ectopic | Percent total | |
|---|---|---|---|---|---|
| Clyman, 1971 | 27 | 41 | 0 | 41 | |
| Garcia, 1972 | 16 | N/A | N/A | | 50–81 |
| Wilson, 1976 | 3 | 67 | 0 | 67 | |
| Gomel, 1980 | 112 | 64 | 1 | 65 | |
| Winston, 1980 | 95 | 59 | 3 | 60 | |
| Diamond, 1977 | 16 | 75 | 0 | 75 | |
| Owens-Pettigrew, 1977 | 10 | 60 | 0 | 60 | |
| Paterson & Wood, 1977 | 9 | 22 | 0 | 22 | |
| Jones-Rock, 1978 | 12 | 75 | 1 | 83 | |
| Siegler, 1979 | 16 | 50 | 1 | 56 | |
| Patton, 1980 | 27 | 70 | 0 | 70 | |
| Total | 343 | 199/327 | 6/205 | | 213/343 |
| Percentage | | 61% | 3%* | 62% | |

*Ectopic pregnancies in total series were 6 of 303 (2%).

al. [91], i.e., 43 percent, and Patton [155a] also found a marked increase in tubal pregnancies following a non-microsurgical approach to tubal reanastomosis; i.e., 2 of 6 pregnancies were ectopic.

The results of microsurgical tubal anastomosis for reversal of tubal sterilization are reported in Table 7-23. These data include reports through 1980. Two review series reported by Winston [233] and Gomel [74] have been included, although these series include those patients reported earlier in 1977. The early report by Clyman [32] appears to have been the first report of microsurgical reanastomosis, yet it failed to achieve the pregnancy levels attained by later microsurgeons. Despite of this slow beginning, the entire group of 343 patients yielded a total pregnancy rate of 62 percent, which compares with the 39 percent rate attained by nonmicrosurgical methods (see Table 7-22). An almost equally remarkable accomplishment was the dramatic decrease in the incidence of ectopic pregnancy when the operating microscope was employed. Only 6 of 205 pregnancies (3 percent) were ectopic in the microsurgical group compared with 16 of 71 pregnancies (23 percent) in the nonmicrosurgical patients.

A number of interesting factors are suggested by the comments included in Table 7-24. Wilson [231] and Winston [233] reported excellent pregnancy results in the reanastomosis of fallopian tubes severed by electrosurgical sterilization methods. The report of 5 successful pregnancies in 8 patients operated on by Winston compares with the earlier report of a similar group of patients who underwent uterotubal implantation resulting in only 1 pregnancy in 10 attempts [227]. Another

**Table 7-24.** Pregnancy following microsurgical and nonmicrosurgical anastomosis techniques

| Technique | No. of patients | Percent uterine pregnancies | Percent total | Ectopic | |
|---|---|---|---|---|---|
| | | | | Percent total | Percent pregnant |
| Nonmicrosurgical | 334 | 34 | 39 | 10 | 23 |
| Microsurgical | 343 | 61 | 62 | 2 | 3 |

significant report was that of Jones and Rock [112], in which a technique of anastomosis utilizing loupes (4.5×) yielded a 75 percent uterine pregnancy rate in 12 patients with only 1 ectopic pregnancy. The question regarding the role of loupes in tubal reanastomosis is as yet unanswered. Finally, it would appear that pregnancy rates have increased with added experience. The best pregnancy results thus far reported are those of Gomel [74] in 47 patients followed longer than 18 months postoperatively. Remarkably, 81 percent of these patients achieved a pregnancy, and only 1 ectopic pregnancy occurred in the group. A comparison of pregnancy results following reanastomosis of the fallopian tube by a nonmicrosurgical and by a microsurgical approaches is briefly presented in Table 7-24.

*Results of Anastomosis for Tubal Pathology*

A major change since the first edition of the *Atlas* has been the introduction of uteroisthmic anastomosis for the treatment of cornual occlusion due to pathologic entities, i.e., salpingitis isthmica nodosa and endometriosis. Both Winston and Gomel deserve credit for establishing this surgical approach, although others suggested the possibility during the 1960s [39]. In 1975, Winston [232] stated: "In view of the poor results following reimplantation and the fact that actual blockage of the intramural portion of the oviduct is probably rare (Peel, 1964), it is likely that a microsurgical anastomosis from the undamaged part of the isthmus to the intramural part of the fallopian tube offers a better chance of pregnancy." Gomel [76], however, stated that "in cornual occlusion of the tubes we have confirmed the findings of Ehrler. The site of occlusion is usually not the intramural portion of the tube, but rather a segment of the isthmus immediately adjacent. In many cases, therefore, a tubouterine implantation may be successfully replaced by an anastomosis."

It would appear that Ehrler, in 1965 [57], was the first to stress the fact that in many cases of cornual occlusion, the intramural segment was patent and the site of occlusion was limited to the uteroisthmic junction. This surgeon proposed that the occluded segment be excised and uteroisthmic anastomosis performed. Unfortunately, Ehrler did not use a microsurgical technique, and his results are difficult to interpret. However, it appears that pregnancy occurred in only 4 of 21 patients, and of these, three had live births [73].

The first successful use of a microsurgical approach to uteroisthmic anastomosis was reported in the rabbit by David, Brackett, and Garcia in 1969 [39]. These surgeons resected the uterotubal junction of rabbit fallopian tubes, a 1.5-cm length of isthmus and cornu, following which a uteroisthmic anastomosis was performed with the aid of a Zeiss operating microscope. Pregnancy occurred in 44 percent (11 of 25) of these rabbits, and in this group, ova implantation in the operated tube was reduced to 41 percent compared with 96 percent in the unoperated tube.

Gomel [76] deserves credit for reporting the first successful treatment of cornual pathology in human females by microsurgical uteroisthmic anastomosis. Most of the attention given to Gomel's earlier report of tubal anastomosis involved the successful reversal of tubal sterilization. However, almost an equal number of patients (14) underwent uteroisthmic anastomosis following resection of the pathologic isthmus or cornual segment. The pregnancy result in this group was excellent. Gomel reported that 7 of 14 patients had an intrauterine pregnancy and ectopic pregnancy occurred in only 1 patient. Tubal patency was achieved in 98.6 percent of these patients. Despite these outstanding results, Gomel concluded, "Nevertheless, the superiority of tubouterine anastomosis over implantation has yet to be proven." Recent reports appear to have established the superiority of this technique [47,130,235].

In a series of 69 patients found to have cornual occlusion of the fallopian tube, Winston [235] performed uteroisthmic anastomosis in 72 percent following resection of the occluded segment. Only 19 patients (28%) required uterotubal implantation. The group of 50 patients undergoing anastomosis can be divided into three separate subgroups including those patients with pure cornual occlusion, those with isthmic tuberculosis, and finally those found to have two areas of tubal occlusion, namely, cornual and fimbrial blocks. The uterine and ectopic pregnancies are listed in Table 7-25. In brief, 52 percent of the 29 patients with pure cornual occlusion had subsequent uterine pregnancies. Of interest, none of the 5 patients found to have isthmic tuberculosis subsequently had uterine pregnancies, although 25 percent of 16 patients undergoing repair of dual tubal blocks did have a uterine pregnancy. Unfortunately, one-third of the pregnancies (2 of 6) in this latter group were ectopic. Gomel [74] expanded his early group to include a

**Table 7-25.** Surgical treatment of pathologic cornual occlusion

| Uteroisthmic anastomosis | No. of patients | Uterine pregnancies | Ectopic | Total pregnancies (%) |
|---|---|---|---|---|
| Isolated cornual occlusion | 18 | 11 | 1 | 67 |
| SIN | 11 | 4 | 0 | 36 |
| Tuberculous salpingitis | 5 | 0 | 0 | 0 |
| Cornual and fimbrial occlusion | 16 | 5 | 2 | 44 |
| Total | 50 | 20 | 3 | |
| Uterotubal implantation | 19 | 3 | 1 | 21 |

Source: R. M. L. Winston and R. A. Margara, Techniques for the Improvement of Microsurgical Tubal Anastomosis. In P. G. Grosighani and B. L. Rubin (eds.), *Microsurgery in Female Infertility*. New York: Grune & Stratton, 1980.

**Table 7-26.** Pregnancy following uterotubal anastomosis in patients with cornual pathology

| Study | No of patients | Uterine pregnancies | Percent uterine | Ectopic pregnancies | Total pregnancies (%) |
|---|---|---|---|---|---|
| Winston and Margara, 1980 | | | | | |
| Pure cornual occlusion[a] | 29 | 15 | 52 | 1 | 55 |
| Cornual and fimbrial occlusion | 16 | 4 | 25 | 2 | 38 |
| Gomel | | | | | |
| 1977 | 14 | 7 | 50 | 1 | 50 |
| 1980 | 38 | 21 | 55 | 2 | 58 |
| Total[b] | 67 | 36 | 54 | 3/39 (8%) | |

[a]Patients with tuberculous salpingitis have been excluded.
[b]Total figures represent a pure group and exclude Winston and Margara's patients who had a double block. This figure also excludes the patients reported by Gomel in 1977, since these patients were included in the 1980 data.

total of 38 patients in whom uterotubal anastomosis was performed following excision of isthmic pathology. In the total group, 21 of 38 patients (55%) had uterine pregnancies postoperatively. Two ectopic pregnancies occurred in this group, however. A comparison of the results of uterotubal anastomoses reported by these two authors is given in Table 7-26.

In summary, 50 to 55 percent of patients found to have pure cornual occlusion of the fallopian tube due either to salpingitis isthmica nodosa, endometriosis, postuterine infection, or polyposis will have uterine pregnancies following resection of the diseased tubal segment and subsequent microsurgical uteroisthmic anastomosis. The ectopic pregnancy rate of 3 of 39 (8 percent) or 3 of 67 (4.5 percent) of total patients is remarkably low. Although not as high as the pregnancy results following reversal of sterilization, this is a better pregnancy rate than had been reported following uterotubal implantation.

*Tubal Length*

It has become clear that the length of the residual oviduct following reanastomosis plays a central role in determining future pregnancy. The excellent pregnancy results achieved in the rabbit by Winston [232] demonstrated that microsurgical reanastomosis can be highly successful when a small segment of oviduct has been

removed. Both Winston and Gomel have studied the effect on pregnancy of removing increasing lengths of rabbit oviduct and have shown a correlation between the length of oviduct removed and subsequent pregnancy (see pages 262–263).

Two clinical studies present data indicating that increased tubal length increases pregnancy. Silber and Cohen [189] recorded the total length of residual oviduct in 25 patients undergoing tubal reanastomosis. Seven patients had residual oviducts that measured 3 cm or less, and none of these women conceived postoperatively. Pregnancy occurred in 43 percent of 7 patients whose residual tube measured 3 to 4 cm, and remarkably, all 11 patients whose residual tube was 4 cm or greater conceived. In contrast, Winston [235] achieved 2 pregnancies in 4 patients whose residual oviduct was less than 2.5 cm and 2 of 7 of those patients whose residual oviduct measured 2.5 to 4.0 cm conceived postoperatively. Overall, in Winston's series, 36 percent of 11 patients with residual oviducts less than 4.1 cm conceived compared with 62 percent of those 24 patients whose residual oviduct was greater than 4 cm.

Gomel [74] has stated that he observed "an inverse relationship between the tubal length of the reconstructed oviduct and the interval between surgery and the occurrence of pregnancy." He found that pregnancy usually occurred within 5 postoperative cycles when the

**Table 7-27.** Types of microsurgical anastomoses

| Type | No. of patients | Uterine pregnancies | Percent uterine | Ectopic | Etiology |
|---|---|---|---|---|---|
| I. Uteroisthmic | | | | | |
|     Gomel, 1977 | 14 | 7 | 50 | 1 | Pathology |
|     Winston, 1980 | 29 | 16 | 55 | 1 | Pathology |
|     Winston, 1980 | 13 | 9 | 69 | 0 | Reversal |
|     Total | 56 | 32 | 57 | 2/34 | |
| II. Uteroampullary | | | | | |
|     Winston, 1977 | 16 | 12 | 75 | 1 | Reversal |
|     Diamond, 1979 | 28 | 21 | 75 | 0 | Reversal |
|     Total | 44 | 33 | 75 | 1/34 | |
| III. Isthmic-Isthmic | | | | | |
|     Winston, 1980 | 14 | 11 | 78 | 0 | Reversal |
|     Siegler, 1979 | 10 | 7 | 70 | 1 | Reversal |
|     Total | 24 | 18 | 75 | 1/19 | |
| IV. Ampullary-Isthmic | | | | | |
|     Gomel, 1979 | 16 | 8 | 50 | 1 | Reversal |
|     Owens, Pickett-Heap, 1977 | 7 | 6 | 86 | 0 | Reversal (Pomeroy) |
|     Siegler, 1979 | 4 | 2 | 50 | 0 | |
|     Winston, 1980 | 14 | 8 | 63 | 1 | |
|     Total | 41 | 24 | 59 | 2/26 | |
| V. Ampullary-Ampullary | | | | | |
|     Winston, 1980 | 18 | 8 | 44 | 0 | Reversal |

oviduct was greater than 6 cm. Among 9 patients who became pregnant in the first postoperative cycle, the longest oviduct was 5.5 cm or greater. In contrast, the interval between surgery and pregnancy averaged 19.1 months in those patients whose residual oviduct measured 4 cm or less. The average time between surgery and subsequent pregnancy in this series was 10.2 months.

A review of reported pregnancies following each of the five types of tubal and uterine anastomosis is presented in Table 7-27. It appears that isthmic-isthmic anastomosis following previous sterilization will result in the highest pregnancy rate, i.e., 75 percent, which is consistent with the animal studies of Eddy and others discussed earlier. In fact, pregnancy results in the absence of the isthmic segment; i.e., uteroampullary anastomosis has also resulted in a 75 percent pregnancy rate in the two studies, suggesting that the function of the isthmic segment is limited in the female.

The most commonly performed ampullary-isthmic reanastomosis utilized following a Pomeroy-type ligation has resulted in a 59 percent (24 of 41) pregnancy rate. Discussion of this apparently low pregnancy result was presented earlier. Finally, it would appear that the lowest pregnancy result following microsurgical tubal reanastomosis has occurred when an ampullary-ampullary reanastomosis was performed. A 44 percent pregnancy rate was reported by Winston, although inadequate data are available to establish the point. It is presently assumed that the decreased length of the ampullary segment is responsible for this low rate, although this has not been proven.

## Uterotubal Implantation

Prior to the introduction of microsurgical technique into oviductal surgery, cornual and proximal isthmic occlusion were treated exclusively by uterotubal implantation. In fact, in the first edition of the *Atlas* it was estimated that 20 percent of infertility operations for tubal disease necessitated uterotubal implantation. This is no longer true, since with the aid of the operating microscope it is now possible to perform uterotubal anastomoses in most of those patients found to have cornual occlusion. The observation by Shirodkar [183] and Ehrler [57], later confirmed by early gynecologic microsurgeons, that cornual occlusion often represents a small area of occlusion near the outer surface at the junction of the isthmic and cornual segments has permitted resection of this small, often 0.5-mm area, and subsequent uterotubal anastomosis. Furthermore, the observation that previously coagulated tubal segments, often with almost complete isthmic destruction, could be successfully repaired by uterotubal anastomosis has also reduced the number of patients requiring uterotubal implantation.

These two primary indications for uterotubal implantation have therefore given way to microsurgical uterotubal anastomosis. Yet there remain patients in whom occlusion of the intramural segment extends almost its entire length. Winston [235] reported that 19 of 60 (32 percent) patients who underwent corrective tubal surgery because of cornual occlusion due to a pathologic process required uterotubal implantation. In this group, 18 patients had an isolated cornual block, an additional 11 patients had bilateral SIN, and 16 had a double block involving cornual and fimbrial occlusion. All these patients were treated by uterotubal anastomosis. Among 19 of these patients, in whom uterotubal implantation was performed by Winston, the pathologic findings were not reported. Siegler and Konlopoulos [188] reported that 11 of 80 (14 percent) patients who underwent microsurgery involving the oviduct had a uterotubal implantation. In this series, only 1 patient had a uterotubal anastomosis. One of us (G.W.P.) has found that the percentage of patients with cornual occlusion who require uterotubal implantation is very low.

### Etiology of Cornual Occlusion

Cornual occlusion may be caused by such pathologic processes as inflammation, endometriosis, or SIN, or it may occur secondary to a sterilization procedure. Rock et al. [168] reported the histologic diagnoses in tubal segments removed from 52 patients who underwent uterotubal implantation. Chronic salpingitis occurred in 21 patients (40%), SIN in 11 (21%), and normal histology in 3. Twelve of the patients (3%) had undergone prior tubal sterilization. Winston [235] noted isthmic tuberculosis in 5 of 60 patients with cornual occlusion, a disease entity rarely encountered in the United States. Endometriosis also may produce occlusion of the cornual segment. Gomel [73] has reported the following remarkable story: "The cause of her cornual occlusion was endometriosis. Following tubocornual anastomosis she achieved a term, live birth. The second pregnancy was a tubal gestation for which a salpingectomy was performed by the gynecologist in attendance. Subsequently, the contralateral tube reoccluded. Upon the patient's insistence, reconstructive surgery was performed for a second time and an anastomosis proved impossible, and an implantation was carried out. This yielded a second child for her." Cornual polyps may also cause occlusion of the distal cornual segment. Inflammation of the cornual segment may be caused by previous illegal abortion, as discussed by Green-Armytage [82], Shirodkar [183], and Moore White [137]. Green-Armytage [82] considered these "ideal cases . . . and will give a 35 to 40 percent pregnancy rate." Moore White [137] also found that cornual occlusion caused by chemical or thermal trauma associated with previous abortion produced excellent pregnancy results following tubal repair by uterotubal implantation.

Although legalized abortion has reduced the number of patients who suffer tubal infection following this procedure, two additional factors are now present. The increasing incidence of gonococcal salpingitis has added a new dimension to the problem: The use of early antibiotic therapy may produce an increasing proportion of infertility patients with cornual occlusion, but with a minimal degree of endosalpingeal disease and pelvic adhesions. This pattern of isolated cornual occlusion caused by an infectious process also has been associated with use of an intrauterine device. The prognosis for ultimate pregnancy in these patients is favorable, however, since so-called pure cornual occlusion due to any cause has a better prognosis for term pregnancy than more severe degrees of pelvic inflammatory disease.

An attempt to distinguish inflammatory and non-inflammatory causes of cornual occlusion is confused by the uncertainty of the etiology of salpingitis isthmica nodosa. Chiari and Heilkunde [29] and Schauta [173] first described this entity in 1884 and 1886. They noted thickening of segments of both tubes, characteristically the isthmic portions. Their microscopic description was that of irregular tubal out-pouching, giving the appearance of multiple lumena. Parsons and Sommers [153a] supported the belief that the nodular process was a form of tubal adenomyosis in which the endosalpingeal mucosa "invaded" the muscularis. However, Woodruff and Paulestein [238] suggested that this process was secondary to chronic salpingitis. Their recent data support the belief that mucosal out-pouching occurs as a result of the postinflammatory healing process. Citing the work of Troell [217], Honore [96] concluded that "SIN is now considered to be an acquired form of diverticulosis distinct from the rare congenital form which affects the midportion of the tube." Honore was led to propose "that SIN is analogous in etiology and pathogenesis to diverticulosis coli, which also affects primarily the sphincter-like sigmoid colon." He went on to state that "as with colonic diverticulosis, the process may take many years to develop and exhibits individual variations in its tempo of evolution and severity." In 6 infertility patients whose proximal tubal segment had been resected, Honore [96] found SIN in 50 percent although, in a large control group of 146 patients in whom salpingectomy had been performed for sterilization, SIN was found in only 1 case for an incidence of 0.6 percent. Finally, a recent report [121] has described a multifactorial etiologic concept in relation to the pathogenesis of SIN. Kontopoulos et al. [21] concluded that inflammation, developmental defects, endosalpingeal metaplasia, and tubal endometriosis may all lead to nodular thickening of the isthmus and intramural portions of both tubes, termed SIN. They also found that 1.2 to 3.5 percent of hysterosalpingograms revealed evidence of SIN [121].

**Table 7-28.** Histologic findings in the excised isthmus

| Finding | No. of specimens |
|---|---|
| No lumen, scar tissue only | 7 |
| Atresia | 2 |
| Distorted, very small lumen; chronic mucosal salpingitis | 16 |
| Distorted, very small lumen; chronic interstitial salpingitis | 33 |
| Distorted, very small lumen; chronic perisalpingitis | 6 |
| Distorted lumen, nodular salpingitis | 2 |
| Tuberculosis | 1 |
| Total | 67 |

Source: A. Grant, Infertility surgery of the oviduct. *Fertil. Steril.* 22:496, 1971.

Despite a clinical impression of bilateral isthmic closure, the pathologist's report of the excised specimen is not always corroborative. This report must be interpreted with unique understanding. Grant [81] reported histologic observations on 67 excised specimens, of which 67 percent were of inflammatory origin (Table 7-28). Mucosal and interstitial involvement was found in 49 of the 67 specimens (73 percent), in contrast to 6 (9 percent) with perisalpingitis and 2 (3 percent) with nodular salpingitis. Only 1 case of tuberculous salpingitis was recorded. Grant noted that obstruction in a number of cases appeared to be a "flap valve" type of block and, in his view, did not represent "tubal spasm." Usually six sections of isthmus were cut. However, in a few cases, as many as 50 sections were made, and evidence of occlusion was found in half the patients who previously had shown no evidence of obstruction.

*Surgical Approach*

The diagnosis of cornual occlusion will usually be made initially by hysterosalpingography and then confirmed during tubal lavage at laparoscopy and again by injection of dye at laparotomy. The honeycomb appearance at hysterosalpingography may identify SIN, and occasionally, x-ray evaluation will note cornual polyps. Most of the time, however, a definite etiology will not be identified during the evaluation phase. At laparoscopy and during laparotomy, bulging or pulsation of the cornual area (Shirodkar sign) will be seen in rhythm to the pressure exerted by the surgeon on the syringe of indigo carmen during attempts to inject dye through the transcervical cannula or transfundal needle. Laparoscopic evaluation of the pelvis offers the ability to evaluate the fimbriae and possible tubal adhesions. The presence of cornual occlusion and fimbrial occlusion with or without tubal adhesions offers a poor prognosis for reconstructive surgery.

At laparotomy, the isthmic segment should be inspected under the operating microscope, and if indicated, uterotubal implantation should be performed with this magnification aid. It is our preference to perform uterotubal anastomosis whenever possible. Therefore, once cornual occlusion is clearly established, the isthmic segment is incised approximately 1 cm from the cornu, as shown in Figure 7-18. This segment is then sliced in repetitive segments closer to the cornu, as described earlier in the section on uterotubal anastomosis (see Fig. 7-18). Following each cut, attempts at lavage via the intrauterine cannula are made and the occluded end is visualized under high magnification. Identification of normal isthmic or cornual mucosa is essential if successful anastomosis is to be performed. Furthermore, injection of the dye through the transcervical cannula will result in a jet stream of fluid exuding from the recently opened cornual segment. If occlusion persists once the surface of the uterus is reached, if probing appears to indicate occlusion well within the intramural segment, if normal mucosa are not apparent, or lastly, if injection of dye does not result in a jet stream but only a small trickle, then uterotubal implantation is selected. This technique is shown in Figure 7-20.

*The Role of the Carbon Dioxide*
*Laser During Uterotubal Implantation*
The carbon dioxide laser can be used during the microsurgical approach to uterotubal implantation shown in Figure 7-20G by substituting the hand-held laser for the microsurgical electrode to remove the occluded cornual segment. Bellina [6] believes that the hand-held carbon dioxide laser adds a refinement to this microsurgical approach by permitting improved hemostatic excision of the cornual segment. Techniques of hemostasis described earlier should be employed when using the laser approach and include use of the tourniquet and injection of dilute Pitressin into the area to be excised. The f50 hand-held carbon dioxide laser unit has been used by Bellina to remove the cornual segment with power density 50,000 W per square centimeter (power 60 watts, spot diameter .125 mm; Fig. 7-20G). The uterine cavity should be distended with fluid to compress the endometrium and to absorb excess laser energy before completing the cylindrical incision. The diameter of the cornual opening may be enlarged to accommodate the distal tubal segment when necessary. The distal tubal segment should then be prepared using the laser beam at power density 800 W per square centimeter (power 2 watts, spot diameter .5 mm) as described earlier in the section on tubal anastomosis. Prior to tubal implantation, laser sites should be irrigated to remove all tissue debris and carbonated matter. A stent is not utilized when performing this microsurgical approach to uterotubal implantation.

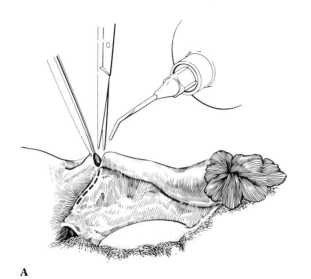

**A**

**Figure 7-20.** Technique of utero-tubal implantation (modified microsurgical approach). **A.** The diagnosis of cornual occlusion has been made by hysterosalpingography and subsequent laparoscopy. At laparotomy, this segment is inspected under high magnification through the operating microscope. Injection of dye is again performed to confirm the diagnosis. Injection of dilute pitressin is made 1 cm from the uterine cornu and this tubal segment cut sharply with straight scissors. The incision into the mesosalpinx, shown by the dotted line, is performed with the fine microelectrode, carefully avoiding damage to subsequent blood vessels. **B.** Since it is preferable to perform utero-isthmic anastomosis whenever possible, the occluded isthmic segment is sliced in segments up to the uterine wall. Tubal lavage is performed to determine patency and the occluded end visualized under high magnification. If occlusion persists once the surface of the uterus is reached and, in reality, once approximately one-half of the intramural segment has been removed, then uterotubal implantation is selected.

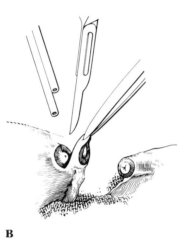

**B**

**C**

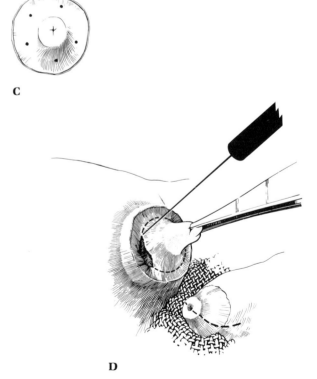

**D**

**C.** Dilute pitressin is injected into the area surrounding the intramural segment, as shown in this drawing. A tourniquet occluding the uterine vessels is occasionally used, however, the combination of careful technique and pitressin usually produces excellent hemostasis. **D.** Excision of the cornual segment is performed under magnification with the microelectrode. The ability of the assistant to visualize this field through the OPMI-7PH, OPMI-6S, or Weck microscopes is invaluable at this point, since suction and wiping with Weck cells permits careful dissection of the entire segment and direct view into the endometrial cavity. This process is very similar to the removal of fibrous fistula. The distal isthmic segment is also visualized under high magnification and a small incision made in the distal end. **E.** The distal isthmic segment is implanted in the intramural opening. Care is taken to ensure that tubal mucosa is in contact with endometrial mucosa. Tubal sutures of 4-0 synthetic absorbable suture or nylon are passed through the new opening and into the uterine wall at the site of the endometrial junction to ensure contact of mucosal surfaces. The author does not use a stent in this technique. **F.** The mesosalpinx is closed with 4-0 synthetic absorbable suture to prevent traction on the implanted segment. Additional 4-0 or 6-0 sutures are placed circumferentially about the tubal mucosa to fix this layer to the uterine serosa. **G.** The hand held carbon dioxide laser can be used to excise the intramural tubal segment during a uterotubal implantation procedure. The usual techniques of hemostasis, which include the tourniquet and pitressin, are employed.

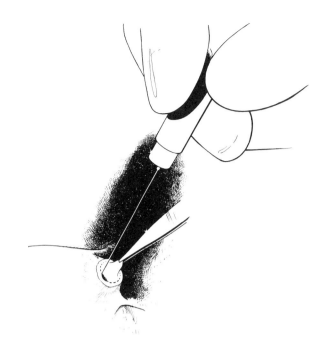

G

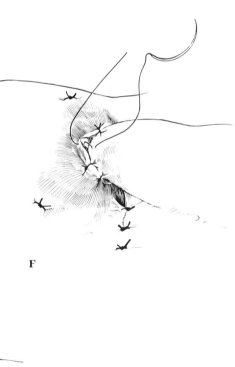

F

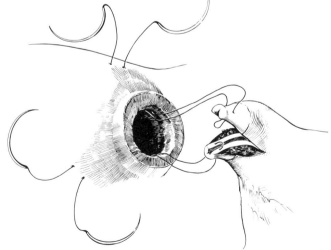

E

**Table 7-29.** Results of tubal implantation using sharp excision of cornu

| Author | No. of patients | Percent tubal patency | Percent pregnant | Percent term pregnancy | Technique |
|---|---|---|---|---|---|
| Moore-White: | | | | | |
| 1951 | 4 | — | 50 | 25 | No splint |
| 1960 | 16 | 75 | 56 | 31 | "Pure" implants |
| | 6 | 0 | 0 | 0 | Mixed procedures |
| Total | 22 | 50 | 41 | 20 | |
| Shirodkar, 1965 | 25 | — | 25 | — | Polyethylene splint, fundal incision |
| Mulligan et al., 1953 | 48 | 38 | 10 | — | Polyethylene splint, fundal incision |
| Rock et al., 1954: | | | | | |
| No splint | 7 | 55 | 29 | 14 | |
| Splint | 42 | 38 | 12 | — | |
| Mulligan et al., 1957 | 41 | 64 | 10 | — | Silastic ring splint, fundal incision |
| Young et al., 1970 | 11 | — | 9 | 9 | Ring splint |
| Horne et al., 1973 | 11 | — | 64 | 46 | Ring splint, dexameth-asone-phenothiazine |
| Garcia, 1968 | 14 | 57 | 14 | — | Ring splint, fundal incision |
| Siegler, 1969 | 12 | — | 8 | — | Polyethylene splint |
| Ingersoll, 1949 | 5 | 60 | 60 | 60 | No splint |
| Palmer, 1952 | 26 | — | 38 | 31 | "Pure" implants; no splint, postoperative oral hydrocortisone |
| Palmer, 1960 | 44 | 75 | 36 | Not reported | Mixed procedures |
| Wheeless, 1977 | 10 | 9 | 10 | 10 | Splint, all patients had prior tubal coagulation |
| Peterson et al., 1977 | 16 | — | 50 | 50 | Original implantation technique |
| Rock et al., 1979 | 26 | — | 15 | 15 | Splint |

**Table 7-30.** Results of tubal implantation using the reamer technique

| Author | No. of patients | Percent tubal patency | Percent pregnant | Percent term pregnancy | Technique |
|---|---|---|---|---|---|
| Holden and Sovak, 1932 | 3 | 66 | 66 | 33 | No splint |
| Pratt et al., 1956 | 5 | — | 80 | — | No splint |
| Hanton et al., 1964 | 22 | 77 | 48 | 48 | No splint |
| Shirodkar, 1960 | 140 | 90 | 35 | — | Ring prosthesis |
| Green-Armytage: | | | | | |
| 1952 | 17 | — | 41 | 34 | |
| 1957 | 38 | — | 42 | 36 | Polyethylene splint rods via cervix |
| 1960 | 43 | — | 40 | — | Splint |
| Johnstone, 1955 | 27 | 55 | 30 | 19 | Fundal incision, splint |
| Wirtz, 1965 | 48 | 83 | 54 | 42 | Modified reamer technique with splint |
| Hellman, 1951 and 1956 | 5 | — | 0 | — | Polyethylene splint |
| Arronet et al., 1969: | | | | | |
| Pure | 24 | — | 46 | — | Polyethylene splint |
| Total | 42 | — | 40 | — | |
| Grant, 1971 | 73 | 55 | 34 | 26 | Splint (later removed through cervix) |
| Rock et al., 1979 | 26 | — | 42 | — | Splint 2–6 months |

## Results

An indepth review of the complications, causes of failure, and pregnancy results associated with uterotubal implantation was presented in the first edition of the *Atlas*. The changing emphasis toward uterotubal anastomosis makes repetition of all this material unnecessary. There are as yet no recorded series of results of uterotubal implantation performed by a microsurgical technique. The results presented in Tables 7-29 and 7-30 reflect the pregnancy results achieved using the techniques of sharp incision and the reamer described previously. An exception was the original technique of implantation reported by Peterson et al. [160].

Until recently, wedge excision of the cornual segment followed by tubal implantation over a prosthesis was used exclusively in Boston, New York, Philadelphia, and Baltimore. The results of this surgical approach were reflected in the pregnancy rates achieved by Mulligan and Rock [141] (10 percent), Garcia [66] (14 percent), Siegler [188] (8 percent) and Rock et al. [169] (15 percent). Moore-White [137] and Palmer [152] reported a 31 percent term pregnancy following an implantation procedure without a prosthesis. The series reported by Horne et al. [97], in which 7 pregnancies occurred in 11 patients, was rather the exception when the collected data on this technique were reviewed.

Two recent studies utilized uterotubal implantation to reverse prior tubal sterilization. Wheeless [227] reported that uterotubal implantation was performed in 10 of 11 patients who had undergone laparoscopic sterilization by electrocoagulation and resection. Pregnancy occurred in only 1 of these patients, despite tubal patency in 9 of the 11 patients. The single patient who underwent end-to-end anastomosis did not conceive postoperatively despite tubal patency. The second report, by Peterson and Behrman [161], used a new technique of uterotubal implantation in which the uterine incision was made in the posterior uterine surface at the level of the ovarian ligaments rather than in the cornual area. These surgeons found that mobilization of the mesosalpinx was easier with this incision, and the blood supply to the oviduct was therefore more easily preserved. Pregnancy occurred in 11 of 16 patients who had bilateral implantation, and interestingly, 3 of 4 patients who had previously undergone tubal coagulation conceived. However, only 3 of 7 patients conceived following a repair of a Pomeroy-type ligation. Later reports by these authors have indicated a lower long-term pregnancy rate in a larger series, however.

The present microsurgical approach to uterotubal implantation appears closer to the reamer technique described earlier [118]. Pregnancy rates reported by the surgeons listed in Table 7-30 are generally higher than pregnancy results following sharp incision of the cornu. A recent report from Johns Hopkins Hospital [168] reviewed all patients who had undergone uterotubal implantation during the years 1942–1976. Among this group of 75 patients, 52 provided adequate documentation for historical review. Of 26 patients in whom a reamer technique was employed, pregnancy occurred in 42 percent, compared to 15 percent when sharp incision was employed. Also of interest was the observation that 64 percent of patients in whom an ampullary implantation was performed by the reamer technique conceived, compared with 27 percent of patients who underwent isthmic implantation by this technique. Overall pregnancy occurred in 29 percent of these 52 patients. A ring prosthesis was employed in all these implantation procedures and was removed 2 to 6 months postoperatively.

The microsurgical implantation technique described above achieves hemostasis by injection of dilute pitressin and by use of the tourniquet technique described earlier. Excision of the cornual segment is performed under direct vision through the microscope utilizing the microelectrode or laser. In this manner it is possible to visualize the endometrial cavity directly. The isthmic segment can then be directly implanted into this opening, as described earlier. A stent is not felt necessary in these patients, and preliminary results with this technique are extremely encouraging.

**Table 7-31.** Incidence of tubal pregnancy

| Population | Incidence |
|---|---|
| Normal female | 0.5–1.0% of pregnancies |
| Prior PID | 1.6% |
| Recurrent tubal pregnancy | 7–27% of pregnancies |
| After infertility surgery* | |
| Salpingolysis | 3% of pregnancies |
| Fimbrioplasty | 5.5% of pregnancies |
| Salpingoneostomy | 35% of pregnancies |
| End-to-end (reversal) | 3.0% of pregnancies |

*Results of microsurgical procedures.

## Tubal Pregnancy

Thus we find that the black thread of tubal pregnancy is woven into the sad story of sterility. . . .

A. GRANT [80]

Ectopic pregnancy may be a causative factor in female sterility, but it may also result from prior attempts by the physician to improve fertility. Extrauterine pregnancy appears to be occurring in increasing numbers, and the traditional number of 1 in 200 live births has reputedly been too low an estimate. Figures of 1 in 69, 1 in 64, and even 1 in 30 live births are becoming commonplace, presumably because of the increasing incidence of tubal infection and/or the use of the IUD [224]. Westrom [224] found that ectopic pregnancy occurred in 1 in 64 live births in patients who had been treated for salpingitis compared with 1 in 145 live births in those patients who had never had a tubal infection. Unmarried patients under 25 years of age who used an IUD for birth control were 6.1 times more likely to develop PID than were females who used other forms of contraception in this study from the University of Lund (Table 7-31).

The significance of ectopic pregnancy to the specialist in infertility becomes relevant when one considers the obstetric future of patients who experience this abnormality. In a representative study [119], 19.4 percent of patients who experienced an ectopic pregnancy had not conceived previously, and an additional 25.1 percent had conceived only once. This 45 percent incidence of low parity in patients who sustained one ectopic pregnancy was confirmed by Schoen and Nowak [174], who found an even higher figure of 65.7 percent in those females who experienced a second tubal pregnancy. Among the females in whom the first pregnancy was ectopic, only 30 percent subsequently produced a live infant, and 12 of the 50 patient (30 percent) under study had a repeat ectopic pregnancy [119]. The chance of recurrent ectopic pregnancy is estimated to be 7.5 to 27 percent in many series [63,174].

Although an ectopic tubal pregnancy can be a cause of sterility, the surgical treatment for tubal disease outlined earlier in this chapter also increases the possibility.

**Table 7-32.** Anatomic sites of 654 ectopic pregnancies

| Site | No. of patients |
|---|---|
| Ovarian | 1 |
| Uterine | 5 |
| Cervical | 1 |
| Cornual | 4 |
| Abdominal | 9 |
| Tubal | 639 |
| Fimbrial | 30 |
| Fimbrial-ovarian | 10 |
| Distal third | 265 |
| Middle third | 245 |
| Proximal third | 79 |
| Interstitial | 8 |

Source: J. L. Breen, A 21-year survey of 654 ectopic pregnancies. Am. J. Obstet. Gynecol. 106:1004, 1970.

Grant [80] has observed a high incidence of ectopic pregnancy in patients attending his Infertility Clinic and established that such patients are 7 to 8 times more likely to have an ectopic pregnancy than other women. These patients are in addition to those who have undergone surgery of the oviduct. The occurrence of tubal pregnancy in this latter group was listed in Table 7-31.

The introduction of microsurgical technique dramatically decreased the incidence of extrauterine pregnancy in patients who have undergone tubal reanastomosis for reversal of sterilization. Our literature review demonstrates an incidence of 10 to 15 percent in the macrosurgical group compared with 3 percent in the microsurgical group (see Table 7-24). Patton observed that ectopic pregnancy occurred in 3 of 10 macrosurgical reversal procedures and has had only 2 ectopic pregnancies thus far in 45 patients who have undergone microsurgical reanastomosis. Microsurgical fimbrioplasty also results in a low incidence of ectopic pregnancy [155]. Patton noted only 1 ectopic pregnancy in 35 patients who had pure microsurgical fimbrioplasty, and a second ectopic pregnancy occurred in 5 additional patients who had a mixed procedure following fimbrioplasty of one tube and salpingostomy of the opposite side. As noted earlier, the uterine pregnancy rate in these patients was 61 percent. In marked contrast to these improved figures are the results reported following microsurgical salpingostomy. Gomel [76] reported that 31 percent of the pregnancies in his series were ectopic, and Swolin [210] found, in a longer follow-up, that forty percent of pregnancies occurred in the tube postoperatively. Recently, Siegler and Konlopoulos [188] found that among 8 pregnancies that occurred following microsurgical salpingoneostomy, 5 were uterine and 3 were ectopic, i.e., 38 percent of pregnancies. Macrosurgical salpingoneostomy was found to result in fewer tubal pregnancies (see Table 7-20). The sites of tubal pregnancy are shown in Figure 7-21 and Table 7-32.

*Historical Background*

Interest in the surgical approach to tubal pregnancy preceded by at least two decades the surgical correction of other tubal disorders. Gabriele Fallopio published his description of the "seminal duct" or "trumpet of the womb" in 1561. Woodruff [238] credited Albucasis with the earliest accurate description of this pathologic entity (extrauterine pregnancy) during the eleventh century. However, Riolan the Younger is given credit for the first description of a tubal pregnancy in 1604. Of more interest was the case of an apparently ruptured tubal pregnancy described by Mauriceau in 1669. This woman died after 3 days of severe abdominal pain, and at autopsy a 6-cm fetus was found within her abdominal cavity. A woodcut of the uterus and tubes removed at autopsy was made by Mauriceau and is frequently published as the earliest recorded case of tubal pregnancy. In 1895, Kelly [115] noted that this patient had actually been treated by the surgeon Benedict Vasal and that Mauriceau had simply made a woodcut of the specimen exhibited after autopsy. Kelly also noted that "it was evident to me that those who accepted this opinion [of tubal pregnancy] had been led into error." He noted that the carving depicts the round ligament leading directly to the dilated, ruptured portion of uterus and thus verifies a cornual pregnancy and not a pregnancy of the uterine tube proper. Most authors accept this as a tubal ectopic pregnancy, since cornual or interstitial pregnancies are considered a form of tubal pregnancy. It is possible, however, that Mauriceau's drawing depicted an anomalous uterine horn that had ruptured during pregnancy.

In 1741, Bronchi suggested a classification of the forms of ectopic pregnancy, and this was simplified by Boehmer in 1752 to include three forms: *gestatio ovarica*, *gestatio tubaria*, and *gestatio abdominalis*. Kelly, in 1895 [115], listed the primary forms of tubal pregnancy as tubouterine or interstitial, isthmic, and ampullar. This differs little from the classification used today, which also includes fimbrial pregnancies (Table 7-32; see also Fig. 7-21).

Kelly credited Lawson and Tait with first use of the term *ectopic gestation*, but Woodruff and Pauerstein [238] gave this credit to Robert Barnes. They did, however, credit Tait with performing, in 1882, the first documented operation for ruptured tubal pregnancy, although others had recommended surgery for extrauterine pregnancy during the preceding 30 years. Charles Briddon receives credit for performing the first operation for ruptured ectopic pregnancy in America in 1883. In 1895, Kelly [115] strongly advised surgical therapy for tubal pregnancy, as did Bovee in 1897 and 1910 [14,15].

**Figure 7-21.** Anatomical sites of tubal ectopic pregnancies. (From R. W. Kistner, *Gynecology: Principles and Practice* (3rd ed). Chicago: Year Book, 1979.)

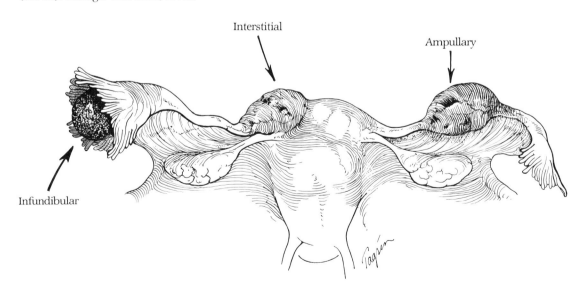

*Etiology*

Insight into the causative factors of tubal pregnancy would be expected to assist the surgeon in an attempt to select, at laparotomy, the surgical technique that would permit a reasonable number of subsequent full-term pregnancies. Unfortunately, this information is not helpful, since clinical data are empirical and, except in cases of severe pelvic inflammatory disease, the etiologic factor is often unknown. The choice of surgical approach is usually related to the surgeon's experience and convenience. Despite this pessimistic viewpoint, it is felt that the subsequent discussion of surgical technique will be clarified by a description of the pathophysiology of this gynecologic entity.

In 1961, Bone and Greene [10] described the relationship between tubal inflammation and ectopic pregnancy as follows: "The most widely accepted theory for the etiology of tubal pregnancy is that of residues of tubal inflammatory disease, usually gonorrheal, but including puerperal, postabortive and postoperative infections. These infections play their etiologic roles in probably one of two ways—either by the production of mechanical obstructive 'pockets' or impairment of propulsive forces of the tube."

They suggested that the residual effects of tubal inflammation might cause tubal obstruction by either extrinsic or intrinsic mechanisms. Extrinsically, this process could produce "peritubal adhesions causing kinking of the tube resulting in narrowing of the tubal lumen." Intrinsic disease of the endosalpinx is evident by microscopic examination of excised tubal specimens. However, the inflammatory reaction caused by the implantation process must be differentiated from residues of prior inflammatory disease. Hellman [89] and Novak and Darner [147] have described the microscopic findings in normal oviducts associated with intrauterine pregnancies and have noted such an inflammatory reaction in these specimens.

Bone and Greene described the etiologic role of follicular salpingitis in tubal pregnancy in their statement that "endosalpingitis with denudation of tubal epithelium may result in adhesions between plical folds of the tubal mucosa. These adhesions produce gland-like spaces and blind pockets in which the fertilized ovum may be trapped and implanted." Thus chronic inflammation and follicular salpingitis are generally considered to be the most important etiologic factors. Bone and Greene found that 38 percent of tubes from 121 patients with tubal pregnancy had residues of antecedent tubal infection. Seventy-seven percent of these patients were white, but other workers have noted a higher incidence of pelvic inflammation in black patients [63]. However, the incidence of documented prior inflammatory disease in black patients having tubal pregnancy is also approximately 35 percent.

The pathologic criteria for identifying prior tubal inflammatory disease are, unfortunately, not as clear-cut as Bone and Greene described. Niles and Clark [144] used the same criteria and found follicular salpingitis in only 2.7 percent of 436 cases of tubal pregnancy. However, they found evidence of an inflammatory process in 40.1 percent of cases, and 28 percent had chronic salpingitis. A control group of 161 specimens from postpartum tubal ligations revealed an 11.8 percent incidence of inflammation and a 7.4 percent incidence of chronic salpingitis.

Two conclusions may be drawn regarding the role of prior tubal inflammation in predisposing to tubal pregnancy. First, pathologic evidence of prior infection can be identified in only one-third of excised tubes. Second, it is evident that present morphologic techniques are inadequate to document a cause-and-effect relationship between tubal infection and tubal pregnancy. Although the mechanism of "ovum trapping" is attractive, it is more likely that abnormalities of tubal physiology such as altered composition of tubal secretions or disturbed innervation produce faulty motility and abnormal patterns of muscular contraction, resulting in delayed ovum transport and tubal implantation. The inflammatory process might disrupt the pacemaker mechanism at the isthmic-ampullar junction, thus supporting Asherman's concept of tubal dyskinesia [3]. The significance of these possibilities is unknown, but it is evident that the etiology of tubal pregnancy is unknown in over 50 percent of cases.

Frankel and Schenck [62], in 1937, advanced the theory that tubal implantation occurred at sites of tubal endometriosis. In a study of 29 patients having postpartum tubal ligation, they noted decidual tissue in 62 percent of the specimens. They examined 16 tubal pregnancy specimens and found that in one "there was a tubal gestation that contained in its decidual tissue demonstrable endometrial glands." Decidual tissue was found adjacent to the implantation site in all tubes, and these workers concluded that "all ectopic pregnancies, tubal or otherwise, occur because of implantation of the fertilized ovum in a locus of endometrial tissue." This conclusion rested on the assumption that decidual tissue was a cause rather than an effect of tubal pregnancy. Pathologic studies of pregnancy changes on the fallopian tube by Novak and Darner [147] and Hellman [89] revealed that decidual change in tubal stromal elements occurs in both intrauterine and ectopic gestation. Most series of tubal pregnancies identify endometriosis at the site of tubal implantation in less than 1 percent of patients [17].

Another theory associates tubal pregnancy with transperitoneal migration of the ovum. This is suggested by finding a corpus luteum in the ovary on the side opposite the involved tube. In 1876, Parry [153] recorded the frequent occurrence of the "contralateral corpus luteum" in cases of tubal pregnancy. Berlind [8] reported in 1960 a study of 48 tubal pregnancies in which a contralateral corpus luteum was found in 50 percent of patients. Obviously, transmigration of the ovum via the uterine or peritoneal cavity is suggested. However, it is possible that the tubal fimbriae envelop the contralateral ovary or that ovum pickup may occur directly from the cul-de-sac.

Anomalous tubal development has also been suggested as a cause of tubal pregnancy. Huffman [98], in 1913, reported such a case in which a rudimentary portion of fallopian tube was attached to the normal tube near its fimbriated end. The miniature segment had normal fimbriae and ostium, but it did not communicate with the lumen of the larger tube. The ectopic pregnancy occurred in this rudimentary segment. Huffman noted that Doran, in 1887, examined 1,000 tubal specimens and found congenital malformations in 0.6 percent of cases. Most reviews of tubal pathology note anomalous tubes in less than 1 percent of cases.

Physiologic malfunction has been suggested by Asherman [3] as a major cause of tubal pregnancy. He proposed tubal dyskinesia to explain the absence of anatomic evidence in tubal pregnancies and ascribed ectopic implantation to altered tubal motility caused by abnormal function of the autonomic nervous system. This theory derives support from recent research describing a pacemaker in the area of the isthmic-ampullar junction and further defines autonomic nervous control of tubal motility. Both alpha- and beta-adrenergic receptors have been demonstrated in human oviducts [1]. Stimulation of alpha receptors has been shown to cause constriction of the oviductal lumen, whereas a dilatation has been observed following beta stimulation. Constricting receptors are activated by norephinephrine, while both the alpha-constricting and beta-dilating receptors are activated by epinephrine. Altered neural control might result in blockage at the isthmic-ampullar junction, thereby causing an ampullar or fimbrial pregnancy. A similar lack of control at the uterotubal junction might produce an isthmic pregnancy. Closure at either junction might occur as a result of (1) closure of the oviductal lumen due to edema of the subserosa and muscularis, (2) partial or complete inhibition of release of contractile activity of the circular muscular fibers at the site of blockage, or (3) variation in the rate and amplitude of tubal muscle contractions (see Aref et al. [1] for review).

A recent histopathologic study from Johns Hopkins Hospital [23] has made an interesting observation regarding the location of a developing tubal ectopic pregnancy. These authors suggest "that although implantation undoubtably occurs on the luminal surface, the growing gestation rapidly penetrates the wall of the tube and subsequently most of its growth occurs in an extratubal location." This observation was based on the careful dissection of 20 tubal ectopic pregnancies as well as an experience with 242 ectopic pregnancies over a 5-year interval. As growth of the ectopic proceeded, "the vast majority of the conceptus develops between the tube and the peritoneum. The mass that results from the gestation and associated hemorrhage looks like a dilated tube, but in most cases it is extraluminal. True dilatation is usually secondary to intratubal hemorrhage."

These observations should assist the surgeon during repair of an unruptured or a minimally ruptured tubal pregnancy. The use of magnification during this type of surgical procedure for conservative repair of an ectopic pregnancy permits the surgeon to evaluate the area of tubal damage and the condition of the tubal mucosa. At times it has appeared to us that the tubal mucosa had been pushed to the side of the ectopic pregnancy, in concert with the preceding observations from Johns Hopkins Hospital. Often in these cases the extent of serosal damage is out of proportion to the mucosal insult, especially when the tubal mass has extended into the mesosalpinx.

A final hypothesis of the etiology of tubal pregnancy relates tubal pregnancy to an abnormality of male semen. Furuhjelm et al. [65] examined the semen from 23 husbands whose wives had had tubal pregnancies and found fewer normal sperm in the affected group. They concluded that "the quality of the semen is inferior in the series of ectopic pregnancies."

Recent studies with prostaglandins [1] make this concept of inferior seminal fluid more tenable. Prostaglandins (Pg) E and F have been shown to exert opposite effects on oviductal contractility, with the PgF group constricting the oviduct and the PgE group negating this effect. Abnormal amounts of PgF might produce an abnormal degree of tubal constriction or at least alter normal motility. Since $PgE_2$ causes relaxation of the isthmus and is probably a prerequisite for ovum transport into the uterus, inadequate amounts of this chemical mediator might result in delayed transport, thus facilitating tubal implantation. However, present evidence does not indicate an etiologic correlation between abnormal prostaglandin levels and tubal pregnancy.

## Choice of Surgical Procedure

The surgeon who encounters a tubal pregnancy must consider a number of factors before deciding on a specific operative procedure. Preoperative discussion, however brief, with the patient and her husband regarding the couple's desire for additional children is of utmost importance. Once the surgeon has entered the abdomen, control of bleeding, of primary concern, is often accomplished quickly by digital pressure on the mesosalpinx. After this has been accomplished, the surgeon must determine the exact location of the pregnancy, the condition of the involved tube, the condition of the opposite tube and ovary, and the importance of other pelvic abnormalities if they exist. The patient's desire for future pregnancy must be considered at this time. This appraisal may occur at the time of laparoscopy or during laparotomy. Five considerations relevant to surgical technique must be weighed in this appraisal:

1. Should the involved tube be removed or conserved?
2. Should ancillary procedures (e.g., plastic procedures on the opposite tube, myomectomy, or appendectomy) be done at the same time?
3. Should a vaginal or abdominal approach be used?
4. Should the ipsilateral ovary be removed?
5. Should the cornual area of the uterus be resected?

CONSERVATIVE SURGICAL APPROACH TO ECTOPIC PREGNANCY
It is this inconsistancy that has prompted us to re-evaluate our objectives in the surgical treatment of ectopic pregnancy. It is no longer sufficient to "point with pride" at a series of 100 ectopic pregnancies with no maternal mortality. Rather in keeping with current views in many areas of obstetric surgery, attempts should be made whenever possible to preserve the affected organ with the aim of preserving the possibility of reproduction. This is particularly true in tubal pregnancy where the high rate of a second ectopic pregnancy in the opposite tube is well known.

W. B. STROMME ET AL., [203]

In approximately 25 percent of patients undergoing laparotomy for tubal pregnancy, the conceptus is found in the remaining oviduct or the contralateral tube is abnormal. If subsequent pregnancy is desired, conservation of the involved tube is indicated. This necessitates expulsion "milking" of the ovisac and placenta from the fimbriae, or linear incision over the distended ampulla or distal isthmus, termed *salpingotomy*. Occasionally, resection of the damaged tubal segment followed by end-to-end reanastomosis will be possible. Uterotubal implantation is no longer indicated, since uterotubal anastomosis at a later time will produce an improved pregnancy result. The conservative surgical procedures for ectopic pregnancy are as follows:

1. Distal tubal pregnancy (see Fig. 7-22):
   a. Expulsion of products of conception: "Milking" the fimbriae
   b. Incision of distal oviduct

**Figure 7-22.** Operative approach to distal tubal pregnancy. **A.** Expulsion of products of conception (milking the tube). Distal tubal pregnancy produces dilatation of the distal ampulla with protrusion of a blood clot from the fimbria. Occasionally, the entire ovisac will be found distending the osteum, in which case it can be expelled by gentle finger pressure. Placental remnants and blood clots, the components of a tubal abortion, may also be expelled by milking the tube. The uterus is held with a curved dever retractor gently placed over the fundus, following which the tubal pregnancy is elevated and the cul-de-sac packed. A Williams or Babcock clamp on the utero-ovarian ligament assists in elevating the ovary and tube. Irrigation of the distal tube with saline and bipolar or monopolar coagulation of bleeding points permit salvage of the entire oviduct. Loupes or the operating microscope are used to visualize this site when available. **B.** Incision of distal oviduct. Milking the tube with gentle finger pressure may fail to remove attached placental fragments or to control excessive bleeding in which case an incision is made in the distal ampulla for a distance of 1 to 2 cm. The uterus has been elevated and the cul-de-sac packed as described earlier. Ocular loupes of magnifications 3.5 to 4.5 power are necessary during this procedure, and the operating microscope very useful. **C.** Incision into the dilated segment is performed under magnification with either a microelectrode or small angled iris scissors. Bleeding sites are coagulated with bipolar or monopolar electrodes, under magnification when available. **D.** Under magnification, the clot is removed from the distal ampulla. Careful removal prevents injury to the mucosal folds. **E.** The incision is closed with 6-0 or 8-0 synthetic absorbable suture material. Care is taken to avoid distortion of the fimbrial architecture. A lacrimal duct probe is easily passed beyond the site of closure, should the surgeon wish to verify patency.

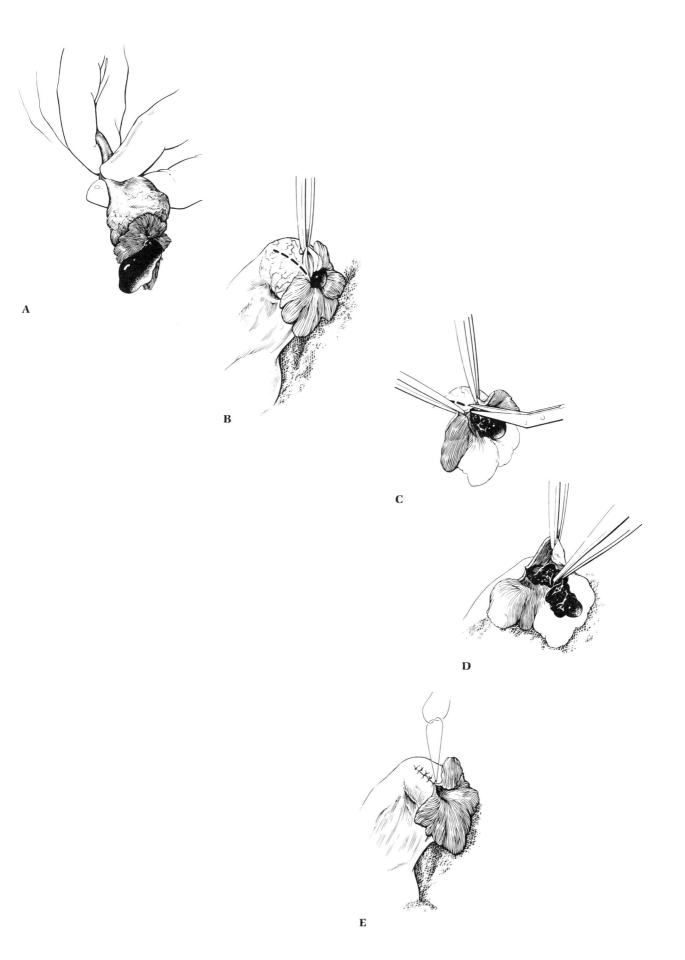

A

B

C

D

E

2. Midsegment and isthmic tubal pregnancy:
   a. Salpingotomy, linear incision (see Fig. 7-23)
   b. Midtubal resection without anastomosis (see Fig. 7-24A through C)
   c. Midtubal resection with reanastomosis (see Fig. 7-24D,E)

**Figure 7-23.** Salpingotomy. **A.** Unruptured pregnancy is shown in the midsegment. Under magnification with loupes or microscope, a linear incision is made along the most distended portion, usually on the antimesentery border; a knife blade or microelectrode on cutting current is used. The electrode is used to coagulate small vessels. Holding sutures are unnecessary when adequate packing is used. **B.** Removal of placental fragments and blood clots is performed carefully under magnification. Gentle separation of these fragments with blunt instruments is initially attempted, and usually results in almost complete removal of the intact clot. Occasionally, sharp excision may be necessary. **C.** Hemostasis is achieved with a fine monopolar or bipolar electrode. Constant irrigation permits cleansing of the musoca and identification of the bleeding sites. Venous ooze is controlled by pressure. A blunt probe, e.g., a Winston probe or glass rod, may then be passed proximally and distally to the site to verify patency. **D.** After hemostasis is complete, the incision is approximated with interrupted sutures of 8-0 or 6-0 synthetic absorbable material placed through the seromuscular layer. The area of repair must be observed for several minutes to make certain that bleeding has been controlled. A small ooze has not been found to be significant.

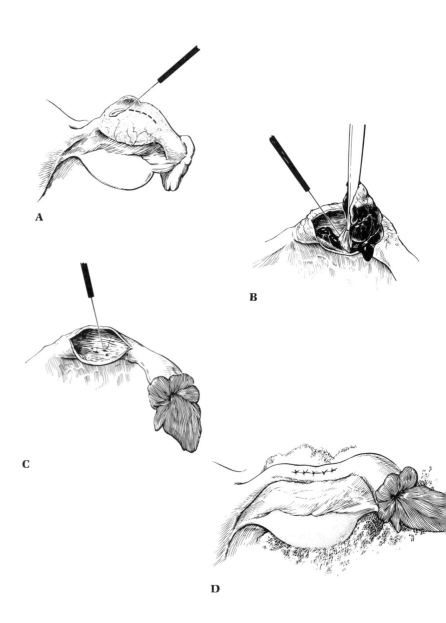

**Figure 7-24.** Midtubal resection, with or without anastomosis. **A.** A ruptured midtubal pregnancy is shown. Fragments of tubal serosa are apparent and repair of this segment is not possible. The dotted line identifies the segment of tube to be removed. Magnification provided by ocular loupes or the operating microscope is helpful to visualize the separation between normal and damaged serosa. **B.** Blood clots are removed from proximal and distal tubal segments as atraumatically as possible. Irrigation of these segments is carefully performed and monopolar or bilpolar coagulation employed for hemostasis. **C.** If magnification is not available, or if the patient's physical condition is unstable, the surgeon should carefully ligate the end of each tubal segment with small gauge suture, such as 4-0 synthetic absorbable material. Preservation of tubal length at this time will lead to improved pregnancy results following subsequent end-to-end anastomosis. **D.** If the patient's condition permits, and if magnification is available, reanastomosis of the cut tubal ends is performed. This is usually an ampullary-isthmic anastomosis; however, dilatation of the isthmic segment with blood clots results in a procedure similar to an ampullary-ampullary anastomosis. Two thin-walled dilated segments are easily reattached with 6-0 or 8-0 synthetic absorbable suture. A single-layer anastomosis has been used occasionally, although if 8-0 suture is employed a two-layer closure is performed. Patency may be demonstrated by transfundal lavage utilizing the Buxton clamp or by passing a blunt probe through the fimbriated end of the oviduct across the line of anastomosis. If preoperative laparoscopy has indicated an ectopic pregnancy amendable to conservative surgery, a transcervial canula (HUI) can be placed at that line and used for tubal hydrotubation during repair.

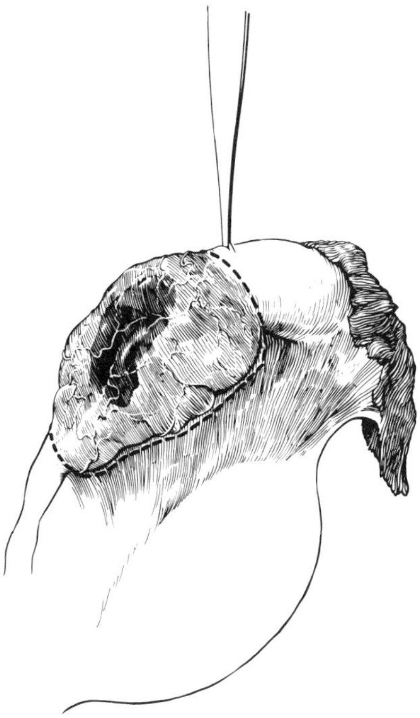

A

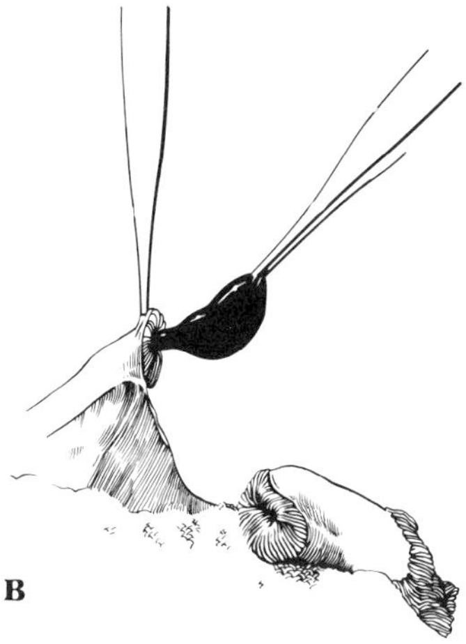

B

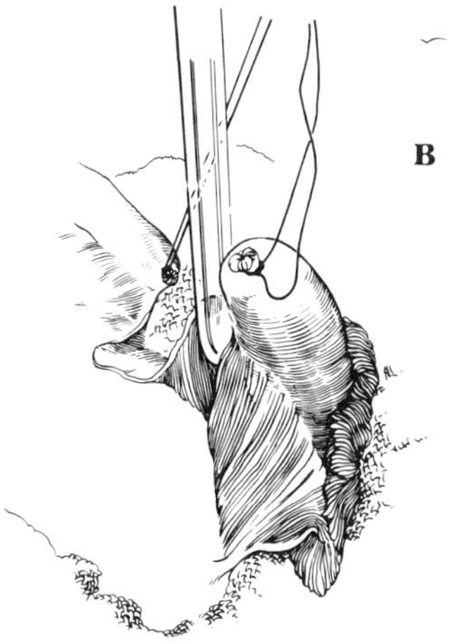

C

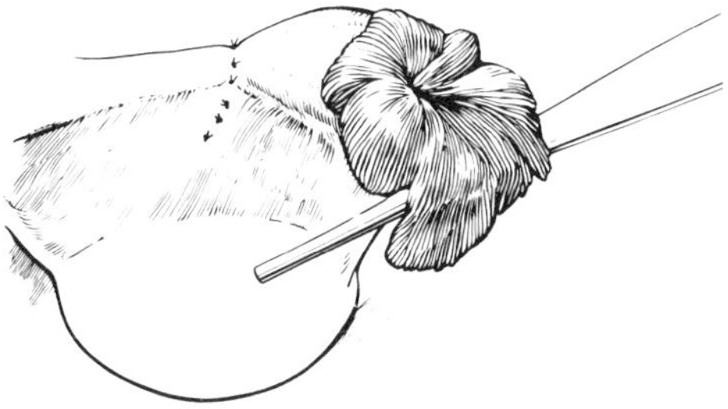

D

A second, more controversial indication for conservative surgery involves those patients of low parity in whom the opposite tube appears functional. Since a second ectopic pregnancy will occur in 10 to 27 percent of patients, it appears reasonable to preserve an involved oviduct should an unruptured ectopic pregnancy amenable to conservative surgery be encountered. Schoen and Nowak [174] studied the obstetric outlook in a group of 75 patients whose first pregnancy was ectopic. Fifty of these patients had adequate follow-up, and only 15 (30%) subsequently produced term infants. In addition, 12 of 50 patients (30%) in this group had recurrent ectopic pregnancies. Most studies of conservative surgery for ectopic pregnancy have noted that recurrent ectopic pregnancy occurs about equally in the conserved and contralateral, presumably normal, tube. Therefore, conservation of the oviduct in the presence of a normal contralateral tube should lengthen the reproductive years of this high-risk population.

The surgeon must also appreciate the difficulty of evaluating the contralateral oviduct when operating on a tubal pregnancy. Seitohik [177] performed postoperative tubal insufflation following surgery for ectopic pregnancy to ascertain the state of the remaining oviduct. This gynecologist found that all patients in whom the opposite tube was thought at surgery to be patent did in fact demonstrate tubal patency by this technique, and 60 percent of those judged to have salpingitis were obstructed. Recently, DeCherney [42] performed 29 hysterosalpingograms on patients who underwent a conservative salpingotomy at the time of tubal ectopic pregnancy and found tubal patency of the operated side in 89 percent of the patients, while only 69 percent of contralateral tubes were patent. Demonstration of contralateral tubal patency at the time of surgery has been recommended by Skulj et al. [190] and is used by the others. Skulj et al. stated that "the instillation of colored fluid into the uterine tubes via the uterine cavity . . . helps distinguish the patent section of the tube from the occluded part. With the exact degree of patency of both oviducts known, the most economical amputation of the damaged part is possible." Although we agree with this concept, in practice, transfundal tubal lavage may be difficult in these patients because evidence of cornual occlusion of the contralateral tube may be the result of uterine blood and decidua. Therefore, this procedure has been used by us only when the information is of considerable importance. The transcervical cannula may be inserted prior to laparotomy if ultrasound has demonstrated an empty uterine cavity. The Buxton clamp and needle technique may be employed intraoperatively. The conservative surgical approach to a distal ectopic pregnancy is presented in Figure 7-22.

Stromme [202] deserves credit for championing the use of conservative surgery in the form of salpingotomy for the treatment of unruptured ectopic pregnancy in the United States. This procedure, which involves a linear incision over the distended midtubal segment, was described again in 1956 by Tompkins [215] and Wexler et al. [226]. Stromme reported a single successful case in 1953 in which salpingotomy was performed in a patient whose opposite tube had previously been removed because of a ruptured tubal pregnancy. Two intrauterine pregnancies then followed this conservative procedure. In 1962, Stromme [203] reported the results of 7 patients who had undergone salpingotomy. Pregnancy occurred postoperatively in 4 of 7 patients, and 3 of the 5 patients who had only a single tube conceived postoperatively. Both Tompkins [215] and Wexler et al. [226] also reported successful pregnancies following salpingotomy. Of interest, in Tompkins' 6 patients who desired future pregnancies, only 1 uterine pregnancy occurred and 2 additional patients sustained repeat ectopic pregnancies. Both ectopic pregnancies occurred in the contralateral tubes, however.

Although Stromme, Tompkins, and others, during the 1950s, were early advocates of a conservative approach to tubal pregnancy, a similar recommendation had been made as early as 1895 [115]. Reports of conservative operations were infrequent during the early part of this century, however. In 1941, Gauss [69] reported 27 conservative operations in 161 ectopic pregnancies, none of which were followed by pregnancy. Caffier [25] reported 10 consecutive operations for ectopic pregnancy. Subsequently, 4 patients had intrauterine pregnancies and only 1 patient had a second tubal pregnancy. In a review of world literature performed in 1956, Wexler and associates [226] reported 21 full-term and 3 recurrent ectopic pregnancies following 79 conservative tubal operations.

*Operative Approach to Mid-Segment or Isthmic Tubal Pregnancy (Figs. 7-23, 7-24).* Two surgical procedures are available to the surgeon confronted with a midtubal ectopic pregnancy. The first, salpingotomy, is useful in the treatment of unruptured midtubal pregnancy. The second, midtubal resection with or without end-to-end anastomosis, is performed when rupture of the midtubal or isthmic segments has occurred, or when control of bleeding is felt to be inadequate. Magnification should be used during these procedures whenever possible. The surgical technique of salpingotomy is shown in Figure 7-23; midtubal or isthmic resection without anastomosis is shown in Figure 7-24 A through C and with anastomosis in Figure 7-24 D.

LAPAROSCOPIC SURGERY FOR ECTOPIC PREGNANCY
An outgrowth of the recent interest in conservative surgical approaches to tubal ectopic pregnancy has been the attempt to perform this surgery by an operative

laparoscopic technique. DeCherney et al. [45] have stated: "We believe that in the proper setting, tubal ectopic pregnancies of small diameter can be successfully treated utilizing laparoscopy alone."

The laparoscopic approach was successfully employed to remove a small (2 cm) isthmic-ampullary pregnancy in 1973 [189]. In a large series of 60 ectopic pregnancies treated by laparoscopy, Bruhat et al. [19] experienced only 3 failures. Linear salpingotomy was performed in 72 percent of these patients. Postoperatively, pregnancy occurred in 72 percent of the group, and repeat ectopic pregnancy was encountered in 12 percent. Although the authors attributed their excellent pregnancy results to the laparoscopic technique, it has been suggested that selection of patients for the laparoscopic approach excluded the more severe cases [45].

Recently, DeCherney et al. [45] reported their experience in 18 patients with ectopic pregnancies in whom a laparoscopic approach was utilized. All patients had met the following criteria: (1) normal pelvic anatomy, including a normal appearing contralateral tube, (2) an ampullary ectopic pregnancy that was unruptured and less than 3 cm in diameter, (3) a gestation less than 8 weeks, (4) stable vital signs, and (5) strong preoperative diagnosis of ectopic pregnancy. The surgical technique employed by this group apparently utilized two punctures. The authors stated that "using a cutting current with Wolf hook scissors, an incision 2 cm or smaller was made on the antimesenteric border of the tube." The products of conception extruded spontaneously during the incision. Bleeding was controlled by high-frequency coagulation. There was one failure in the series, not included in the numbers.

Among the patients reported by the group from Yale [45], 16 attempted conception following laparoscopic removal of an ectopic pregnancy. In the first postoperative year, 3 of 8 patients became pregnant. In the second year, an additional 5 patients conceived, for a total pregnancy rate of 50 percent. There were no repeat ectopics in this small group.

The major weakness in the report by DeCherney et al. [45] was, of course, the presence of a normal contralateral oviduct. Postoperative pregnancy may have occurred in the normal tube rather than in the one operated on. This point was approached in a second series of 15 patients operated on for ectopic pregnancy by the Yale group [46] in whom the contralateral oviduct had been previously removed or was occluded. Three patients were treated with a linear salpingotomy, performed via the laparoscope, and 2 of these women had a uterine pregnancy postoperatively. One patient had a repeat ectopic pregnancy.

In summary, the laparoscopic approach to an unruptured tubal ectopic pregnancy is one of linear salpingotomy performed utilizing a high-frequency cutting current. This approach is similar to that utilized by us during a microsurgical salpingotomy and described earlier, with the exception that tissue damage is better controlled under loupe or microscopic magnification (see Fig. 7-23). The most difficult aspect of a laparoscopic approach involves the inability to achieve complete hemostasis at the site of placental attachment on the inferior tubal wall. Under magnification, this site can be clearly identified and bleeding controlled with point electrocoagulation. This is the most tedious aspect of a laparoscopic approach, and it results from the difficulty of everting the tubal edges during operative laparoscopy as the pregnancy remnants or clot are being removed. The ability to hold the tube and electrocoagulate the placental site requires extreme dexterity.

At present, we prefer a microsurgical approach to unruptured tubal ectopic pregnancies in which a laparotomy is performed and salpingotomy is carried out. Excellent intratubal hemostasis is achieved in this manner and the tubal edges may be approximated with 8-0 or 6-0 synthetic absorbable sutures. It is possible that an operative laparoscopic approach using the carbon dioxide laser may permit more exact hemostasis and lead to increased utilization of this approach. At present, however, the laser approach remains experimental.

**Table 7-33.** Incidence of pregnancy following conservative surgery for tubal pregnancy

| Author | No. of patients | Percent pregnant | Percent term pregnancy | Percent ectopic pregnancy | Comment |
|---|---|---|---|---|---|
| Skulj et al., 1964 | 92 | — | 25 | 1.1 | 10 of the 23 pregnancies in patients with only 1 remaining tube |
| Stromme et al., 1962: | | | | | |
|   Single tube | 7 | 57 | — | 0 | |
|   Total | 15 | 60 | — | 0 | |
| Tompkins, 1956 | 6 | 50 | 19 | 33 | |
| Timonen and Nieminen, 1967: | | | | | |
|   Radical | 558 | 49.3 | 27.2 | 11.5 | |
|   Conservative | 185 | 53 | 23.8 | 12.4 | |
| Vehaskari, 1960: | | | | | |
|   Radical | 219 | 48 | 35 | 8 | |
|   Conservative | 88 | 49 | 30 | 16 | |
| Wexler et al., 1956 | 79 | 29 | 26 | 4 | Collected series Europe and United States |
| Jarvinen et al., 1972 | 41 | 18 | 14 | 7 | Single remaining tube |
| Grant (literature review), 1962 | 141 | 25 | 19 | 6 | Single remaining tube |
| Bukovsky, 1979 | 23 | 70 | — | 1 | Opposite tube functional |
| DeCherney, 1979 | 48 | 58 | 39 | 18 | |
| DeCherney, 1980 | 9 | 56 | 56 | 0 | Termed microsurgery |
| Janecek, 1978 | 6 | 50 | 50 | 0 | End-to-end with prosthesis |
| Stangle, 1978 | 4 | 50 | 50 | 0 | End-to-end loupes |
| Patton, 1982 | 17 | 53 | 47 | 11 | Single remaining tube |

**Table 7-34.** Incidence of pregnancy after conservative and radical tubal surgery

| Operation | Percent term pregnancy | Percent extrauterine pregnancy | Percent abortion | Percent total pregnancies | Total cases |
|---|---|---|---|---|---|
| Tubal section | 36.1 | 18.1 | 13.3 | 61.4 | 83 |
| Expression of ovisac | 24.1 | 24.1 | 20.7 | 65.5 | 29 |
| Tubal resection | 17.6 | 8.8 | 11.8 | 38.2 | 68 |
| Reimplantation | 20.0 | 20.0 | 0.0 | 40.0 | 5 |
| Total conservative operations | 27.0 | 15.7 | 14.1 | 53.0 | 185 |
| Total radical operations | 29.2 | 11.5 | 10.6 | 49.3 | 558 |

*Note:* The percentage of total pregnancies may be less than the sum of the three types since a few patients with term pregnancy also had an extrauterine pregnancy.

Source: S. Timonen and U. Nieminen, Tubal pregnancy: Choice of operative method of treatment. *Acta Obstet. Gynecol. Scand.* 46:327, 1967.

RESULTS

Our literature review is presented in Table 7-33. The early work of Stromme was updated in 1975. However, the pregnancy rate in these recent data was difficult to ascertain. Three recent retrospective studies by DeCherney et al. (Yale) [46], Buchovsky et al. (Tel Aviv) [20], and Sherman (Tel Aviv) [184] are included as well as small personal studies of conservative surgery for ectopic pregnancy by DeCherney et al. [42,44] and Stangel et al. [198] in which a modified microsurgical technique was employed to remove the ectopic. A series of conservative microsurgical procedures performed by the author (G.W.P.) is also included.

A large Scandinavian series of 1,067 tubal pregnancies was reported by Timonen and Nieminen in 1967 [214], of which 185 patients were treated conservatively. The various procedures included tubal section, expression of fertilized ovum, tubal resection, and tubal implantation. *Tubal section* (termed *salpingotomy* in this text) refers to a longitudinal incision of the ampulla with removal of the conceptus through this opening. Expression (milking) of the fertilized ovum was performed when fimbrial pregnancy was encountered. *Tubal resection* refers to excision of the involved segment with end-to-end anastomosis. Implantation also involved resection of the involved tubal segment accompanied by uterotubal implantation, a technique rarely performed today. Polyethylene catheters were used frequently by Timonen and Nieminen [214] following reconstruction. Selection of patients for conservative surgery was based on age and desire for subsequent pregnancy, and the procedure was employed "if the other tube had previously been removed or was seriously damaged." Their data are presented in Table 7-34.

Longitudinal tubal section, salpingotomy, was performed in 44.6 percent of this series, usually on unruptured tubes. A polyethylene splint was utilized in over half these cases, a technique not employed by other surgeons or by us. Tubal resection was performed in 73.5 percent of patients with tubal rupture and accounted for 36.7 percent of all conservative operations. The postoperative pregnancy rate in these patients was difficult to evaluate, since no data regarding the contralateral tube were included. Penicillin-hydrocortisone solution, 4 ml daily, was distilled through a plastic catheter into the pelvic cavity following surgery by these Scandinavian authors.

Table 7-34 lists the pregnancy yield reported by Timonen and Nieminen. In the group of 250 women who had not conceived prior to surgery, 90 (36 percent) were treated conservatively. Forty-nine of these patients did conceive postoperatively and 26.8 percent had term pregnancies. However, 18.9 percent had recurrent tubal pregnancies. Repetitive tubal pregnancy was particularly high following expression of the ovisac from the fimbria in this study, although this has not been observed by others [44,45,203].

Timonen and Nieminen [214] reported subsequent pregnancies in about 50 percent of patients undergoing radical or conservative surgery for tubal pregnancy. Term pregnancies occurred in over half the patients in both groups, and recurrent ectopic pregnancies were noted in 11.5 percent after radical surgery compared with 15.7 percent following conservative surgery. These results are similar to the collected data for all procedures reported in 1962 by Grant [80]. He recorded a 43 percent postoperative pregnancy rate, with 22 percent term and 9 percent recurrent ectopic. Vehaskari [221] reported 30 to 35 percent term and 9 percent recurrent tubal pregnancy rates after radical surgery, compared with a similar number of term pregnancies but a 15 percent rate of recurrent tubal pregnancy after conservative surgery. In a collected series of patients undergoing surgery on a remaining tube, Grant found subsequent pregnancy in 25 percent. Uterine gestation occurred in 19 percent and recurrent tubal pregnancy in 6 percent.

Recently, DeCherney et al. [44] evaluated 98 patients who had an ectopic tubal pregnancy. Forty-eight conservative procedures were compared with a similar control group of 50 patients who underwent salpingectomy or salpingo-oophorectomy. The conservative operative procedure was that of salpingotomy, as described by Stromme. Overall, uterine pregnancies occurred in 40 percent of patients, and recurrent ectopic pregnancies occurred in 10 percent. Recurrent ectopic pregnancies occurred in 18 percent of the conservative group (9 of 48), and 30 percent (19 of 48) subsequently had viable pregnancies. Unfortunately, those patients with uterine abortion were not included in these statistics. Six patients underwent salpingotomy in the single remaining tube. Four of the patients (66 percent) had uterine pregnancies without a recurrent ectopic. In the radical group reported by DeCherney et al., ectopic pregnancies occurred in 6 of 50 patients (12 percent) and viable pregnancies in 21 of 50 (42 percent). In a small personal series reported in 1980, DeCherney and Naftolin [43] presented the outcome of 9 patients who had undergone a conservative procedure by microsurgical technique. In all patients, a salpingotomy was performed through a 2.5-cm linear incision. This authors stated "that neither an operating microscope nor operating loupes were used except in the first two cases." The suture material utilized was 4-0 and 6-0 Vicryl. Of interest in this surgical technique, however, was the use of Rheomacrodex placed in the abdominal cavity at the conclusion of surgery. Apparently these 9 patients were selected from a total of 53 ectopic pregnancies that occurred during this same interval. Four of the 9 patients had a ruptured ectopic pregnancy, compared with 5 in whom the pregnancy was unruptured. Overall, pregnancy occurred in 5 of these 9 patients without a recurrent ectopic. Bellina [6] has used the carbon dioxide laser during a microsurgical approach to linear salpingostomy to incise the tubal serosa over the gestational sac. This surgeon reports that successful pregnancies have followed 6 such microsurgical procedures.

The most optimistic reports have been published in Israel by Bukovsky [20] in 1979 and Sherman [184] in 1982. Among 116 ectopic pregnancies operated on in Tel Aviv (1972–1977 [20]), 45 were unruptured, and of these, conservative surgery was performed on 23 patients. Ten patients had a history of previous PID, and 2 had experienced prior ectopic pregnancies. The surgical procedure was a linear salpingotomy, similar to that described by Stromme [203]. Postoperative pregnancies occurred in 14 of 20 patients who desired pregnancy (70 percent), and only 1 ectopic pregnancy occurred in this group (5 percent), and it occurred in a contralateral oviduct. A recent report by Sherman from this same hospital found a conception rate of 81 percent and a recurrent ectopic rate of 7.8 percent in 154 women following surgery for ectopic pregnancy.

The role of end-to-end tubal anastomosis in the conservative treatment of an oviduct damaged by ectopic pregnancy has not been established, although Ingersol [101] described this approach in detail in 1962 and Hallet [27] also suggested the usefulness of this approach. No clinical data pertaining to its benefit have been published until recently, however. In 1976, Stangel et al. [197] described a modified microsurgical approach to anastomosis for unruptured ampullary or midtubal pregnancy. Postoperatively, both patients who underwent this procedure conceived. The status of the contralateral tube was described as "extensive adhesions tightly binding the fimbria and tube on the contralateral side to the pelvic side wall." Stangel et al. stated that an operating loupe was used at first, but this aid was subsequently found to be unnecessary. In a later report [198], Stengel et al. stated that an operating loupe of magnification 4 or 6× was utilized during these procedures and that 6-0 and 8-0 nylon sutures were employed. Postoperatively, 2 of 4 patients who underwent reanastomosis by Stangel et al. had intrauterine pregnancies, and neither had a recurrent ectopic pregnancy. Tubal patency had been noted postoperatively in all 4 patients who underwent this procedure. A second report of end-to-end anastomosis has been published in the French Literature by Janecek and DeGrandi [106]. The technique used in this series of 6 unruptured ampullary tubal pregnancies consisted of excision of the damaged tubal segment followed by end-to-end anastomosis over a polyethylene wire. Early hydrotubation was performed by these authors, and postoperative hysterosalpingography performed six months following the surgical procedure demonstrated tubal patency in all 6 cases. Three patients had uterine pregnancies following this procedure. No data on the contralateral tube were presented; presumably, it was normal.

**Table 7-35.** Surgical approach to ectopic pregnancy*

| Technique | Patients | Pregnancy | Ectopic |
|---|---|---|---|
| Removal of tube | | | |
|   Normal opposite tube | 14 | 8 (57%) | 1 |
|   Abnormal opposite tube | 11 | 3 | 2 |
| Total | 25 | 11 (44%) | 3 |
| Conservation of remaining tube | | | |
|   End to End | 1 | 1 | 0 |
|   Milking | 2 | 1 | 0 |
|   Salpingotomy | 14 | 7 | 1 |
| Total | 17 | 9 (53%) | 1 |

*Personal results 1976–1982 (G.W.P.).

Patton operated on 51 patients who had an ectopic pregnancy during the years 1976–1982. The involved oviduct was removed in 25 of these women, and postoperatively, pregnancy occurred in 11. Eight patients experienced an intrauterine pregnancy and three had recurrent ectopic pregnancies. In 14 of the 25 patients in whom the opposite oviduct was judged to be normal, pregnancy occured in 8 patients (57%), and only one was an ectopic pregnancy (see Table 7-35).

In the last four years of this study, many patients with an ectopic pregnancy were referred to the author for possible conservation of the involved tube because of his interest in infertility surgery. The number of patients who underwent a conservative operation during these years thus increased from a 40 percent incidence in the years 1976–1978 to a 59 percent incidence during the 1979–1981 interval. In 1982, 64 percent of 11 ectopic pregnancies were treated by a conservative operation. The benefit of conservative microsurgery for ectopic pregnancy was evaluated in 17 patients in this series who had a single remaining oviduct at the time of surgery. In all of these patients, magnification by an ocular loupe or Zeiss operating microscope was employed. Nine pregnancies occurred in these patients (53%), and one of them was a tubal ectopic pregnancy. Of particular interest, 10 of these 17 patients were operated on for a second tubal pregnancy by this microsurgical approach, and postoperatively, 5 conceived of which only 1 conception resulted in a third ectopic pregnancy (Table 7-35).

In summary, clinical data have established that pregnancy will occur after conservative surgery for tubal gestation. The merits of the three operative procedures—(1) "milking" the fimbriae, (2) salpingotomy, and (3) tubal resection combined with end-to-end anastomosis—have been established, but not clarified. Unfortunately, most series of conservative operations for ectopic pregnancy have included numbers of patients in whom the contralateral oviduct was normal or at least patent. In each of the large series reported in Table 7-33, small numbers of patients had only a single tube at the

**Table 7-36.** Pregnancy after surgery on contralateral tube
(following salpingectomy or salpingo-oophorectomy on involved tube)

| Operation | No. of patients | Percent pregnant | Percent term pregnancy | Percent recurrent ectopic pregnancy |
|---|---|---|---|---|
| Salpingolysis on contralateral tube | 52 | 48 | 25 | 20 |
| Salpingostomy on contralateral tube | 15 | 34 | 20 | 7 |
| Total | 67 | 41 | 24 | 17 |

Source: Modified from A. Vehaskari, The operation of choice for ectopic pregnancy with reference to subsequent fertility. *Acta Obstet. Gynecol. Scand.* 39(Suppl. 3):3, 1960.

time of conservative surgery. In general, the results in these few patients have been favorable. Stromme [203] achieved pregnancy in 4 of 7 such patients, and Decherney and Kase [42] reported similar results in 4 to 6 patients. Patton achieved pregnancy in 9 of 17 such patients with only a single recurrent ectopic pregnancy. Interestingly, recurrent ectopic pregnancy is as likely to occur in the opposite, presumably normal oviduct as in the conservatively operated tube.

CONTRALATERAL TUBAL SURGERY

This discussion relates to the decision to perform a *reparative* procedure on the opposite tube after either removing the involved tube or performing a conservative procedure for tubal pregnancy. The preceding section dealt with surgery of the oviduct directly involved in the ectopic pregnancy. Many surgeons have performed fimbriolysis and salpingostomy on the contralateral tube if it appeared diseased at the time of salpingectomy for tubal pregnancy. However, few data are available regarding the prognosis for this type of surgery.

Vehaskari [221], in 1960, presented the surgical treatment and subsequent fertility of a series of 366 patients with ectopic pregnancy. Sixty-seven of these patients underwent salpingectomy and contralateral tubal surgery. Table 7-36 summarizes the pregnancy yield in these patients. Salpingectomy with contralateral salpingolysis resulted in 25 percent subsequent term pregnancies. This is essentially the same as the incidence following salpingectomy alone. Recurrent ectopic pregnancy occurred in 20 percent of this group, a rate similar to the 27 percent reported by Franklin in which many patients had residual scarring from prior pelvic infections. Whether salpingolysis improved the chance of subsequent pregnancy in these patients is a moot point. Somewhat more impressive are the results of salpingostomy and salpingectomy. A rate of 20 percent for term pregnancy after salpingostomy is about average, as is the 7 percent for recurrent ectopic pregnancy.

Vehaskari also performed tubal section, expression of the ovum, and evacuation of a hematocele in 31 additional patients. Postoperative fertility in this group is of little significance, since in many cases, both tubes were present and had undergone mixed operative procedures.

The patients reported by Vehaskari may be divided into two groups. The first are those patients with ectopic pregnancy in whom the contralateral tube appeared normal and unilateral salpingectomy was performed. Postoperatively, 48 percent conceived, 35 percent had term pregnancies, and 8 percent had recurrent tubal pregnancies. The second, presumably less favorable, group included those patients in whom the uninvolved tube appeared abnormal and in whom reconstructive surgery was performed together with conservative surgery on the involved tube. Pregnancy occurred in 49 percent of this group, with 30 percent going to term; however, 16 percent had a recurrent tubal gestation.

The introduction of microsurgical technique into the field of infertility has markedly altered the surgeon's approach to salpingolysis and repair of tubal disease. The emphasis on meticulous hemostasis, an integral part of microsurgery, makes the surgeon hesitant to perform extensive tubal surgery when operating on an ectopic pregnancy. The use of monopolar and bipolar electrodes permits resection of adhesions under magnification provided by an ocular loupe, but salpingostomy and myomectomy are not indicated at this time.

Despite these recent favorable results, the question of performing contralateral tubal repair of salpingolysis at the time of salpingectomy or conservative surgery for tubal pregnancy is unsettled. If the operator is an experienced infertility surgeon and is able to utilize ocular loupes, instruments such as glass rods and a monopolar microelectrode, as well as a bipolar forceps, then resection of adhesions is practical.

Recently, Sherman et al. [184] reported that reconstructive procedures, including lysis of adhesions and tuboplasty, were carried out in a group of 45 patients who underwent either radical or conservative surgical treatment for ectopic pregnancy. Thirty-nine of these patients were included in the study group, and of these, pregnancies occurred in 52 percent. This represented 20 of 114 (18 percent) of all pregnancies. In contrast, 48 percent did not conceive, and these 19 patients represented 51 percent of the infertile patients (19/37). This was a unique series of patients and pregnancy occurred in an unusually high incidence of total patients (114 of

151). Of interest, 58 percent of ectopic pregnancies were unruptured at the time of surgery.

Under these circumstances, resection of minimal fimbrial adhesions may also be performed. Microsurgical fimbrioplasty or salpingostomy is not performed at this time, however. If these instruments are not available, and if the operator is not an experienced microsurgeon, it is recommended that surgery of the opposite tube be delayed. It is recommended that the surgical approach to the remaining abnormal tube be made under optimal conditions. These conditions, including preoperative hydrocortisone and use of the operating microscope, combined with surgical assistance, are best achieved during a second laparotomy scheduled shortly after the end of the menses. The advantage of these carefully controlled conditions outweighs the risk of a second general anesthetic.

VAGINAL APPROACH

In 1897, Bovée [14] reported 6 cases of ruptured tubal pregnancy and advocated a vaginal approach by a posterior colpotomy for surgical removal of the ruptured tube. He stated that "for those cases in which hemorrhage has stopped . . . no other route is as safe, quick and efficient." Other surgeons before Bovée, including Kelly [115], had utilized vaginal colpotomy for removal of a tubal pregnancy. Of interest, however, was a subsequent report by Bovée, in 1910, in which he stated that "shortly after reading that paper [1897] I was horrified by a fatal result for which I concluded the route and manner of operating were absolutely responsible. . . . During the following six years I lost three other patients in whom I employed this method." All deaths were related to profound hemorrhage, and Bovée concluded that only very stable patients without hemorrhage and in whom good exposure was obtained should be treated vaginally [14]. Cherney [28] reported the use of colpotomy in the management of tubal pregnancy and advocated this approach. However, in his series of 203 tubal pregnancies, only 54 were treated by colpotomy alone. Cherney concluded that "it is believed in our clinic that the vaginal approach is preferred." It should be noted, however, that laparotomy was required in 63 percent of patients following colpotomy.

It is our opinion that the use of vaginal colpotomy as a diagnostic technique has been replaced by laparoscopy or culdoscopy. Furthermore, the question of fertility following partial salpingectomy performed through a colpotomy incision has not been evaluated. From a theoretical standpoint, it could be expected that manipulation of the tube and ovary via colpotomy might result in cul-de-sac adhesions, with tubal and ovarian fixation. If subsequent fertility is not desired and the posterior colpotomy is being utilized for diagnosis, an attempt at removal through this incision may be warranted, particularly if the involved tube is easily mobilized and bleeding is minimal.

CORNUAL RESECTION

When removing the tube, it has been common to excise the distal half of the interstitial portion of the tube and thereby minimize the possibility of recurrence of pregnancy in the tubal stump. However, Woodruff and Pauerstein [238] recently reviewed the advantages and disadvantages of cornual resection in patients with tubal pregnancy and concluded that interstitial pregnancy is rare after homologous salpingectomy and that cornual resection is not guaranteed protection against ipsilateral interstitial pregnancy.

At the Boston Hospital for Women (now part of the Brigham and Women's Hospital), cornual resection was often performed at the time of salpingectomy. A wedge of superficial myometrium was excised, including the cornual portion of the tube. Care was taken not to enter the endometrial cavity. Placenta accreta and uterine rupture have been reported [238] following deep cornual excision and Fulsher [64] reported 6 cases of interstitial pregnancy occurring after cornual resection. Kalchman and Meltzer [114] reviewed 75 cases of interstitial pregnancy, of which 20 percent followed cornual resection.

We do not accept the criticism that cornual resection results in increased blood loss, since blood loss depends on individual surgical technique. It has been shown [12] that the luminal diameter of the uterine artery is about 1.9 mm during pregnancy, but is reduced to 1.0 mm in the nonpregnant condition. A horizontal mattress suture may be placed beneath the excision site and tightened following excision to prevent bleeding. In our experience, this procedure is not usually associated with marked blood loss unless the ascending uterine vessel has not been ligated.

From a theoretical standpoint it is clear that one cannot remove the entire interstitium without entering the uterine cavity. The latter is carefully avoided, which means leaving a small segment of the interstitial tube in situ. Theoretically, this segment could be the site of recurrent ectopic pregnancy. However, since at least half of this segment is removed, the number of recurrent ipsilateral pregnancies should be relatively small.

This issue has been confused by those who assume that cornual excision has failed if any postoperative interstitial pregnancies occur. Rather, one should expect a *reduction* in this number, and the series of Fulsher [64], Kirschner [116], and Kalchman [119] revealed fewer interstitial pregnancies following wedge excision than after simple salpingectomy.

In summary, although cornual wedge excision was recommended in the first edition, we now feel that it is rarely indicated today. Rather, increased care is exercised during removal of the involved oviduct flush with the uterus in order that blood vessels in the mesosalpinx are not severely damaged. Blood supply to the involved ovary is thereby conserved.

**Table 7-37.** Results obtained with salpingectomy versus salpingo-oophorectomy

| Surgeon | No. of patients | Percent pregnant | Percent term pregnancy | Percent tubal pregnancy | Comment |
|---|---|---|---|---|---|
| Bender, 1956 | | | | | |
| Salpingectomy | 187 | 42 | — | 7 | Salpingo-oophorectomy performed on most severe cases |
| Salpingo-oophorectomy | 51 | 56 | — | 8 | |
| Douglas et al., 1969 | | | | | |
| Salpingectomy | 78 | 42.3 | 33.3 | — | |
| Salpingo-oophorectomy | 28 | 53.5 | 35.7 | 113 | |
| Franklin et al., 1973 | | | | | |
| Salpingectomy | 251 | 38 | — | 41 | 29% gross inflammatory disease |
| Salpingo-oophorectomy | 67 | 38.6 | — | 59 | 43% gross inflammatory disease |

IPSILATERAL OOPHORECTOMY

According to Jeffcoate [109], "The conclusion may be that it sometimes pays to put all the eggs into one basket." This statement reflects the convincing argument advocated by Jeffcoate and others that removal of the ipsilateral ovary at the time of salpingectomy for tubal pregnancy should increase postoperative fertility by permitting all ovulated ova easy access to a normal fallopian tube. The theoretical disadvantage relates to loss of ovarian function by a subsequent pathologic entity that might destroy the remaining ovary. While the chances of this occurrence would seem extremely low, a controlled prospective study comparing fertility after salpingectomy versus salpingo-oophorectomy has not been reported. Cooper reviewed the cases at the Boston Hospital for Women (now part of the Brigham and Women's Hospital) and found a slight increase in the incidence of pregnancy in patients treated by salpingo-oophorectomy. However, that was a retrospective study and the number of patients was too small to make a statistically valid conclusion.

As in the discussion of cornual resection, one encounters a lack of objective data regarding the value of ipsilateral oophorectomy. Recently, removal of the ovary in patients with a severely diseased adenexa due to inflammatory disease was carried out in 9 patients [216]. Remarkably, 7 of these patients became pregnant postoperatively. The creditable postoperative fertility rates following ovarian removal underscore the value of this procedure, since these patients should be less fertile than those with less pelvic disease.

The available data are obviously intrinsically biased, since oophorectomy is usually performed because of extension of the disease process. If pelvic adhesions are extensive, patients undergoing salpingo-oophorectomy would be expected to have a lower subsequent fertility rate than those without adhesions who have salpingectomy only (see Table 7-37). In his series, Franklin noted that 43 percent of patients undergoing salpingo-oophorectomy had evidence of pelvic infection, compared with 29 percent of those having salpingectomy only [63]. Franklin noted, "Thus the similarity in subsequent fertility rate and the disparity in the rate of repeat ectopic pregnancy in this population following salpingectomy versus salpingo-oophorectomy were attributable to a dissimilarity in the character of the populations studied."

Bender [17] published a series in which postoperative pregnancy occurred in 58 percent of patients undergoing salpingo-oophorectomy, compared with 42 percent following salpingectomy alone. Douglas and associates [52] also noted an increased pregnancy rate—53.5 percent—following salpingo-oophorectomy, compared with 42.3 percent after salpingectomy. However, the term pregnancy yield was not statistically different. The series by Franklin revealed equal postoperative fertility following these two procedures, but increased recurrent ectopic pregnancies in the salpingo-oophorectomy group.

A new element in this discussion involves the future role of in vitro fertilization (IVF) or injection of the ovum into an occluded oviduct. Conservation of the ovary in these patients may facilitate ovum capture by laparoscopy. There are as yet no data relating to the use of IVF in patients who have had prior ectopic pregnancies. However, the recent excellent results from the Norfolk Clinic suggest the future use in these patients. We recommend that ipsilateral oophorectomy not be carried out unless absolutely necessary.

PRESENT SURGICAL APPROACH

The occurrence of a tubal pregnancy severely affects the future reproductive ability of that individual. The incidence of this pathologic entity is increasing and will be encountered by all involved in the practice of obstetrics and gynecology. This involves physicians of varying surgical skill and expertise in the area of reparative tubal surgery. Although other types of tubal pathology may be referred to an expert in microsurgery for tubal repair, the handling of an ectopic pregnancy may occur in an emergency situation, and therefore, the approach to this entity must be familiar to all involved.

The patient and her husband should be informed preoperatively of the effects of tubal pregnancy on her reproductive potential and of the types of surgery that are possible prior to surgical intervention. The patient may choose to retain her potential for future childbearing and thus undergo a conservative operation if it is surgically feasible. If future childbearing is not desired, the risk of recurrent tubal pregnancy warrants elective sterilization at the time of laparotomy. The following discussion represents our present approach to tubal pregnancy in patients desiring additional children.

Diagnosis suggested by clinical history and supported by a serum assay for the beta subunit of HCG and by ultrasonography is then verified by laparoscopy, unless the patient is in hemorrhagic shock. An intrauterine cannula is not employed when the possibility of an intrauterine pregnancy exists. In those patients in whom ectopic pregnancy is highly suspicious, the procedure is carried out with the patient in the supine position utilizing a two-puncture technique. Laparotomy rather than vaginal colpotomy is advised in patients desiring future pregnancy. Cornual resection is no longer recommended routinely with salpingectomy. Ipsilateral oophorectomy was often performed at the time of salpingectomy. However, increasingly this ovary is left in situ when partial midtubal resection without anastomosis is performed. In these patients, future tubal reanastomosis remains possible. In addition, the possibility of future in vitro fertilization influences our decision to conserve the ovary in younger patients.

If the ectopic pregnancy occurs in a patient who has had a previous salpingectomy, or if the opposite tube appears diseased or even occluded, and finally, if an unruptured ectopic pregnancy is found that can easily be removed in the presence of a normal opposite tube, conservative surgery is advocated. Linear salpingotomy—a horizontal incision over the dilated tubal segment—may permit removal of the products of conception and clot without tubal destruction (see Fig. 7-23). A second procedure involving extrusion of a distal ampullary pregnancy through the fimbriated segment by milking the tube with one's finger or by making a small linear incision into the distal ampulla under magnification (shown in Fig. 7-22) also permits salvage of the oviduct. The problem of midsegment reconstruction immediately after resection of a severely damaged tubal segment is unsettled. Increasing expertise with microsurgical tubal reanastomosis following prior sterilization has expanded the usefulness of this approach. A second factor relates to the diameter of the tubal lumen encountered during tubal pregnancy. The surgeon will find that the blood clot has dilated the tubal lumen beyond the area of tubal damage. End-to-end anastomosis in these patients, therefore, is similar to an am-

pullary-ampullary anastomosis procedure despite extension of the area into the distal isthmus. Lumen diameters are usually at least 0.5 cm and often larger. We employ loupes (2.5 ×) or the Zeiss OPMI-6S operating microscope and 8-0 synthetic absorbable suture material for this purpose. It is frequently possible to pass a small probe across the suture line following anastomosis, although transfundal tubal lavage utilizing a Buxton clamp also may be performed. The reader should be aware, however, that when we perform emergency surgery for ectopic pregnancy, the operation is performed in an operating room in which the nursing staff is familiar with infertility surgery. Our instruments and magnification aids are all available at a moment's notice. This procedure is illustrated in Figure 7-24.

In those patients not thought to be candidates for end-to-end anastomosis at the time of resection of an ectopic pregnancy, either because of an unstable vascular system, difficulty in visualizing the tubal lumen, or limitation of the surgeon's ability, it is recommended that the smallest possible segment of tube be resected. This permits repair by end-to-end anastomosis by a microsurgical approach at a later date under optimal circumstances. Uterotubal implantation is no longer recommended for the treatment of tubal ectopic pregnancies, except in the rare instance of an intramural pregnancy. Under these circumstances, the procedure should be carried out secondarily.

Transfundal tubal lavage is performed when possible. We have not used dextran 70 during this procedure, although it has been recommended by others [108, 197]. Uterine suspension is rarely performed. Appendectomy is occasionally performed if the patient's general condition is good. These patients are placed on dexamethasone and promethazine before and after surgery. We have not used postoperative hydrotubation, although it has also been recommended [81,214].

## The Future

### In Vitro Fertilization

Louise Joy Brown was born July 25, 1978 in Oldham General Hospital near Manchester, England. This birth marked the beginning of a new era in human reproduction. It was the first recorded case in which a human egg had been taken from a woman's ovary, had been fertilized externally, and then had been implanted in the woman's uterus and had developed to term. This success gave hope to those couples suffering from severe, irreparable forms of oviductal occlusion. At the time of Louise Brown's birth, research on external fertilization had been suspended for about 5 years in the United States. In March of 1979, the Ethical Advisory Board in Washington, D.C., established to review this concept, reported that research on external fertilization and subsequent implantation "would be acceptable from an ethical standpoint." The first clinic in the United States

**Table 7-38.** Results of in-vitro fertilization

| | | 1980 | | | | | Phase I—1981 | | | | | Phase II—1981 | | | | |
|---|---|---|---|---|---|---|---|---|---|---|---|---|---|---|---|---|
| | | No. | %A | %B | %C | %D | No. | %A | %B | %C | %D | No. | %A | %B | %C | %D |
| A | Laparoscopies | 41 | | | | | 31 | | | | | 24 | | | | |
| B | Fertilizable eggs | 19 | 46 | | | | 26 | 84 | | | | 22 | 92 | | | |
| C | Eggs fertilized | ND* | ND | ND | | | ND | ND | ND | | | 21 | 88 | 95 | | |
| D | Transfers | 13 | 32 | 68 | ND | | 12 | 39 | 46 | ND | | 19 | 79 | 86 | 90 | |
| E | Pregnancies | 0 | 0 | 0 | ND | 0 | 2 | 6 | 8 | ND | 17 | 5 | 21 | 23 | 24 | 26 |

*ND = not determined.

Source: H. W. Jones et al. The program for in-vitro fertilization at Norfolk. *Fertil. Steril.* 38:14, 1982.

for the study and practice of in vitro fertilization (IVF) was established at Eastern Virginia Medical School in Norfolk, Virginia by Drs. Georgianna and Howard Jones in 1979. Although a report by Jones et al. in March of 1981 indicated that there had been no successful transfers at that time, one year later, in March of 1982, pregnancy had occurred in 7 patients [110], and by the end of 1983, 105 pregnancies had been achieved. In the early months of 1984 at least eleven centers in the United States reported successful pregnancies after IVF.

The steps involved in the process of in vitro fertilization are as follows:

1. Selection of patient couple, i.e., with occluded tubes, low sperm count, or unexplained infertility
2. Regulation of ovulation, i.e., normal cycles versus controlled cycles
3. Evaluation of follicular size and timing of oocyte development
4. Laparoscopic removal of oocyte
5. Preparation of egg and sperm
6. Fertilization of the egg and early incubation
7. Transfer of the developing ovum into uterus
8. Monitoring of luteal phase and early pregnancy
9. Monitoring of late pregnancy and timing of delivery

An extensive discussion of these steps is beyond the scope of this text. An exciting aspect of this technique is its wide scope and application. At this writing, couples with occluded oviducts, low sperm counts, and unexplained infertility have benefited from the process.

A roundtable discussion held at the 38th Annual Meeting of the American Fertility Society in March of 1982 included Doctors Steptoe, H. Jones, and Lopata, perhaps the three most active scientists in the field of IVF. Doctors Howard and Georgianna Jones had utilized Pergonal and HCG to control ovulation in patients undergoing IVF. During a 3-month interval prior to March of 1982, this group had obtained eggs for fertilization in a group of 24 patients, and fertilization and transfer were carried out in 19. Pregnancy resulted in 5 patients, for a 21 percent success rate (Table 7-38). Dr. H. Jones also reported a markedly increased success rate when multiple eggs were obtained at laparoscopy,

**Table 7-39.** Norfolk series 1–12: Pregnancies by number of concepti and day of transfer (at least one preovulatory oocyte per transfer)

| | Transfer—day 3 | | |
|---|---|---|---|
| Concepti transferred | No. | Pregnancy | Pregnancy/ transfer |
| 1 | 116 | 26 | 22 |
| 2 | 122 | 30 | 25 |
| 3 | 44 | 14 | 32 |
| 4 | 23 | 10 | 43 |
| 5 | 8 | 3 | 38 |
| 6 | 3 | 1 | 33 |
| Total | 316 | 84 | 27 |

Source: H. W. Jones, In Vivo Fertilization. In S. J. Behrman, R. W. Kistner and G. W. Patton (eds.), *Progress in Infertility* (3rd ed.). Boston: Little, Brown, in preparation.

subsequently fertilized, and transferred back into the uterine cavity. The concept of multiple embryo transfer has become standard practice (Table 7-39).

Steptoe (111) presented the results he and Edwards had obtained during their studies of in vitro fertilization in a recent series of 110 cases and in their entire series of 630 patients. In the large group of 630 patients who had undergone a laparoscopy, there were apparently 104 pregnancies. Approximately one-third of these pregnancies, however, ended in a spontaneous abortion. An approximate 20 percent success rate was achieved by these physicians, both in the recent and in the larger series. Steptoe and Edwards, once strong proponents of utilizing natural cycles during IVF, appear to be experimenting with the use of Clomid to control ovulation.

The greatest number of patients undergoing in vitro fertilization was reported by Dr. Lopata from his clinic in Melbourne. In 1980, almost 140 patients underwent laparoscopic oocyte retrieval, and a similar number were studied in 1981. Again, this group has also found an approximate 20 percent success rate, although one-half these pregnancies were lost early in gestation. It is important to realize that during the early stages of development, none of these three centers achieved a 20 percent pregnancy rate. This latter figure, therefore, rep-

**Table 7-40.** A life table for intrauterine mortality in the human (per 100 ova exposed to risk of fertilization)

| Week after ovulation | Death (expulsion of dead embryos) | Survivors |
|---|---|---|
| | 16 (not fertilized) | 100 |
| 0 | 15 (failed to cleave) | 84 (fertile) |
| 1 | 27 | 69 (implanted) |
| 2 | 5.0 | 12 |
| 6 | 2.9 | 37 |
| 10 | 1.7 | 34.1 |
| 14 | 0.5 | 32.4 |
| 18 | 0.3 | 31.9 |
| 22 | 0.1 | 31.6 |
| 26 | 0.1 | 31.5 |
| 30 | 0.1 | 31.4 |
| 34 | 0.1 | 31.3 |
| 38 | 0.2 | 31.32 |
| Live births (including birth defects) | | 31 |
| Natural wastage | | 69 |

Source: H. Leridon, *Human Fertility: The Basic Components*. Chicago: Univ. Chicago Press, 1977. Copyright © by The University of Chicago.

resents the best success thus far reported. This is typified by the report from Wood and others [237], in Melbourne, who achieved 9 pregnancies in 103 patients undergoing laparoscopy for oocyte retrieval. This study ended in October of 1980, and certainly, pregnancy results subsequent to that time would be expected to be higher.

The future success of in vitro fertilization appears to depend on technical ability to master the steps in this procedure listed above, as well as the ability to increase the success level beyond 20 percent. Pierre Soupart [195,196] prepared a table and a discussion relevant to this point prior to his recent death. This material was taken from data collected by Leridon [124] in 1977 on the incidence of blighted human ova, together with data on fetal mortality, and a "life table of intrauterine morality" was constructed (Table 7-40). The table shows a remarkably high natural rate of embryonic loss. In fact, following a single exposure to fertilization, failure to fertilize occurred at 16 percent of individuals; 52 percent of pregnancies were then lost during the first 3 months; and only 31 percent achieved a live birth—for a natural pregnancy wastage rate of 69 percent.

The preliminary results of Lopata, Jones, and Wood suggested that the recovery, fertilization, and transfer of multiple oocytes during a single cycle may resulted in marked improvement in the success rate of IVF. Certainly the life table presented in Table 7-40 represents the natural course of an individual oocyte, thus lending support to the concept that the transfer of two or three fertilized eggs back into the uterine cavity should improve the chance of a viable infant. Data to support this hypothesis, are shown in the results reported from Norfolk (Table 7-39).

*Low Tubal Ovum Transfer*
In October of 1980, Kreitman and Hodgen [122], work-

ing at the National Institutes of Health in Bethesda, Maryland, reported results of an experimental procedure termed *low tubal ovum transfer*. This technique was proposed as an alternative to in vitro fertilization and involved "aspiration of the ovum from the dominant follicle of the monkey during laparoscopy immediately preceding the expected date of ovulation," with subsequent "injection into the lumen of the occluded fallopian tube 1.0 to 2.0 cm above the uterotubal junction." The monkeys had previously undergone bilateral tubal resection and ligation of the ampullary region of each tube. Successful ovum collection occurred in 77.5 percent (31 of 40) of the monkeys at the time of laparoscopy. However, 20 of these oocytes were judged to be immature on the basis of morphologic criteria. Pregnancy occurred in 16.1 percent (5 of 31) of the animals in which collection was successful, and 3 of 5 pregnancies arose from eggs judged to be immature. None of the 5 pregnancies was ectopic.

Certainly this technique opens the possibility of a new form of treatment in the patient whose tubes are irreparably damaged, particularly the large group of women with recurrent fimbrial occlusion who have undergone previous salpingostomy. Improvement in the technique of ovum capture in the female, developed by Steptoe and Edwards [200] and others [126,237], should permit early evaluation of the transfer technique in the human. The overwhelming concern must be the possibility of ectopic pregnancy. In the monkey study, normal fallopian tubes were ligated. However, this will not be the case in the female who has had a failed salpingostomy.

*Tubal Transplants and Pedicle Grafts*
Innovative attempts at tubal transplantation took place during the latter part of the 1970s, following Winston's success in the rabbit in 1974. Two studies described allografts in three patients by macrosurgical and mi-

crosurgical techniques. Unfortunately, all three grafts were rejected. Three additional studies described surgical techniques that transferred a segment of one tube to the other adnexa. Two of these procedures were pedicle grafts and the third a true tubal homotransplant. All three procedures resulted in pregnancy.

Two surgeons attempted allografts in human volunteers during the 1970s. In the first, Cohen [34] developed a technique for vascularized transplantation of the fallopian tube in the pig and the ewe and then performed this procedure on 2 female patients. In each case, the diseased right fallopian tube of the recipient was replaced with a vascular tubal transplant from a donor. Vascular patency was achieved, but immunologic rejected occurred in both patients prior to pregnancy. The surgical technique employed by Cohen utilized an operating loupe providing $2\times$ magnification.

The second report of a tubal allograft was published in 1978 by Wood and his associates [237] in Melborne. A single patient underwent an allograft from a compatible donor following the loss of both oviducts associated with two ectopic pregnancies. A microsurgical approach was utilized and initial tubal function was achieved. However, rejection occurred at 3 months. Immunosuppressive therapy with prednisone and Immurane was utilized. Pregnancy did ensue prior to rejection.

In 1979, Shapiro and Haning [181] reported the first successful use of a fimbrial pedicle graft to the opposite tube. Not a true tubal transplant, this innovative procedure transferred a pedicle graft involving the left fimbria to the right ampullary segment. Both ovaries were secured in the midline. A microsurgical tubal anastomosis was performed, and conception occurred 18 months postoperatively. Recently, Falk et al. [59] also recorded the use of a pedicle graft, in this case the right tube and ovary, which were then transferred to the left tube by means of a microsurgical tubal anastomosis. Unfortunately, an ectopic pregnancy occurred, necessitating removal of the pedicle graft.

A true homotransplantation of a fallopian tube was recently reported by DeCherney and Naftolin [143]. In this patient, the left fimbrial segment was removed and a vascular transplant performed to the right uterine vessels followed by microsurgical tubal anastomosis. Subsequently, tubal patency was established; pregnancy occurred, but it resulted in a spontaneous abortion.

Although use of an allograft from a healthy donor is not as yet practical because of immunologic rejection, the use of a pedicle graft, as described by Shapiro, or a tubal homotransplant, as described by DeCherney, may be found useful by the infertility surgeon in selected cases. Certainly, the pedicle graft technique described by Shapiro provides a simpler surgical approach. Homotransplantation, although theoretically more satisfactory, clearly involves a greater risk of vascular rejection.

## References

1. Aref, I., and Hafez, E. S. Utero-oviductal motility with emphasis on ova transport. *Obstet. Gynecol. Surv.* 28:679, 1973.
2. Arronet, G. H., Eduljee, S. Y., and O'Brien, J. R. A nine-year survey of fallopian tube dysfunction in human infertility: Diagnosis and therapy. *Fertil. Steril.* 20:903, 1969.
3. Asherman, J. G. Etiology of ectopic pregnancy: A new concept. *Obstet. Gynecol.* 6:619, 1955.
4. Bagley, G. P. Mulligan hood removed through the laparoscope. *Obstet. Gynecol.* 39:950, 1972.
5. Barsky, A. J., and Blinick, G. Use of cartilage grafts to maintain patency of fallopian tubes. *Plast. Reconstr. Surg.* 11:87, 1953.
5a. Behrman, S. J., and Kistner, R. W. (eds.). *Progress in Infertility* (2nd ed.). Boston: Little, Brown, 1975.
6. Bellina, J. Reconstruction of the Fallopian Tube. In A. H. Andrews and T. Polanyi (Eds.), Microscopic and Endoscopic Surgery with the $CO_2$ Laser. Boston: John Wright PS6, 1982. P. 254.
7. Bender, S. Fertility after tubal pregnancy. *J. Obstet. Gynecol. Br. Comm.* 63:400, 1956.
8. Berlind, M. The contralateral corpus luteum: An important factor in ectopic pregnancies. *Obstet. Gynecol.* 16:51, 1960.
9. Blandau, R. J. Comparative aspects of tubal anatomy and physiology as they relate to reconstructive procedures. *J. Reprod. Med.* 21:7, 1978.
10. Bone, N. L., and Greene, R. R. Histologic study of uterine tubes and tubal pregnancy. *Am. J. Obstet. Gynecol.* 82:1166, 1961.
11. Bonney, V. The fruits of conservation. *J. Obstet. Gynaecol. Br. Comm.* 44:1, 1937.
12. Borell, V., and Fernstrom, I. Adnexal branches of uterine artery: Arteriographic study in human subjects. *Acta Radiol.* 40:561, 1953.
13. Bourne, A. Discussion of the treatment of acute salpingitis. *Br. Med. J.* 2:399, 1923.
14. Bovee, J. W. Deductions based largely upon a series of seventy cases of ectopic pregnancy treated surgically. *Am. J. Obstet. Gynecol.* 61:583, 1910.
15. Bovee, J. W. The vaginal route in operation for ruptured tubal pregnancy. *J.A.M.A.* 29:1294, 1897.
16. Boys, F. The prophylaxes of peritoneal adhesions. *Surgery* 11:118, 1942.
17. Breen, J. L. A 21-year survey of 654 ectopic pregnancies. *Am. J. Obstet. Gynecol.* 106:1004, 1970.
18. Bronson, R. A., and Wallach, E. Lysis of periadenexal adhesions for correction of infertility. *Fertil. Steril.* 28:617, 1977.
19. Bruhat, M. A., Manhes, H., Mage, G., and LucPouly, J. Treatment of ectopic pregnancy by means of laparoscopy. *Fertil. Steril.* 33:411, 1980.
20. Buchovsky, I., Langer, R., Herman, A., and Caspi, E. Conservative surgery for tubal pregnancy. *Obstet. Gynecol.* 53:709, 1979.
21. Buckman, R. F., et al. A physiologic basis for the adhesion-free healing of deperitonealized surfaces. *J. Surg. Res.* 21:67, 1976.

22. Buckman, R. F., Woods, M., Sargent, L., and Gervin, A. S. A unifying pathogenetic mechanism in the etiology of intraperitoneal adhesions. *J. Surg. Res.* 20:1, 1976.

23. Budowich, M., et al. The histopathology of the developing tubal ectopic pregnancy. *Fertil. Steril.* 34:169, 1980.

24. Burrage, W. L. The remote results of conservative operations on the ovaries and tubes. *Am. J. Obstet.* 41:195, 1900.

25. Caffier, P. Die konservative Operation des schuangeren eileifers. *Arch. Gynaekol.* 173:261, 1941.

26. Castallo, M. A. Experimental recanalization of the fallopian tubes in the rhesus monkey. *Fertil. Steril.* 1:435, 1950.

27. Chalier, A. Quoted by S. L. Israel. *Fertil. Steril.* 2:505, 1951.

28. Cherney, W. B., Wilbanks, C., and Peete, C. H. The management of ectopic pregnancy by colpotomy. *South. Med. J.* 55:568, 1962.

29. Chiari, J. B. Z. *Heilkunde* 8:457, 1887; quoted by E. Rics, Nodular forms of tubal disease. *J. Exp. Med.* 11:26, 1897.

30. Choate, W. J., Just-Viera, J. O., and Yeager, G. H. Prevention of experimental peritoneal adhesions by dextran. *Arch. Surg.* 88:249, 1964.

31. Clyman, M. J. Silastic hoods in tuboplasty: A new approach to their removal. *Fertil. Steril.* 19:537, 1968.

32. Clyman, M.J. Tubal Reconstructive Surgery for Infertility. In A. I. Sherman (ed.), *Pathways to Conception.* Springfield, Ill.: Charles C Thomas, 1971.

33. Cognat, M. Presentation d' une prosthese-drain destince a la chirurgic tubulaire pour sterilite. *Bull. Fed. Soc. Gynecol. Obstet. Fr.* 23:4, 1971.

34. Cohen, B. Preliminary experiences with vascularized fallopian tube transplants in the human female. *Int.J. Fertil.* 21:147, 1976.

35. Cohen, E. M., and Katz, M. The significance of the convoluted oviduct in the infertile women. *J. Reprod. Med.* 21:31, 1978.

36. Comminos, A. C. Salpingostomy: Results of two different methods of treatment. *Fertil. Steril.* 28:1211, 1977.

37. Crane, M., and Woodruff, D. Factors influencing the success of tuboplastic procedures. *Fertil. Steril.* 19:80, 1968.

38. Crane, M., and Woodruff, D. Factors influencing the success of tuboplastic procedures. *Obstet. Gynecol. Surv.* 24:458, 1969.

39. David, A., Brackett, B. G., and Garcia, C. R. Effects of microsurgical removal of the rabbit uterotubal junction. *Fertil. Steril.* 20:250, 1969.

40. David, A., Garcia, C. R., and Czernoblisky, B. Human hydrosalpinx. *Am. J. Obstet. Gynecol.* 105:400, 1969.

41. David, A., Serr, D. M., and Czernoblisky, B. Chemical composition of human oviduct fluid. *Fertil. Steril.* 24:435, 1973.

42. DeCherney, A., and Kase, N. The conservative surgical management of unruptured ectopic pregnancy. *Obstet. Gynecol.* 54:451, 1979.

43. DeCherney, A., and Naftolin, F. Homo-transplantation of the human fallopian tube: Report of a successful case and description of a technique. *Fertil. Steril.* 34:14, 1980.

44. DeCherney, A. H., Polan, M. L., Kurt, H., and Kase, N. Microsurgical technique in the management of tubal ectopic pregnancy. *Fertil. Steril.* 34:324, 1980.

45. DeCherney, A. H., Romero, R., and Naftolin, F. Surgical management of unruptured ectopic pregnancy. *Fertil. Steril.* 35:21, 1981.

46. DeCherney, A. H., Maheaux, R., and Naftolin, F. Salpingostomy for ectopic pregnancy in the sole patent oviduct: Reproductive outcome. *Fertil. Steril.* 37:619, 1982.

47. Diamond E. A comparison of gross and microsurgical techniques for repair of cornual occlusion in infertility: A retrospective study. *Fertil. Steril.* 32:370, 1979.

48. Diamond, E. Microsurgical reconstruction of the uterine tube in sterilized patients. *Fertil. Steril.* 28:1203, 1977.

49. Diamond, E. Microsurgical Study of the Blood Supply to the Uterine Tube and Ovary. In J. Phillips (ed.), *Microsurgery in Gynecology.* Downey, Calif.: American Association of Gynecological Laparoscopists. 1981.

50. Diamond, E. Lysis of postoperative pelvic adhesions in infertility. *Fertil. Steril.* 31:287, 1979.

51. DiZerega, G. S., and Hodgia, G. D. Prevention of post-surgical tubal adhesions: Comparative study of commonly used agents. *Am.J. Obstet. Gynecol.* 136:173, 1980.

52. Douglas, E. S., Shingleton, H. M., and Crist, T. Surgical management of tubal pregnancy: Effects on subsequent fertility. *South. Med.J.* 62:954, 1969.

53. Eddy, C. A. Experimental Tubal Microsurgery. In P. G. Crosignani and B. L. Rubin (eds.), *Microsurgery in Female Infertility.* New York: Grune & Stratton, 1980, p. 21.

54. Eddy, C. A., Antonini, R., and Pauerstein, C. J. Fertility following microsurgical removal of the ampullary isthmic junction in rabbits. *Fertil. Steril.* 28:1090, 1977.

55. Eddy, C. A., Hoffman, J. J., and Pauerstein, C. J. Pregnancy following segmental isthmic reversal of the rabbit oviduct. *Experimentia* 32:1194, 1976.

56. Ellis, H. The course and prevention of postoperative intraperitoneal adhesions. *Surg. Gynecol. Obstet.* 133:497, 1971.

57. Ehrler, P. Anastomose intramurale de la trompe. *Bull. Fed. Soc. Gynecol. Obstet. Fr.* 17:866, 1965.

58. Falk, V. Treatment of acute non-tuberculosis salpingitis with antibiotics alone and in combination with glucocorticoids. *Acta Obstet. Gynecol. Scand.* [Suppl.] 44:1, 1965.

59. Falk, R. J., Elliott, J. J., Gianfertoni, J., and Rifka, S. M. Tuboovarian transposition for multifacal obstructive tubal disease. *Fertil. Steril.* 33:564, 1980.

60. Feldman, Y. M., and Riccardi, N. B. Incidence and Epidemiology of Sexually Transmitted Diseases. In *Sexually Transmitted Disease.* New York: Science and Medicine, 1979.

61. Ferguson, A. H. President's address. *Med. Fortnight* 24:527, 1903.

62. Frankel,J. M., and Schenck, S. B. The endometrial theory of ectopic pregnancy. *Am. J. Obstet. Gynecol.* 33:393, 1937.

63. Franklin, E., Zeiderman, A. R., and Laemmle, P. Tubal ectopic pregnancy: Etiology and obstetric and gynecologic sequelae. *Am.J. Obstet. Gynecol.* 117:220, 1973.

64. Fulsher, R. Tubal pregnancy following homolateral salpingectomy. *Am. J. Obstet. Gynecol.* 78:355, 1959.

65. Furuhjelm, M.,Jonson, B., and Lagergren, C. C. A contribution to the aetiology of ectopic pregnancy. *Acta Obstet. Gynecol. Scand.* 41:313, 1962.

66. Garcia, C. R. Surgical Reconstruction of the Oviduct in the Infertile Patient. In S. J. Behrman and R. W. Kistner (eds.), *Progress in Infertility* (1st ed.). Boston: Little, Brown, 1968.

67. Garcia, C. R. Reconstruction of Previously Ligated Fallopian Tubes. Presented at the 11th Annual Meeting of the American Fertility Society, New York, April 1972.

68. Garcia, C. R. Sixth Annual Postgraduate Course on Infertility Surgery. Presented at the 12th Annual Meeting of the American Fertility Society, San Francisco, April 1973.

69. Gauss, C. J. Erhaltung der Tube beitubargraviditat. *Wein. Klin. Wochenschr.* 54:877, 1941; quoted by D. J. Wexler, *Fertil. Steril.* 7:241, 1956.

70. Geist, S. H., and Goldberger, M. A. A study of the intramural portion of normal and diseased tubes with special reference to the question of sterility. *Surg. Gynecol. Obstet.* 41:646, 1925.

71. Gepfert, J. R. Studies on reconstruction of fallopian tube. *Am. J. Obstet. Gynecol.* 38:256, 1939.

72. Gepfert, J. R. Reconstruction of the oviducts in the human. *Am. J. Obstet. Gynecol.* 45:1030, 1943.

73. Gomel, V. Clinical Results of Infertility Microsurgery. In P. G. Crosignani and B. L. Rubin (eds.), *Microsurgery in Female Infertility.* New York: Grune & Stratton, 1980.

74. Gomel, V. Microsurgical reversal of female sterilization: A reappraisal. *Fertil. Steril.* 33:587, 1980.

75. Gomel, V. Salpingostomy by microsurgery. *Fertil. Steril.* 29:380, 1978.

76. Gomel, V. Tubal reanastomosis by microsurgery. *Fertil. Steril.* 28:59, 1977.

77. Gomel, V., and McComb, P. Microsurgery in Gynecology. In S. Silber (ed.), *Microsurgery.* Baltimore: Williams & Wilkins, 1979.

78. Gomel, V. Profile of women requesting reversal of sterilization. *Fertil. Steril.* 30:39, 1978.

79. Gouillioud, P. De la salpingostomie. *Lyons Med.* 53:13, 1900.

80. Grant, A. The effect of ectopic pregnancy on fertility. *Clin. Obstet. Gynecol.* 5:861, 1962.

81. Grant, A. Infertility surgery of the oviduct. *Fertil. Steril.* 22:496, 1971.

82. Green-Armytage, V. B. Tubo-uterine implantation. *J. Obstet. Gynaecol. Br. Comm.* 64:47, 1957.

83. Green-Armytage, V. B. Discussion on modern methods of salpingostomy. *Proc. R. Soc. Med.* 53:10, 1960.

84. Greenhill, J. P. Evaluation of salpingostomy and tubal implantation for treatment of sterility. *Am. J. Obstet. Gynecol.* 33:39, 1937.

85. Grobstein, C. External human fertilization. *Sci. Am.* 240:57, 1979.

86. Hafez, E. S. E., and Evans, T. W. *Human Reproduction.* New York: Harper & Row, 1973.

87. Hallet, J. G. Ectopic pregnancy in perspective. *Postgrad. Med.* 44:100, 1968.

88. Hedberg, E., and Spetz, S. O. Acute salpingitis. *Acta Obstet. Gynecol. Scand.* 37:131, 1958.

89. Hellman, L. M. The morphology of the human fallopian tube in the early puerperium. *Am. J. Obstet. Gynecol.* 57:154, 1949.

90. Hellman, L. M. The use of polyethylene in human tubal plastic operations. *Fertil. Steril.* 2:498, 1951.

91. Hodari, A. A., Vibhasire, S., and Isaac, A. Y. Reconstructive tubal surgery for midtubal obstruction. *Fertil. Steril.* 28:620, 1977.

92. Holden, F. C., and Sovak, F. W. Reconstruction of the oviducts: An improved technique with report of cases. *Am. J. Obstet. Gynecol.* 24:684, 1932.

93. Holtz, G. Prevention of postoperative adhesions. *J. Reprod. Med.* 24:141, 1980.

94. Holtz, G., and Baker, E. R. Inhibition of peritoneal adhesion re-formation after lysis with thirty-two percent dextran 70. *Fertil. Steril.* 34:394, 1980.

95. Holtz, G., Baker, E. R., and Tsai, C. Effect of thirty-two percent dextran 70 on peritoneal adhesion formation and reformation after lysis. *Fertil. Steril.* 33:660, 1980.

96. Honore, L. Salpingitis isthmica nodosa in female infertility and ectopic tubal pregnancy. *Fertil. Steril.* 29:164, 1978.

97. Horne, H. W., et al. The prevention of postoperative pelvic adhesions following conservative operative treatment for human infertility. *Int. J. Fertil.* 18:109, 1973.

98. Huffman, O. V. A theory of the causes of ectopic pregnancy. *J.A.M.A.* 61:213, 1913.

99. Hulka, J. F. Tubal Damage in Elective Sterilization. In J. M. Phillips (ed.), *Microsurgery in Gynecology.* Downey, Calif.: American Association of Gynecologic Laparoscopists, 1977.

100. Hulka, J. F., and Ulberg, L. C. Reversibility of clip sterilization. *Fertil. Steril.* 26:1132, 1975.

101. Ingersoll, F. M. Operation for tubal pregnancy. *Clin. Obstet. Gynecol.* 5:853, 1962.

102. Ingersoll, F. M. Plastic operation on the fallopian tube. *N. Engl. J. Med.* 241:686, 1949.

103. Israel, S. L. Total linear salpingostomy. *Fertil. Steril.* 2:505, 1951.

104. Jacobson, L. Laparoscopy in the diagnosis of acute salpingitis. *Acta Obstet. Gynecol. Scand.* 43:160, 1964.

105. Jacobson, L., and Westrom, L. Objectivized diagnosis of acute pelvic inflammatory disease. *Am. J. Obstet. Gynecol.* 105:1088, 1969.

106. Janecek, P., and DeGrandi, P. Chirurgic restauratrice D' emblee dans le traitement des grossesses extrauterinis. *J. Gynecol. Obstet. Biol. Reprod.* 7:1261, 1978.

107. Jarvinen, P. A., Nummi, S., and Pietila, K. Conservative operation treatment of tubal pregnancy with postoperative daily hydrotubations. *Acta Obstet. Gynecol. Scand.* 51:169, 1972.

108. Jarvinen, P. A., Nummi, S., and Pietila, K. Conservative operative treatment of tubal pregnancy. *Fertil. Steril.* 15:634, 1964.

109. Jeffcoate, T. N. A. Salpingectomy or salpingoophorectomy. *Obstet. Gynaecol. Br. Comm.* 62:214, 1955.

110. Jones, H. W., et al. The program for in-vitro fertilization at Norfolk. *Fertil. Steril.* 38:14, 1982.

111. Jones, H. W. Symposium on In Vitro Fertilization. Presented at the American Fertility Society Meeting, Las Vegas, March, 1982.

112. Jones, H. W., and Rock, J. A. On the reanastomosis of fallopian tubes after surgical sterilization. *Fertil. Steril.* 29:702, 1978.

113. Kahn, E. Plastic rings to retain the patency of a newly formed ostium. *Fertil. Steril.* 4:80, 1953.

114. Kalchman, G. G., and Meltzer, R. M. Interstitial pregnancy following homolateral salpingectomy. *Am. J. Obstet. Gynecol.* 96:1139, 1966.

115. Kelly, H. A. Extrauterine Pregnancy. In Richard C. Norris (ed.), *An American Textbook of Obstetrics*. Philadelphia: Saunders, 1895.

116. Kirschner, R., and Kimball, H. W. Interstitial pregnancy following unilateral salpingectomy. *J.A.M.A.* 175:1180, 1961.

117. Kistner, R. W. Endometriosis and infertility. *Clin. Obstet. Gynecol.* 22:112, 1979.

117a. Kistner, R. W. *Principles and Practice of Gynecology* (2nd ed.). Chicago: Yearbook, 1971.

118. Kistner, R. W., and Patton, G. W. *Atlas of Infertility Surgery* (1st ed.). Boston: Little, Brown, 1975.

119. Kitchen, J. S., et al. Ectopic pregnancy: Current clinical trends. *Am. J. Obstet. Gynecol.* 34:870, 1974.

120. Kleppinger, R. K. Ovarian cyst penetration via laparoscopy. *J. Reprod. Med.* 21:16, 1978.

121. Kontopoulos, V. G., Wang, C. F., and Siegler, A. The impact of salpingitis isthmica nodosa on infertility. *Fertil. Family* 34:5, 1979.

122. Kreitmann, O., and Hodgen, G. D. Low tubal ovum transfer: An alternative to in-vitro fertilization. *Fertil. Steril.* 34:375, 1980.

123. Kuo, Y. P., and Lim, R. K. S. On the mechanism of the transportation of the ova: II. Rabbit and pig oviduct. *Chin. J. Physiol.* 2:389, 1928.

124. Leridon, H. *Human Fertility: The Basic Components*. Chicago, Ill.: University of Chicago Press, 1977.

125. Lisa, J. R., Gioia, J. D., and Rubin, I. C. Observations on the interstitial portion of the fallopian tubes. *Surg. Gynecol. Obstet.* 99:159, 1954.

126. Lopata, A., Johnston, I. W. H., Hoult, I. J., and Speirs, A. I. Pregnancy following intrauterine implantation of an embryo obtained by in-vitro fertilization of a preovulatory egg. *Fertil. Steril.* 33:117, 1980.

127. Lopata, A. Fifteenth Annual Postgraduate Course in In Vitro Fertilization. Presented at the American Fertility Society Meeting, Las Vegas, March 1982.

128. Martin, F. H. Ovarian transplantation and reconstruction of fallopian tubes. *Chicago Med. Rec.* 25:1, 1903.

129. Mazuji, M. D., and Fahdli, H. A. Peritoneal adhesions: Prevention with povidone and dextran 75. *Arch. Surg.* 91:872, 1965.

130. McComb, P., and Gomel, V. Cornual occlusion and its microsurgical reconstruction. *Clin. Obstet. Gynecol.* 23(3):1229, 1980.

131. McComb, P., and Gomel, V. The effect of segmental ampullary reversal on the subsequent fertility of the rabbit. *Fertil. Steril.* 31:83, 1979.

132. McComb, P., and Gomel, V. The influence of fallopian tube length on fertility in the rabbit. *Fertil. Steril.* 31:673, 1979.

133. McCormack, W. Sexually Transmitted Diseases: Incidence and Epidemiologic Considerations. In *Sexually Transmitted Disease*. New York: Science and Medicine, 1979.

134. McCormick, W. G., and Torres, J. A method of pomeroy tubal ligation reversal. *Obstet. Gynecol.* 47:623, 1976.

135. McCormick, W. G., Torres, J., and McCanne, L. R. Tubal reanastomosis: An update. *Fertil. Steril.* 31:689, 1979.

136. Moghissi, K. S. Human fallopian tube fluid: I. Protein composition. *Fertil. Steril.* 21:821, 1970.

137. Moore-White, M. Evaluation of tubal plastic operations: Classification of tubal disease. *Int. J. Fertil.* 5:237, 1960.

138. Morikawa, H., et al. Physiologic study of the human mesotubarium ovarica. *Obstet. Gynecol.* 55:493, 1979.

139. Mulligan, W. J. Results of salpingostomy. *Int. J. Fertil.* 11:424, 1966.

140. Mulligan, W. J., and Rock, J. Surgical Treatment of Infertility. In J. Meigs and S. Sturgis (eds.), *Progress in Gynecology* (vol. 3). New York: Grune & Stratton, 1957.

141. Mulligan, W. J., Rock, J., and Easterday, C. L. Use of polyethylene in tuboplasty. *Fertil. Steril.* 4:5, 1953.

142. Murray, E. Peritoneal factor in sterility. *Clin. Obstet. Gynecol.* 5:836, 1962.

143. Neuwrith, R. S., and Khalaf, S. M. Effect of thirty two percent dextran 70 on peritoneal adhesion formation. *Am. J. Obstet. Gynecol.* 121:420, 1975.

144. Niles, J. H., and Clark, J. F. Pathogenesis of tubal pregnancy. *Am. J. Obstet. Gynecol.* 105:1230, 1969.

145. Novak, E. R., Jones, R. H., and Jones. G. E. S. *Novak's Textbook of Gynecology* (8th ed.). Baltimore: Williams & Wilkins, 1973.

146. Novy, M. J. Reversal of Fimbriectomy Sterilization. Presented at the *PARFR Conference on the Reversability of Sterilization*, San Francisco, December, 1977.

147. Novak, E., and Darner, H. L. The correlation of uterine and tubal changes in tubal gestation. *Am. J. Obstet. Gynecol.* 49:295, 1925.

148. Okamura, H., et al. A morphologic study of mesotubarium ovarica in the human. *Obstet. Gynecol.* 49:197, 1977.

149. Ory, H. W. Ectopic pregnancy and intrauterine contraceptive devices: New perspectives. *Obstet. Gynecol.* 57:137, 1981.

150. Owen, E. R., and Picket-Heaps, A. A. The microsurgical basis of fallopian tube reconstruction. *Aust. N.Z. J. Surg.* 47(3):300, 1977.

151. Palmer, R. Les resultats du traitement chirurgical des obturations tubaires. *Bull. Fed. Soc. Gynecol. Obstet. Fr.* 4:197, 1952.

152. Palmer, R. Salpingostomy: A critical study of 396 personal cases operated upon without polyethylene tubing. *Proc. R. Soc. Med.* 53:357, 1960.

153. Parry, J. S. *Extrauterine Pregnancy*. Philadelphia: Lea & Febriger, 1876.

153a. Parsons, L., and Sommers, A. C. *Gynecology* (1st ed.). Philadelphia: Saunders, 1962.

154. Parsons, L., and Ulfelder, H. *An Atlas of Pelvic Operations* (2nd ed.). Philadelphia: Saunders, 1968.

155. Patton, G. W. Pregnancy outcome following microsurgical fimbrioplasty. *Fertil. Steril.* 37:150, 1982.

155a. Patton, G. W. Unpublished data, 1977–1980.

156. Patton, G. W. Unpublished data, 1978–1980.

157. Patton, G. W. Unpublished data, 1981.

158. Patton, G. W., and Kistner, R. W. Surgical Reconstruction of the Oviduct. In S. J. Behrman and R. W. Kistner (eds.), *Progress in Infertility* (2nd ed.). Boston: Little, Brown, 1975.

159. Peel, J. Utero-tubal implantation. *Proc. R. Soc. Med.* 57:26, 1964.

160. Peterson, E. P., Musich, J. K., and Behrman, S. J. Uterotubal implantation and obstetric outcome after previous sterilization. *Am. J. Obstet. Gynecol.* 128:622, 1977.

161. Peterson, E. P., Ayers, J., and Soto, C. Uterotubal implantation—A reappraisal (abstract). *Fertil. Steril.* 39:401, 1983.

162. Pfeffer, W. H. Adjuvants in tubal surgery. *Fertil. Steril.* 33:245, 1980.

163. Polishuk, W. Z., and Aboulafia, Y. Dextran in prevention of peritoneal adhesions. *Isr. J. Med. Sci.* 3:806, 1967.

164. Polk, W. M. The conservative surgery of the female pelvic organs. *Trans. Cong. Am. Phys. Surg.* 3:182, 1894.

165. Replogle, R. L., Johnson, B. A., and Gross, R. E. Prevention of postoperative intestinal adhesions with combined promethazine and dexamethasone therapy. *Ann. Surg.* 163:580, 1966.

166. Riouz, J. E., and Yuzpe, A. A. Evaluation of female sterilization procedures. *Curr. Prob. Obstet. Gynecol.* 11:9, 1979.

167. Rock, J. A., et al. Factors influencing the success of salpingostomy techniques for distal fimbrial obstruction. *Obstet. Gynecol.* 52:591, 1978.

168. Rock, J. A., et al. Pregnancy outcome following uterotubal implantation: A comparison of the reamer and sharp cornual wedge excision techniques. *Fertil. Steril.* 31:634, 1979.

169. Rock, J., Mulligan, W. J., and Easterday, C. L. Polyethylene in tuboplasty. *Obstet. Gynecol.* 3:21, 1954.

170. Roland, M. Spiral Teflon splint for tuboplasty involving fimbria. *Obstet. Gynecol.* 36:359, 1970.

171. Roland, M., and Leisten, D. Tuboplasty in 130 patients. *Obstet. Gynecol.* 39:57, 1972.

172. Ryan, G. B., Grobety, J., and Majno, G. Postoperative peritoneal adhesions. *Am. J. Pathol.* 65:117, 1971.

173. Schauta, A. F. *Gynaekologie* 33:27, 1888; quoted in E. Ries, Nodular forms of tubal disease. *J. Exp. Med.* 11:26, 1897.

174. Schoen, J. A., and Nowak, R. J. Repeat ectopic pregnancy. *Obstet. Gynecol.* 45:542, 1975.

175. Schroeder, C. Die excision von ovarian Tumoren mit Erhaltung des Ovarium. *Zentralbt. Gynaekol.* 8:716, 1884.

176. Seki, K., et al. Comparison of two techniques of suturing in microsurgical anastomosis of the rabbit oviduct. *Fertil. Steril.* 28:1218, 1977.

177. Shikata, J., and Yamaoka, I. The role of topically applied dexamethasone in preventing peritoneal adhesions: Experimental and clinical studies. *World J. Surg.* 1:389, 1977.

178. Seitz, H. M., Schenker, J. G., Epstein, S., and Garcia, C. R. Postoperative intraperitoneal adhesions: A double blind assessment of their prevention in the monkey. *Fertil. Steril.* 24:935, 1973.

179. Shapiro, S. S. Personal communication to G. W. Patton, 1981.

180. Shapiro, H. I., and Adler, D. H. Excision of an ectopic pregnancy through the laparoscope. *Am. J. Obstet. Gynecol.* 117:290, 1973.

181. Shapiro, S. S., and Haning, R. V. Tubal anastomosis of a fimbrial segment pedicle graft. *Fertil. Steril.* 32:477, 1979.

182. Shirodkar, V. N. *Contributions to Obstetrics and Gynecology.* London: Livingston, 1960.

183. Shirodkar, V. N. Factors influencing the results of salpingostomy. *Int. J. Fertil.* 2:361, 1966.

184. Sherman, D., et al. Improved fertility following ectopic pregnancy. *Fertil. Steril.* 37:497, 1982.

185. Siegler, A. M. Classifying tuboperitoneal operations for infertility. *Contemp. OB-GYN* 14:111, 1979.

186. Siegler, A. M. Salpingostomy: Classification and report of 115 operations. *Obstet. Gynecol.* 34:339, 1969.

187. Siegler, A. M. Surgical treatment of tuboperitoneal causes of infertility since 1967. *Fertil. Steril.* 28:1019, 1977.

188. Siegler, A. M., and Konlopoulos, V. An analysis of macrosurgical and microsurgical techniques in the management of the tuboperitoneal factor in infertility. *Fertil. Steril.* 32:377, 1979.

189. Silber, S., and Cohen, M. R. Microsurgical techniques for tubal reanastomosis. *Int. J. Fertil.* 14:141, 1969.

190. Skulj, V., et al. Conservative operative treatment of tubal pregnancy. *Fertil. Steril.* 15:634, 1964.

191. Skutsch, F. Beitrag sur operativen Therapie der Tubenerkrankum. *Zentralbl. Gynaekeol.* 13:565, 1889.

192. Soderstrom, R. M. Unusual uses of laparoscopy. *J. Reprod. Med.* 15:77, 1975.

193. Solomons, B. The end results of salpingostomy in chronic salpingitis with special regard to pregnancy. *J. Obstet. Gynecol. Br. Comm.* 34:218, 1927.

194. Solomons, B. The conservative treatment of pathological conditions of the fallopian tube. *J. Obstet. Gynecol. Br. Comm.* 43:619, 1936.

195. Soupart, P. In Vitro Fertilization and Embryo Transfer. In D. Goldstein and J. Leventhal (eds.), *Current Problems in Obstetrics and Gynecology* (vol. 3). Chicago: Yearbook, 1979.

196. Soupart, P. Present Status of In Vitro Fertilization of the Human Egg. Presented at the 15th Annual Postgraduate Course on In Vitro Fertilization during the American Fertility Society Meeting in Las Vegas, March 1982.

197. Stangel, J. J., Reyniak, J. V., and Stone, M. L. Conservative surgical management of tubal pregnancy. *Obstet. Gynecol.* 48:241, 1976.

198. Stangel, J. J., Reyniak, J. V., and Stone, M. L. Conservative surgical management of tubal pregnancy with tubal reconstruction. *Surg. Forum* 28:577, 1977.

199. Steptoe, P. C., and Edwards, R. G. Birth after the reimplantation of a human embryo. *Lancet* 2:336, 1978.

200. Steptoe, P. C., and Edwards R. G. Laparoscopic recovery of preovulatory human oocytes after priming of ovaries with gonadotrophins. *Lancet* 1:683, 1970.

201. Steptoe, P. C., Edwards, R. G., and Purdy, J. M. Clinical aspects of pregnancies established with cleaving embryo grown in vitro. *Br. J. Obstet. Gynaecol.* 87:757, 1980.

202. Stromme, W. B. Salpingotomy for tubal pregnancy. Report of a successful case. *Obstet. Gynecol.* 1(4):472, 1953.

203. Stromme, W. B., McKelvey, J. L., and Adkins, C. D. Conservative surgery for ectopic pregnancy. *Obstet. Gynecol.* 19:294, 1962.

204. Sunden, B. The results of conservative treatment of salpingitis diagnosed at laparotomy and laparoscopy. *Acta Obstet. Gynecol. Scand.* 38:286, 1959.

205. Sweeny, W. J. The interstitial portion of the uterine tube—Its gross anatomy, coarse and length. *Obstet. Gynecol.* 19:3, 1962.

206. Sweet, R. L. Diagnosis and management of acute salpingitis. *J. Reprod. Med.* 19:21, 1977.

207. Swolin, K. Fertilitatoperationen: Teil I. Literatur und methodik. *Acta Obstet. Gynecol. Scand.* 46:234, 1967.

208. Swolin, K. Fertilitat superationen: Teil II. Material und results. *Acta Obstet. Gynecol. Scand.* 46:234, 1967.

209. Swolin, K. Fifty fertility operations: I. Literature and methods. *Obstet. Gynecol. Surv.* 23:382, 1968.

210. Swolin, K. Electromicrosurgery and salpingostomy: Long term results. *Am. J. Obstet. Gynecol.* 121:418, 1974.

211. Ten-Beige, B. S., and Lok, T. T. Plastic surgery of closed tubes with chorion-amnion. *Fertil. Steril.* 7:232, 1954.

212. Throwbridge, E. H. The treatment of abdominal adhesions by the use of the electro-surgical knife. *N. Engl. J. Med.* 201:1183, 1929.

213. Tietze, C. Extrauterine pregnancy. *Br. Med. J.* 2:302, 1966.

214. Timonen, S., and Nieminen, U. Tubal pregnancy: Choice of operative method of treatment. *Acta Obstet. Gynecol. Scand.* 46:327, 1967.

215. Tompkins, P. Preservation of fertility by conservative surgery for ectopic pregnancy. *Fertil. Steril.* 7:448, 1956.

216. Trimbus-Kemper, T. C., Trimbos, J. B., and vanHall, E. V. The management of infertile patients with unilateral tubal pathology by paradoxical oophorectomy. *Fertil. Steril.* 37:623, 1982.

217. Troell, S. Diverticula of the walls of the fallopian tubes. *Acta Obstet. Gynecol. Scand.* 49:17, 1970.

218. Umezaki, C., Katoyama, K. P., and Jones, H. W. Pregnancy rates after reconstructive surgery of the fallopian tubes. *Obstet. Gynecol.* 43:418, 1974.

219. Urquhart, J. Effect of the veneral disease epidemic on the incidence of ectopic pregnancy. Implications for the evaluation of contraceptives. *Contraception* 19:455, 1979.

220. Utian, W. H., Goldfarb, J. M., and Starks, G. C. Role of dextran 70 in microtubal surgery. *Fertil. Steril.* 31:79, 1979.

221. Vehaskari, A. The operation of choice for ectopic pregnancy with reference to subsequent fertility. *Acta Obstet. Gynecol. Scand.* 39(Suppl.3):3, 1960.

222. Viberg, L. Acute inflammatory conditions of the uterine adenexae. *Acta Obstet. Gynecol. Scand.* 43(Suppl.4):5, 1964.

223. Westrom, L. Effect of acute pelvic inflammatory disease on fertility. *Am. J. Obstet. Gynecol.* 121:707, 1975.

224. Westrom, L., Bengtson, L. P., and Mardh, P. A. IUD and PID estimations of the risk of acquiring pelvic inflammatory disease in women using intra-uterine contraceptive devices as compared to non-users. *Lancet* 2:221, 1976.

225. Westrom, L., and Mardh, P. A. Epidemiology, Etiology, and Prognosis of Acute Salpingitis: A Study of 1,457 Laparoscopically Verified Cases. In D. Hobson and K. K. Holmes (eds.), *Nongonococcal Urethritis and Related Infections.* Washington: American Society for Microbiology, 1977. Pp. 84–90.

226. Wexler, D. J., Kohn, A., and Birnberg, C. H. Conservative tubal surgery in ectopic pregnancy. *Fertil. Steril.* 7:241, 1956.

227. Wheeless, C. R. Problems with tubal reconstruction following laparoscopic sterilization using the electrocoagulation and resection technique. *Fertil. Steril.* 28:723, 1977.

228. Williams, G. F. J. Followup after sterilization. *Lancet* 1:1426, 1968.

229. Williams, G. F. J. Fallopian tube surgery for reversal of sterilization. *Br. Med. J.* 1:559, 1973.

230. Williams, J. W. Contribution to the normal and pathological histology of the fallopian tubes. *Am. J. Med. Sci.* 102-377, 1891.

231. Wilson, P. C. M. Microsurgical repair of fallopian tubes. *Med. J. Aust.* 1:1013, 1976.

232. Winston, R. M. L. Microsurgical reanastomosis of the rabbit oviduct and its functional and pathological sequelae. *Br. J. Obstet. Gynaecol.* 82:513, 1975.

233. Winston, R. M. L. Microsurgical tubocornual anastomosis for reversal of sterilization. *Lancet* 5:284, 1977.

234. Winston, R. M. L., and Brown, J. C. M. Pregnancy following autograft transplantation of fallopian tube and ovary in the rabbit. *Lancet* 8:494, 1974.

235. Winston, R. M. L., and Margara, R. A. Techniques for the Improvement of Microsurgical Tubal Anastomosis. In P. G. Grosighani and B. L. Rubin (eds.), *Microsurgery in Female Infertility.* New York: Grune & Stratton, 1980.

236. Wood, C., et al. Microvascular transplantation of the human fallopian tube. *Fertil. Steril.* 29:607, 1978.

236a. Wood, C., et al. Clinical features of eight pregnancies resulting from in vitro fertilization and embryo transfer. *Fertil. Steril.* 38:22, 1982.

237. Wood, C., et al. A clinical assessment of nine pregnancies obtained by in vitro fertilization and embryo transfer. *Fertil. Steril.* 35:502, 1981.

238. Woodruff, J. D., and Pauerstein, C. J. *The Fallopian Tube.* Baltimore: Williams & Wilkins, 1969.

239. Yaffe, H., Beyth, Y., Reinhartz, T., and Levij, I. S. Foreign body granulomas in peritubal and periovarian adhesions: A possible cause for unsuccessful reconstructive surgery in infertility. *Fertil. Steril.* 33:277, 1980.

240. Young, P. E., Egan, J. E., Barlow, J. J., and Mulligan, W. J. Reconstructive surgery for infertility at the Boston Hospital for Women. *Am. J. Obstet. Gynecol.* 108:1092, 1970.

The most common indication for ovarian surgery in infertility is endometriosis [8]. However, lysis of periovarian adhesions subsequent to pelvic inflammatory disease and wedge resection for sclerocystic (polycystic) ovarian syndrome are performed frequently in an effort to aid conception [21]. Unfortunately, ovarian surgery may occasionally produce infertility. Inopportune and excessive resection of follicular and corpus luteum cysts may seriously diminish the amount of ovarian cortex and its supply of primordial follicles. Similarly, extensive periovarian and peritubal adhesions may result from such surgery if adequate attention is not given to meticulous tissue approximation and hemostasis. It is hoped that increased use of diagnostic procedures, such as laparoscopy, will reduce unnecessary ovarian surgery. These same anatomic deformities may also occur subsequent to ovarian resection for dermoid cysts or other benign neoplastic tumors. It is important, therefore, to emphasize three major facets of ovarian surgery: (1) conservation of ovarian cortex, (2) reconstruction with precise tissue approximation, and (3) complete hemostasis. These facets, as well as those involving surgery of the oviduct (Chap. 7), have been advanced by the addition of microsurgical technique. Magnification, usually provided by loupes, and fine monopolar and bipolar electrocoagulation are thankful additions to surgery involving the ovary.

**Resection of Benign Cysts**

The ovary is freed from any attachments to omentum or bowel and is brought into the operative field. Follicular and corpus luteum cysts are usually free of adhesions, whereas inflammatory cysts and endometrioses are frequently adherent to the tube and the posterior leaf of the broad ligament. A ruptured corpus luteum cyst, however, may be adherent to the tube and the posterior leaf of the broad ligament. Dermoid cysts are usually not adherent to adjacent structures, but they may be fixed in the cul-de-sac if leakage has occurred.

Figure 8-1 shows the technique of resection of benign cysts. Figure 8-2 shows an alternative method of ovarian reconstruction that is particularly advantageous when a large amount of thin cortex remains after excision of the cyst. The use of magnification provided by the ocular loupe improves the surgeon's ability to excise the cyst and permits electrocoagulation of small bleeding vessels without damage to the surrounding ovary.

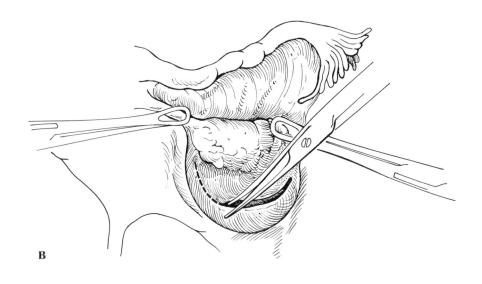

**B**

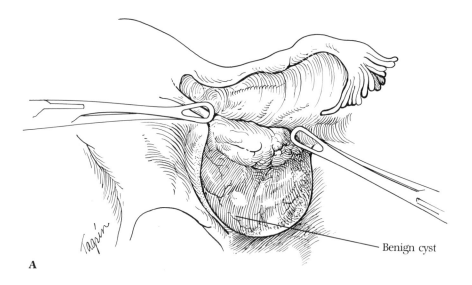

**A**

Benign cyst

**Figure 8-1.** Resection of benign cysts. **A.** William clamps are placed on the uteroovarian ligament and the cephalad portion of the ovary near the infundibulopelvic ligament. Magnification is provided by loupes. **B.** An incision is made over the dome of the cyst through the thin tunica albuginea. **C.** Using the knife handle, the cyst is separated from the ovarian capsule and removed intact. **D.** Using sharp dissection with curved or angular scissors, or electrosurgical excision with a fine cutting electrode, the cyst is freed from the hilar portion of the ovary. A few small blood vessels in this area may require ligation with 6-0 Vicryl or 6-0 PDS suture.

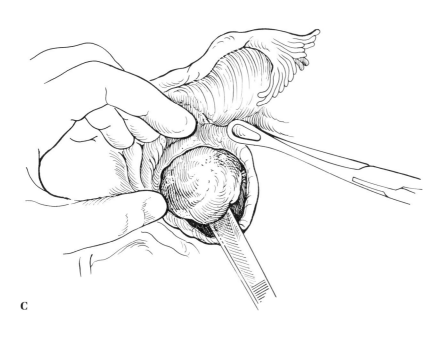

C

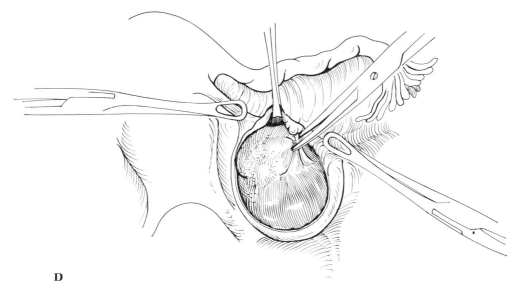

D

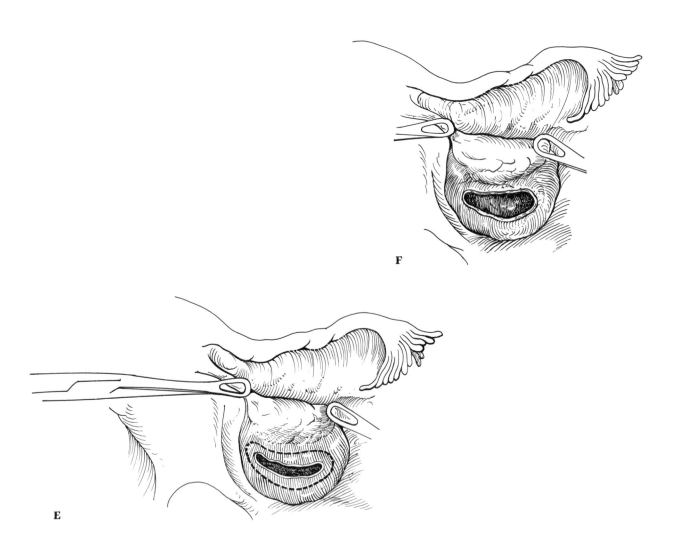

**Figure 8-1 (continued)**
**E.** An elliptical excision of the excess thinned ovarian cortex
is performed. **F.** The excess thinned cortex is removed. **G.**
The cortex is approximated with interrupted sutures of 6-0
Vicryl or PDS. (Continuous sutures do not produce adequate
hemostasis and may result in ovarian hematoma.) **H.** The
intraovarian dead space is reduced by placement of mattress
sutures near the ovarian hilus. **I.** Completion of ovarian reconstruction.

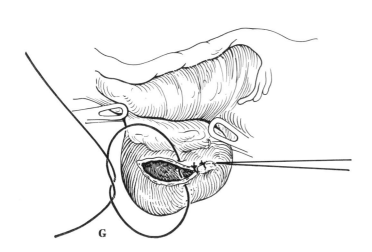

G

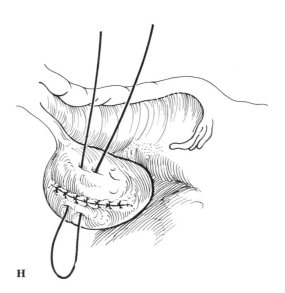

H

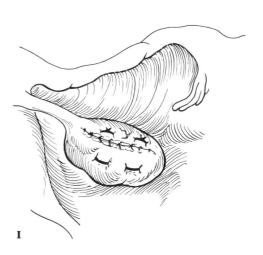

I

At the conclusion of the operation, and just prior to closure of the peritoneum, the ovary should be reinspected to be certain of complete hemostasis. A gentle spray of saline from a syringe will remove adherent blood clots and permit the operator to note oozing or actively bleeding surfaces.

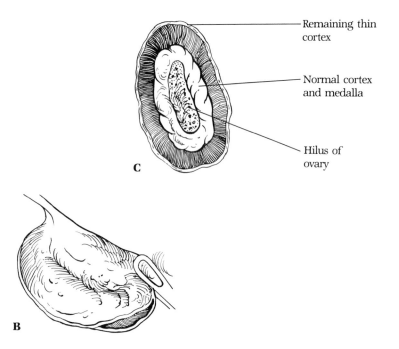

Remaining thin cortex

Normal cortex and medalla

Hilus of ovary

C

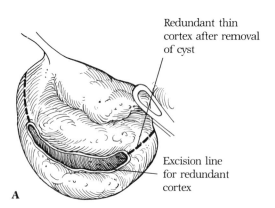

Redundant thin cortex after removal of cyst

Excision line for redundant cortex

**Figure 8-2.** Infolding technique of ovarian reconstruction. **A.** Excision line of redundant thin cortex after removal of ovarian cyst. **B.** Redundant cortex has been excised and ovary trimmed to normal size. **C.** View looking into the resected ovary showing relationships of hilus, normal cortex, and thinned cortex. **D.** Ovarian cortex at the uterine and tubal poles is turned in and sutured in place with 4-0 Vicryl or PDS. **E.** Anterior and posterior margins of cortex are similarly turned in to the hilus. **F.** Ovarian cortex is approximated with interrupted sutures of 6-0 Vicryl or PDS. One or more mattress sutures are placed to diminish dead space and improve hemostasis. **G.** View from crown of ovary showing reconstructed ovary with two mattress sutures in place. **H.** Lateral view of reconstructed ovary.

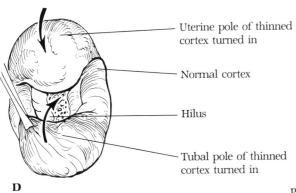

Uterine pole of thinned cortex turned in

Normal cortex

Hilus

Tubal pole of thinned cortex turned in

**D**

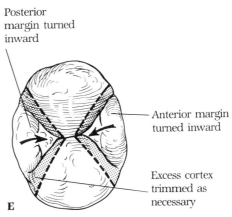

Posterior margin turned inward

Anterior margin turned inward

Excess cortex trimmed as necessary

**E**

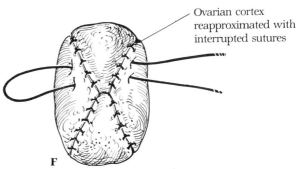

Ovarian cortex reapproximated with interrupted sutures

**F**

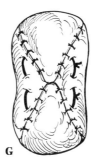

**G**

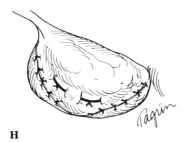

**H**

## Wedge Resection for Sclerocystic Ovarian Syndrome

### Indications

Ovulation may be produced in most patients with sclerocystic ovarian syndrome by the administration of clomiphene citrate [13]. In some patients, human chorionic gonadotropin is necessary to effect the ovulatory process. This is given in a single dose of 10,000 I.U. 4 days after the last dose of clomiphene. Human chorionic gonadotropin simulates the action of luteinizing hormone and produces rupture of the mature follicle. In a few patients with sclerocystic ovarian syndrome, a slight elevation of 17-ketosteroids is found, in a range of 15 to 25 mg per 24 hours. This suggests an excess production of adrenal androgens, and ovulation in these patients is effected by the administration of dexamethasone (125 mg three times daily) together with clomiphene.

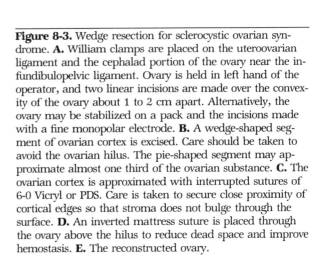

**Figure 8-3.** Wedge resection for sclerocystic ovarian syndrome. **A.** William clamps are placed on the uteroovarian ligament and the cephalad portion of the ovary near the infundibulopelvic ligament. Ovary is held in left hand of the operator, and two linear incisions are made over the convexity of the ovary about 1 to 2 cm apart. Alternatively, the ovary may be stabilized on a pack and the incisions made with a fine monopolar electrode. **B.** A wedge-shaped segment of ovarian cortex is excised. Care should be taken to avoid the ovarian hilus. The pie-shaped segment may approximate almost one third of the ovarian substance. **C.** The ovarian cortex is approximated with interrupted sutures of 6-0 Vicryl or PDS. Care is taken to secure close proximity of cortical edges so that stroma does not bulge through the surface. **D.** An inverted mattress suture is placed through the ovary above the hilus to reduce dead space and improve hemostasis. **E.** The reconstructed ovary.

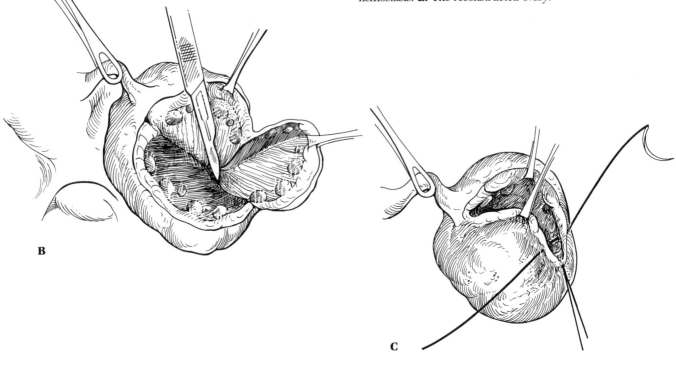

There is no doubt that wedge resection of the ovaries in properly selected cases results in a normal ovulatory process and subsequent pregnancy [21]. Since the advent of clomiphene, however, the number of patients needing this surgical procedure has markedly diminished. However, there remain a few patients, possibly those whose ovaries have been subjected to abnormal gonadotropin stimulation for long periods of time, who apparently ovulate after clomiphene but in whom pregnancy does not occur. Leventhal [17] has suggested that "intraovarian" ovulation occurs in these patients and that ovum release from the thickened capsule is probably not possible. We have noted this in a few patients who apparently responded to clomiphene but in whom pregnancy did not occur after six or seven consecutive cycles of therapy. Subsequent wedge resection apparently was responsible for pregnancy.

We now recommend that ovarian wedge resection be performed on patients who *apparently* ovulate following the use of clomiphene, clomiphene plus human chorionic gonadotropin, or clomiphene plus hydrocortisone, but in whom pregnancy does not occur. In some of these patients, ovarian enlargement and cortical thickening may progress during such therapy and the ovary may become more recalcitrant if hormonal treatment continues. Prolonged medical management in such patients is more radical than wedge resection.

Many of the timeworn criteria for wedge resection need to be reevaluated. In the original paper by Stein and Leventhal [21], the size of the ovary was emphasized as being an important criterion for selection. However, numerous investigators have found no relationship between the response to surgery and the size of the ovaries or the results of 17-ketosteroid assays or other laboratory determinations [7].

## Mechanism of Action

The precise mechanism by which wedge resection of the ovary brings about ovulation is not clear. It has been suggested that the surgical procedure inflicts severe trauma on the ovary and there follows a transient but drastic reduction in ovarian output of hormones (both androgens and estrogens). The vicious cycle of constant positive estrogen feedback is eliminated, at least temporarily. The demand for constant gonadotropin release is eliminated, and a process of pituitary regrouping and reorganization is permitted. Gonadotropins accumulate, exhausted ovarian enzymes are reconstituted, the hypothalamic cyclic center resumes its normal rhythm, and cyclic menstrual activity follows [9].

## Technique

Figure 8-3 shows the technique of wedge resection. We do not support the theory that a portion of the ovarian hilus needs to be excised in order to bring about subsequent ovulation. As a matter of fact, such a procedure frequently results in excessive bleeding from the hilar vessels and may predispose to ovarian senescence. Use of loupes (2.5×) is recommended during this procedure. Monopolar current may be used to cut the wedge, and bipolar electrocoagulation is employed for hemostasis.

If other procedures are carried out in the pelvis at the time, it is again important to reinspect each ovary before closing the peritoneum to be absolutely certain of complete hemostasis.

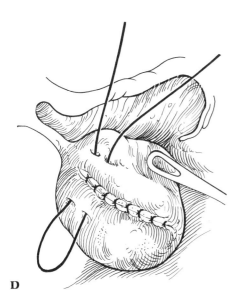

**D**

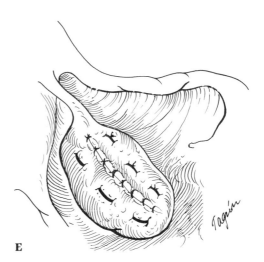

**E**

### Endometriosis

*Correlation with Infertility*

There exists a definite correlation between infertility and endometriosis, and Rubin [19] stated that the expectation of pregnancy when this disease is present is about half that in the general population. Thus, compared with the usual incidence of infertility, approximating 15 percent, the incidence of infertility approximates 30 to 40 percent in patients with endometriosis. However, if no other cause for infertility exists, conservative surgical procedures will result in subsequent pregnancy in 40 to 90 percent of patients. Acosta and coworkers [1] reported a pregnancy rate of 45.7 percent, and Spangler and coworkers [20] cited a 52 percent rate following conservative surgery. Kelly and Rock [10] reported endometriosis to be the causative factor of tuboovarian adhesions in 24 percent of 143 women who had culdoscopy

**Figure 8-4.** Classification of Endometriosis. (Kistner, Siegler and Behrman.) **A.** Stage I. **B.** Stage II, A. **C.** Stage II, B. **D.** Stage III. **E.** Stage IV. (From R. W. Kistner, Endometriosis and infertility. *Clin. Obstet. Gynecol.* 22:101, 1979.)

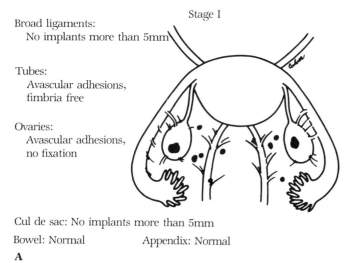

Stage I

Broad ligaments:
   No implants more than 5mm

Tubes:
   Avascular adhesions, fimbria free

Ovaries:
   Avascular adhesions, no fixation

Cul de sac: No implants more than 5mm

Bowel: Normal          Appendix: Normal

**A**

Stage II, A

Broad ligaments:
   No implants more than 5mm

Tubes:
   Avascular adhesions, fimbria free

Ovaries:
   Endometrial cyst 5cm or less—A1 stage; over 5cm—A2; ruptured—A3

A1

A2

A3

Cul de sac: No implants more than 5mm

Bowel: Normal          Appendix: Normal

**B**

because of infertility, and we have reported that endometriosis is found in one-third of "infertility laparotomies" [14]. If studies of an infertile patient show ovulation to be occurring regularly, the oviducts to be patent, the endometrium to be normal, and the post-coital test to be adequate, endometriosis should be considered and diagnostic procedures instituted.

There are several factors that influence the pregnancy rate:

1. Extent of the disease. Acosta et al. [1] reported a 75 percent pregnancy rate in mild cases, 50 percent in moderate cases, and only 33 percent in severe cases. Figure 8-4 illustrates the extent of disease by a classification suggested by Kistner, Siegler, and Behrman [12].

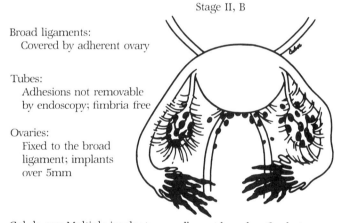

Stage II, B

Broad ligaments:
    Covered by adherent ovary

Tubes:
    Adhesions not removable by endoscopy; fimbria free

Ovaries:
    Fixed to the broad ligament; implants over 5mm

Cul de sac: Multiple implants, no adherent bowel or fixed uterus

Bowel: Normal          Appendix: Normal

C

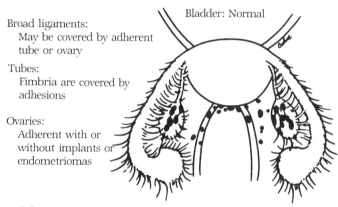

Stage III

Bladder: Normal

Broad ligaments:
    May be covered by adherent tube or ovary

Tubes:
    Fimbria are covered by adhesions

Ovaries:
    Adherent with or without implants or endometriomas

Cul de sac: Multiple implants, no adherent bowel or fixed uterus

Bowel: Normal          Appendix: Normal

D

Stage IV
(Usually combined with stage I, II, III)

Bladder: Implants

Uterus:
    May be fixed and adherent posteriorly

Cul de sac:
    Covered by adherent bowel or fixed retrodisplaced uterus

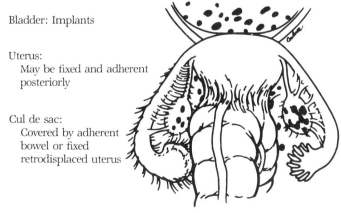

Bowel: Adherent to the cul-de-sac, uterosacral ligaments or corpus

Appendix: May be involved

E

2. Age of the patient. Over age 35, the pregnancy rate is 25 percent or less.
3. History of previous surgery for endometriosis and existence of other pelvic pathologic changes, such as peritubal adhesions, diminish the possibility of subsequent pregnancy.
4. Duration of infertility prior to surgery. The highest pregnancy rates occur in patients who have been infertile 3 years or less. The lowest rates (less than 25 percent) occur when the duration of infertility exceeds five years.
5. Length of follow-up after surgery. About 35 percent of patients become pregnant in the first year after surgery; an additional 15 to 20 percent become pregnant within the next 2 years. The precise factors responsible for this prolonged delay are unknown. However, we have noted luteal phase insufficiency in almost 25 percent of patients immediately following conservative surgery for endometriosis [14]. If this remains untreated, it could be a factor in the delay of conception.

The exact cause of the infertility in patients with endometriosis is unknown. The oviducts are usually patent, but perisalpingeal and perioophoritic adhesions are frequently found, with an adherent, retroverted uterus. The endometrium is usually normal, and biopsy specimens show secretory endometrium with progestational maturity. If other pathologic conditions such as submucous myomas and endometrial polyps are excluded, we believe that the most important factor responsible for infertility is an inadequacy of tuboovarian motility secondary to fibrosis and scarring. This results in imperfect ovum acceptance by the fimbriae. A classification of pelvic endometriosis recently proposed by the American Fertility Society is presented in Figure 8-5.

Patient's name _____

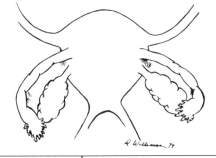

| Stage I (mild) | 1–5 |
| Stage II (moderate) | 6–15 |
| Stage III (severe) | 16–30 |
| Stage IV (extensive) | 31–54 |

Total _____

| | | | | |
|---|---|---|---|---|
| **Peritoneum** | Endometriosis | <1 cm | 1–3 cm | >3 cm |
| | | 1 | 2 | 3 |
| | Adhesions | Filmy | Dense w/ partial cul-de-sac obliteration | Dense w/ complete cul-de-sac obliteration |
| | | 1 | 2 | 3 |
| **Ovary** | Endometriosis | <1 cm | 1–3 cm | >3 cm or ruptured endometrioma |
| | R | 2 | 4 | 6 |
| | L | 2 | 4 | 6 |
| | Adhesions | Filmy | Dense w/ partial ovarian enclosure | Dense w/ complete ovarian enclosure |
| | R | 2 | 4 | 6 |
| | L | 2 | 4 | 6 |
| **Tube** | Endometriosis | <1 cm | >1 cm | Tubal occlusion |
| | R | 2 | 4 | 6 |
| | L | 2 | 4 | 6 |
| | Adhesions | Filmy | Dense w/ tubal distortion | Dense w/ tubal enclosure |
| | R | 2 | 4 | 6 |
| | L | 2 | 4 | 6 |

Associated pathology:

**Figure 8-5.** Classification of Endometriosis: American Fertility Society. (From The American Fertility Society: Classification of endometriosis. *Fertil Steril* 32:633, 1979. Reproduced with the permission of the publisher, The American Fertility Society.)

*Diagnosis*

The diagnosis may be suggested by the history, corroborated by the pelvic examination, and verified by culdoscopy, biopsy, and laparoscopy. On pelvic examination, the finding of tender, nodular uterosacral ligaments in conjunction with a fixed uterine retroversion is almost pathognomonic. Biopsy of suspect lesions in the vagina, perineum, umbilicus, or cervix will prove the presence of endometriosis in those areas. Investigation of the cul-de-sac may be performed by culdoscopy or posterior culpotomy if the rectum is not too adherent. Laparoscopy is recommended if the cul-de-sac is obliterated. It should be recalled that small areas of endometriotic tissue removed at laparotomy may show only endometrial stroma with hemorrhage and hemosiderin-laden macrophages. This should be sufficient for diagnosis in most cases, but in order to aid the pathologist, tiny blue spots, or "powder burns," should be tagged with a suture for easy identification.

The nodularity of the cul-de-sac so common in endometriosis may be produced in rare instances by metastatic ovarian carcinoma, bowel cancer, or calcified mesotheliomas. A gastric carcinoma with ovarian metastases may occasionally produce nodularity in the cul-de-sac. Rarely, cul-de-sac irregularity may be produced by infestation with *Enterobius vermicularis*. Calcified particles of splenic tissue have been reported in the cul-de-sac subsequent to rupture of the spleen and should be included in the differential diagnosis of cul-de-sac nodules.

Bidigital rectovaginal and bimanual abdominopelvic examination must be performed in order to palpate adequately the uterosacral ligaments, the posterior surface of the uterus, and the ovaries. The ovaries are often fixed in or lateral to the cul-de-sac, so that they can be palpated rectally. The pelvic examination should be repeated during the first 24 hours of the next menstrual period or during the second or third day of flow. To facilitate the thoroughness of the examination, the bladder must be empty and the rectum emptied by enemas.

Laboratory studies are not of particular diagnostic value, but occasionally, moderate leukocytosis and an elevated erythrocyte sedimentation rate are present.

Gross or microscopic blood in the urine or feces at the time of menstruation is highly suggestive of perforating endometriosis of the bladder mucosa or rectosigmoid. Cystoscopic and sigmoidoscopic examination may aid in establishing the diagnosis, and biopsy of bladder or sigmoid lesions is occasionally necessary. In specific instances, x-ray study of the colon may be of value in detecting lesions above the reach of the sigmoidoscope.

The differential diagnosis includes such diverse lesions as adenomyosis, pelvic inflammatory disease, nonspecific adhesions, and ovarian carcinoma.

Adenomyosis may produce similar symptomatology but usually occurs in older, multiparous patients. The adenomyotic uterus may be symmetrically enlarged, nodular, and tender, but the cul-de-sac is usually normal. In pelvic inflammatory disease, the pelvic examination frequently reveals bilateral tender broad-ligament masses that are characteristically doughy or fluctuant. Laboratory findings indicate the presence of an inflammatory process, and objective and subjective improvement follows proper antibiotic and conservative therapy. Nonspecific adhesions frequently occur after previous surgical intervention, especially appendectomy or incomplete surgery for pelvic infection. Ovarian carcinoma may be detected by laparoscopy or laparotomy, with biopsy or aspiration of ascitic fluid. The presence of a persistent pelvic mass, especially if solid, in the adnexal area is an absolute indication for abdominal exploration.

*Hormonal Treatment*

The optimum treatment for endometriosis is prolonged cessation of menstruation [14]. If pregnancy can be accomplished, this is recommended as primary therapy. If culdoscopy or laparoscopy reveal ovarian endometriosis without anatomic deformity of the ovary or tube, pseudopregnancy for 6 months utilizing norgestrel with ethinyl estradiol (Ovral) or norethynodrel with mestranol (Enovid-E) is suggested. Endoscopy repeated at the end of 6 months usually reveals no evidence of endometriosis. If no other cause for infertility exists, pregnancy may be expected to occur in about 50 percent of these patients within 1 year of cessation of therapy.

Prolonged hormonal therapy is applicable in the following patients:

1. Unmarried patients with maximal symptoms and minimal palpable findings. Extension of the disease may be prevented and subsequent fertility preserved.
2. Patients with recurrent disease after a previous conservative operation. Pregnancies have been noted subsequent to hormonal treatment in patients to whom hysterectomy had been suggested.

Short-term hormonal therapy is indicated in the following situations:

1. Prior to conservative surgery. Areas of endometriosis will enlarge and appear hemorrhagic, making identification and excision simpler and more complete. Six to 8 weeks of therapy is adequate.
2. Subsequent to conservative therapy (in order to inhibit ovulation and prevent reactivation of remaining areas of endometriosis). Twelve to 24 weeks of therapy is adequate. Postoperative pseudopregnancy is utilized only when the disease is extensive and if all areas of endometriosis cannot be excised.

Results of treatment by various investigators have been uniform. About 85 percent of patients show improvement during the period of therapy and for varying times thereafter. In patients treated primarily with progestins, that is, without previous surgery, remissions have lasted as long as 6 years [14]. In those patients who did not improve or whose symptoms were aggravated by surgery, either adenomyosis or pelvic inflammatory disease was subsequently found coexisting with the endometriosis. Patients who have recurrent endometriosis after preliminary surgery present a serious challenge to the gynecologist or surgeon. Prolonged pseudopregnancy has been of particular value in these patients, and therapy should be continued for 12 to 24 months to secure optimum results.

A summary of the results of prolonged administration of these steroids for endometriosis can be made: (1) they are effective inhibitors of ovulation and produce a decidual reaction in areas of endometriosis; (2) about 85 percent of the patients are improved during therapy and for varying periods thereafter; and (3) no abnormalities of endometrial, ovarian, or pituitary function, except for occasional luteal phase insufficiency, have been observed during the posttreatment period, and subsequent pregnancies have occurred without incident in a high percentage of patients. Ulfelder, in a discussion of the various approaches presently available [23], stated: "At present it appears that hormone therapy for endometriosis will be the most widely applicable form of management in the future."

The use of an antigonadotropic steroid, Danocrine, has been reported by Dnowski and Cohen [6] to result in pregnancy in 46 percent of 99 patients treated with this preparation. If patients with good fertility potential (excluding male and tubal factors) are evaluated, the corrected pregnancy rate is 72 percent.

*Surgical Treatment*
In contemplating surgical treatment of endometriosis, one should remember that functioning ovarian tissue is necessary for the continued activity of the disease. Therefore, successful treatment of endometriosis depends on a knowledge of when it is reasonably safe or desirable to maintain ovarian function and when it is necessary to destroy it. It is obvious that ovarian function should be preserved in treating the very early, and perhaps symptomless, lesions, and hysterectomy should be performed only when the ovaries are destroyed by endometriosis. Unfortunately, the majority of cases will fall between these two extremes and may present problems in surgical judgment seldom encountered in any other pelvic disease. As our knowledge of the life history of endometriosis has increased, there has been a definite tendency to become more conservative, particularly in the treatment of the infertile patient. In general, it is believed that one should err on the side of conservatism;

this belief is based on the fact that endometriosis (1) usually progresses slowly over a period of years, (2) is not, and rarely becomes, malignant, and (3) regresses at the menopause.

Early implantations on the surface of the peritoneum should be excised. Electrocoagulation is not recommended because of the possibility of subsequent adhesions to the small intestine or the adnexal structures. Small endometrial cysts on the ovary may be excised or a major portion of one or both ovaries may be resected. Small endometrial implants on the intestines should be excised. To aid in the prevention of recurrence, conservative operations should be accompanied by correction of uterine displacements, relief of cervical obstruction, and removal of any other concomitant pelvic pathologic conditions. Endometriosis coexisting with uterine myomas, ovarian cysts, or other pelvic abnormalities may be insignificant, but on the other hand, the extent or location of these may make conservative surgery hazardous. Decisions cannot always be made prior to laparotomy, and the patient should be so informed.

The use of magnification provided by loupes (2.5 or 4.5×) permits careful definition of endometrial implants and assists in excision without damage to surrounding tissue. The operating microscope has been utilized less often because of the difficulty viewing sites of endometrial implants beneath the ovary and on the broad ligament. Another change in the corrective surgical approach to endometriosis has been the use of microelectrosurgery and carbon dioxide laser surgery. The microelectrode can be utilized to carefully excise endometrial implants when magnification is employed and is also useful for excision of ovarian endometriosis. Bellina [3] has utilized the carbon dioxide laser in the surgical treatment of pelvic endometriosis, and it is perhaps here that the laser technique finds its greatest value.

CONSERVATIVE SURGERY (OVARIAN RESECTION)
If childbearing function is to be preserved, operative procedures should be as conservative as possible. All surgical procedures should be preceded by a thorough curettage, and every patient should have had a cytologic examination to exclude possible malignancy of the cervix.

The approach should usually be through a transverse suprapubic incision. However, if the ovarian masses are large, a midline incision may be necessary. Thorough exploration of the pelvic and abdominal organs should be performed routinely, and the decision reached as to whether conservative or radical surgery is preferable.

Because of recurrent bleeding and fibrosis associated with the process of endometriosis, the ovaries are frequently adherent to the posterior leaf of the broad ligament and must be carefully displaced from this site before resection is possible. The use of loupe magnification is invaluable at this time.

When the disease is extensive, the uterus is usually fixed in third-degree retroversion, with both ovaries adherent to the uterus or the posterior leaf of the broad ligament and to the rectosigmoid. When this situation exists, it is frequently safer to displace the ovaries by gentle finger dissection than by sharp dissection with a knife or scissors. In extensive endometriosis, the ureter is frequently displaced medially and may be immediately adjacent or adherent to the fixed ovary. Knife or scissors dissection might inadvertently injure or divide the ureter.

If the ovarian masses are large, as with bilateral endometriomas, it is advisable to finger dissect both ovarian masses first and then elevate the uterus from its fixed position.

In order to free the uterus, it is frequently necessary to place upward traction on the rectosigmoid so that its attachment to the back of the uterus and cervix may be identified. The rest of the surgical technique is shown in Figure 8-6.

**Figure 8-6.** Ovarian resection for endometriosis. **A.** A transverse incision *(broken line)* is made on the posterior aspect of the uterus just above the insertion of the uterosacral ligaments, and the attached rectosigmoid is displaced. **B.** William clamps are placed at both ends of the ovary, and all areas of endometriosis are excised. **C.** Babcock clamps are placed on the reflected ovarian edges, and the endometriotic cyst is dissected free with scissors. **D.** The ovaries are reconstructed with interrupted sutures of 4-0 and 6-0 Vicryl or PDS. Several mattress sutures are placed to eliminate dead space. An omental graft is sutured in place over the denuded area behind the uterus. The uterosacral ligaments are plicated in the midline with interrupted sutures of 0 chromic catgut.

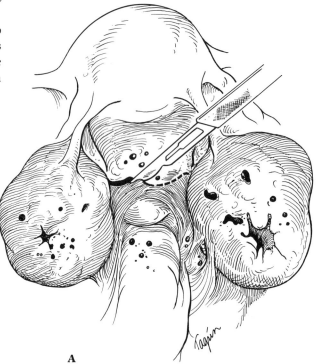

A

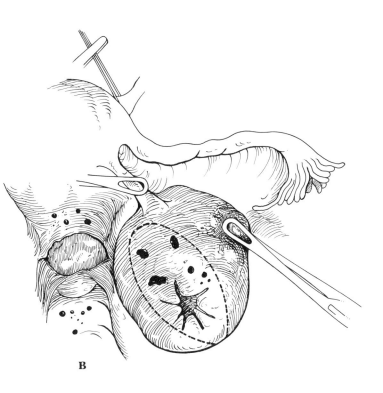

**B**

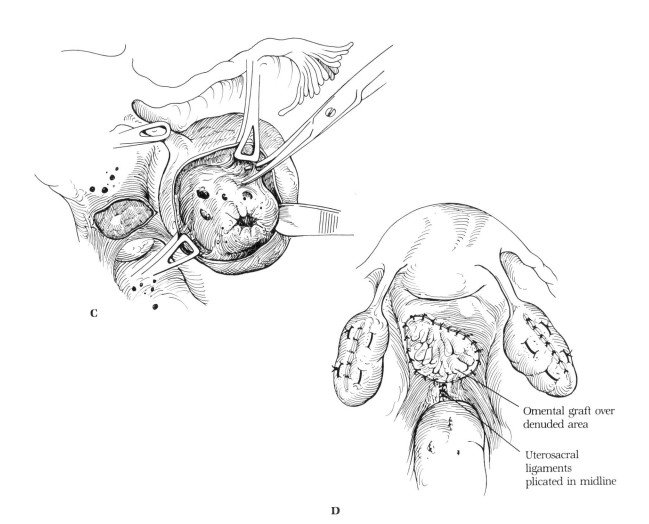

**C**

Omental graft over
denuded area

Uterosacral
ligaments
plicated in midline

**D**

327

Occasionally, the ovary is intimately attached to the lateral peritoneum immediately over the course of the ureter. In this case, the posterior peritoneum is opened at the level of the promontory of the sacrum in the same way as for a presacral neurectomy. We usually perform the presacral neurectomy first, so that the posterior peritoneum may be left open until all steps of the operations have been concluded. This prevents ureteral damage during mobilization of the fixed ovaries. Allis clamps are then placed on the edge of the peritoneum and the right ureter is identified on the lateral flap. The left ureter lies below the superior hemorrhoidal vessels and is somewhat more difficult to locate. A right-angle clamp is then used to tease the ureter free from the peritoneum in the area where the ovary is attached. After this has been accomplished, the ovary may be mobilized by sharp dissection. Since the contents of endometriomas are irritating to the peritoneum and bowel serosa, several packs are placed above the pelvis to protect these structures.

Small areas of endometriosis are frequently found deep in the substance of the ovary and these are excised. Occasionally, the major portion of the ovarian substance has been completely destroyed or replaced by endometriosis, and at the conclusion of the resection, only a small fragment of ovarian cortex at the hilus remains. This should not be an absolute indication for oophorectomy, since we have observed pregnancies in women who have had a unilateral salpingo-oophorectomy and three quarters of the remaining ovary removed. In the ovarian reconstruction, the operator should attempt to reapproximate the cortical surface as closely as possible in order to prevent adhesion of omentum or small intestine to the ovary.

Areas of endometriosis on the posterior surface of the uterus and cervix or on the anterior surface of the rectosigmoid should be excised as completely as possible. This frequently results in large areas of denudation of the peritoneum and raw, oozing surfaces in the cul-de-sac. While it is possible to cover these areas by reflecting the redundant sigmoid inferiorly and suturing it to the posterior aspect of the uterus, this results in obliteration of the cul-de-sac. In order to preserve the anatomic configuration of the cul-de-sac, we feel that it is advantageous to cover the raw surface with an omental graft. We have had the opportunity to observe these grafts at second operations and have found them to be intact and free of adhesions to the adnexal structures or intestines.

At the conclusion of the ovarian resection, the entire oviduct should be carefully inspected, and adhesions of the fimbriated portion of the distal oviduct to the ovary should be freed. Ligation of small blood vessels on the oviduct is accomplished with 6-0 Vicryl. If the bowel lumen is entered, closure of the submucosal and seromuscular layers is done in the usual two-layer manner. After all areas of endometriosis have been excised, the edges of available peritoneum are closed with fine catgut. All denuded areas should be covered with peritoneal or omental grafts.

In conservative operations for endometriosis, a uterine suspension and presacral neurectomy are usually performed. We feel that it is important, from the viewpoint of subsequent fertility, to ensure the anatomic normality of the cul-de-sac, and this is best accomplished by anterior uterine suspension.

Plication of the uterosacral ligaments is an adjunctive procedure to uterine suspension and improves the posterior deflection of the cervix, thus aiding anterior positioning of the uterus. In many cases, the denuded area over the rectosigmoid is adequately peritonealized by plication of the uterosacral ligaments. This is accomplished with three interrupted sutures of 0 Vicryl, the first suture being placed just at the insertion of the uterosacral ligaments and two sutures just below the first. After this has been completed, the sigmoid colon fits nicely into the arc of the uterosacral ligaments. When plicating the uterosacral ligaments care must be taken not to place the sutures too far laterally, because of the possibility of kinking or obstructing the ureter. Since we advise doing the presacral neurectomy before the ovarian and cul-de-sac resections, it is frequently advantageous to leave the posterior peritoneum open until this has been concluded. The ureters will then be easily visualized during these dissections and reconstructions (see Fig 8-1).

If subsequent pregnancy is not a prime factor, or if there is evidence of extensive involvement of other pelvic structures, such as bowel or ureter, a hysterectomy and bilateral salpingo-oophorectomy may be indicated.

Since leiomyomas of the uterus are found in about 15 percent of the patients with endometriosis, single or multiple myomectomy should be carried out as part of the conservative approach (see Chap. 4). It has been our practice to do a presacral neurectomy whenever the uterus is not removed. Even if the patient has not had dysmenorrhea or pelvic pain preceding surgery, these symptoms may develop postoperatively. The presacral procedure should be extensive, with excision of all nerve tissue between the right ureter and the superior hemorrhoidal vessels. In addition, we frequently remove a part of the uterosacral ligaments at their insertion into the uterus, thus accomplishing pelvic denervation.

An appendectomy is performed at the time of surgery because functioning endometriosis of the appendiceal serosa has been noted in many patients. Endometriosis of the terminal ileum is seen only rarely and may be treated by superficial excision. If the muscularis and mucosa are involved, resection and end-to-end anastomosis should be performed.

Pseudopregnancy is induced for a minimum of 3 months after operation; then concerted efforts toward conception are made. About 50 percent of women so treated will become pregnant if no other cause for infertility exists. One author has reported the incidence of pregnancy to be as high as 90 percent following conservative surgery, but this seems to be an exceptionally high success rate and may depend on patient selection [8].

USE OF THE CARBON DIOXIDE LASER DURING
EXCISION OF ENDOMETRIOSIS

The carbon dioxide laser appears particularly useful during the surgical excision of pelvic endometriosis. The shallow depth of injury procured by the laser beam appears to permit the safe excision of endometrial implants from bowel serosa and peritoneal surfaces overlying the ureter. The following technique has been described by Bellina [3]. Implants of endometriosis that occur on the uterosacral ligaments and other serosal surfaces can be vaporized and removed by the carbon dioxide laser at low power densities of 200–400 W per square centimeter* (power .5–1 watt, spot diameter .5 mm). The hand-held unit or the micromanipulator attached to the operating microscope may be used for this purpose. Rapid movement of the laser beam is used to completely remove the lesion, often revealing normal stroma beneath the lesion. Remarkably, this technique of superficial excision of endometrial implants has been used safely to remove endometriosis from the bowel and large vessel surfaces. The laser beam may occasionally be used in the pulse mode (TM .05–.1 second) to destroy endometrial implants. Bellina prefers to utilize the micromanipulator to rapidly sweep the beam over all endometrial implants. As noted earlier during the discussion of salpingolysis (p. 232), a silver-surfaced mirror permits the surgeon to reflect the laser beam into the ovarian fossa and difficult-to-reach areas that cannot be visualized directly (Fig. 8-7). Reflecting the laser beam in this manner is one of the unique features of laser surgery and is particularly useful during surgical excision of ovarian endometriosis (Fig. 8-8).

Ovarian endometriosis can be completely removed using the carbon dioxide laser. Small endometrial cysts (less than 2 cm) may be destroyed by first excising the outer exposed surface and then photocoagulating the internal walls of the cysts with a power density of 400 W per square centimeter (power 1, spot diameter .5 mm).

*Power Density (PD) equals power in watts times 100 divided by the square of the spot diameter (in millimeters).

**Figure 8-7.** Demonstration of the use of a front silver surfaced mirror to direct the laser energy beneath the ovary to resect adhesions in a patient with stage IV endometriosis. (Courtesy of Joseph H. Bellina, M.D., Ph.D.)

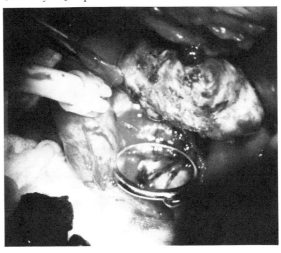

**Figure 8-8.** The laser beam controlled by the micromanipulator has been reflected by a dental mirror under the ovary to cut adhesions and to vaporize implants of endometriosis.

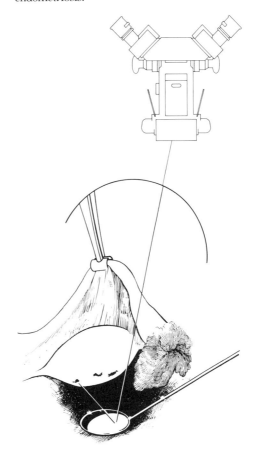

Bellina does not close this defect and during evaluation with secondlook laparoscopy has rarely found adhesions to these surfaces. Larger endometriomas are similarly removed using the carbon dioxide laser to destroy endometrial tissue. However, the large defect in the ovarian surface is approximated with 4-0 synthetic absorbable suture material. All carbonized tissue should be thoroughly removed by irrigation prior to completion of surgery.

One remarkable feature of the carbon dioxide laser technique is the ability to remove areas of endometriosis of the surface of the bowel without extensive damage. Bellina has excised areas of endometriosis in the large intestine of 7 patients utilizing the carbon dioxide laser and cutting mode at a power density of 10,000 W per square centimeter (power 25 watts, spot diameter .5 mm). The sigmoid colon was the involved site in all these cases, and the implant of endometriosis was excised from the serosal surface without penetrating the mucosal layer. The serosal layer was then closed with interrupted sutures. In one of these cases the bowel wall was completely transected, producing a defect 3 cm in diameter. This defect was closed primarily without a diverting colostomy and primary healing ensued. Factors that appear to have contributed to the success of this approach are the use of magnification with careful inspection of the layers of bowel wall involved, and also limited tissue necrosis because of adjustment of the laser beam to produce mainly a cutting effect.

*Results*

Analysis of our results during the last 20 years reveals a pregnancy rate of 50.8 percent in 186 patients treated by pseudopregnancy alone. These patients' only abnormality, as determined by endoscopy, was surface ovarian endometriosis without endometriomas or tuboovarian adhesions. The pregnancy rate subsequent to surgical treatment of ovarian endometriomas, with or without peritoneal endometriosis involving the bladder, uterus, cul de sac, or lateral pelvic wall, was 76 percent in 232 patients. It should be noted, however, that postoperative pseudopregnancy was used in these patients only if all areas of endometriosis could not be excised at the time of surgery. Furthermore, 96 percent of these patients were under 32 years of age, and no other factors contributing to infertility were present. The incidence of pregnancy following surgical therapy in 106 patients who were found to have ovarian and peritoneal endometriosis complicated by tuboovarian, uteroovarian, or sigmoidoovarian adhesions was, however, only 38 percent [15].

We have recently reviewed 100 patients who were treated with Danocrine alone and Danocrine plus surgery [2]. Danocrine was administered to patients classified as stage I and stage IIA in a dose of 800 mg daily, and patients in stages IIB, III, and IV were treated by surgery plus preoperative and, occasionally, postoperative Danazol. Fifty-six patients were infertile, and in those patients with stage I and stage II endometriosis, treatment with Danazol alone resulted in a 50 percent corrected pregnancy rate. Nine of 11 pregnancies occurred in patients with stage I disease. In contrast, 44 percent of those patients treated with combined therapy conceived postoperatively, and remarkably, 57 percent (4 of 7) of patients with stage IV disease obtained a pregnancy.

It is interesting that in selected series, surgery alone appears to result in a higher pregnancy rate, even in patients with mild endometriosis (stage I), than does treatment with Danocrine for conventional pseudopregnancy. Kistner reported that in 524 patients treated between the years 1955 and 1975, 232 had endometriosis without significant adhesions and 76 percent conceived postoperatively [14]. In contrast, the pregnancy rate following surgery in 106 patients with endometriosis and severe adhesions was 38 percent. Buttram [4] has also noted the advantage of surgical treatment of all stages of endometriosis in the infertile patient. Among 127 patients found to have endometriosis as their only pelvic pathology, pregnancy occurred postoperatively in 58 percent. However, when these patients were divided into stages—mild, moderate, and severe—pregnancy occurred in 73 percent, 56 percent, and 40 percent, respectively. In addition, 86 percent of these pregnancies occurred within a 15-month interval following surgery.

There were 56 patients in Buttram's group who had mild endometriosis, and 78 percent had been trying to conceive for at least 2 years preoperatively. Following conservative surgery, 73 percent of this group was pregnant within a 15-month interval. Both this study and that of Kistner suggest the value of conservative surgical excision in those infertile patients found to have mild endometriosis (stages I or IIA). This is by no means a universal recommendation, however, and "the management of each case of endometriosis presents its own diagnostic and therapeutic challenge to the clinician" [2]. The decision whether to utilize Danazol alone or Danazol plus conservative surgery, or lastly, conservative surgery alone, must rest with the individual physician and patient.

## Extirpative Surgery

The treatment of choice for extensive endometriosis in women who no longer desire pregnancy is total hysterectomy and bilateral salpingo-oophorectomy. It has not seemed reasonable to leave the ovaries in situ if the uterus is removed for this disease, since ovulation continues in cyclic fashion and remaining areas of endometriosis may be stimulated to grow by endogenous estrogen and progesterone. In experimental endometriosis in monkeys, the most extensive growth has been obtained by the cyclic administration and withdrawal of estrogen and progesterone. This is exactly the situation that exists when functioning ovaries are preserved. When there is extensive bladder, bowel, or ureteral endometriosis, hysterectomy and bilateral salpingo-oophorectomy will effect a cure.

Large bilateral ovarian endometrial cysts with extensive peritoneal endometriosis and numerous pelvic adhesions or with marked invasion of the rectosigmoid and rectovaginal space constitute the most urgent indications for radical removal of all involved pelvic organs, regardless of the age of the patient. Failure to castrate in the presence of marked endometriosis of the bowel is undoubtedly the most hazardous of all attempts at conservative surgery because of the dangers of subsequent intestinal obstruction [22].

From the operative standpoint, early or moderately advanced endometriosis offers no unusual difficulties, but extensive endometriosis may present technical problems. In contrast to pelvic inflammatory disease (particularly that due to gonorrheal infection), endometriosis produces pelvic adhesions without planes of cleavage. Therefore, much of the dissection must be done with sharp instruments, and the dangers of damage to adherent structures are increased. This hazard may be diminished by the use of preoperative pseudopregnancy.

A hysterectomy and bilateral salpingo-oophorectomy can usually be accomplished in patients with large endometrial cysts and extensive pelvic adhesions, even those with marked invasion of the rectovaginal septum. This may be facilitated by incising the posterior peritoneum above the insertion of the uterosacral ligaments. The endopelvic fascia and rectosigmoid may then be reflected and the danger of fistula is minimized. At times it may be necessary to leave a considerable portion of the growth attached to the bowel or other pelvic structures, but these remnants will regress following ablation of the ovaries.

## References

1. Acosta, A. A., Buttram, V. C., Jr., Besch, P. K., Malinak, R. L., Franklin, R. R., and Vanderheyden, J. D. A proposed classification of endometriosis. *Obstet. Gynecol.* 42:19, 1973.
2. Barbieri, R. L., Evans, S., and Kistner, R. W. Danazol in the treatment of endometriosis: Analysis of 100 cases with a 4-year follow-up. *Fertil. Steril.* 37:737, 1982.
3. Bellina, J. H. Personal communication, 1982.
4. Buttram, V. C., Jr. Conservative surgery for endometriosis in the infertile female: A study of 206 patients with implications of both medical and surgical therapy. *Fertil. Steril.* 31:117, 1979.
5. Buttram, V. C., Jr., and Betts, J. W. Endometriosis. *Curr. Probl. Obstet. Gynecol.* 2(11):3, 1979.
6. Dnowski, W. P. and Cohen, M. R. Antigonadotropin (Danazol) in treatment of endometriosis: Evaluation of post treatment fertility and 3-year follow-up data. *Am. J. Obstet. Gynecol.* 130:41, 1978.
7. Goldzieher, J. W. Polycystic Ovarian Disease. In S. J. Behrman and R. W. Kistner (eds.), *Progress in Infertility* (2nd ed.). Boston: Little, Brown, 1975.
8. Green, T. H. Symposium on endometriosis. *Clin. Obstet. Gynecol.* 9:269, 1966.
9. Kase, N. Steroid synthesis in abnormal ovaries: III. Polycystic ovaries. *Am. J. Obstet. Gynecol.* 90:1268, 1964.
10. Kelly, J. V., and Rock, J. Culdoscopy for diagnosis in infertility. *Am. J. Obstet. Gynecol.* 72:523, 1959.
11. Kistner, R. W. Unpublished data, 1982.
12. Kistner, R. W. Endometriosis and infertility. *Clin. Obstet. Gynecol.* 22:101, 1979.
13. Kistner, R. W., Induction of Ovulation with Clomiphene Citrate. In S. J. Behrman and R. W. Kistner (eds.), *Progress in Infertility* (2nd ed.). Boston: Little, Brown, 1975.
14. Kistner, R. W. Endometriosis and Infertility. In S. J. Behrman and R. W. Kistner (eds.), *Progress in Infertility* (2nd ed.). Boston: Little, Brown, 1975.
15. Kistner, R. W. Management of endometriosis in the infertile patient. *Fertil. Steril.* 26:1151, 1975.
16. Kistner, R. W., Siegler, A. M., and Behrman, S. J. Suggested classification for endometriosis: Relationship to infertility. *Fertil. Steril.* 28:1008, 1977.
17. Leventhal, M. L. Personal communication, 1969.
18. Norwood, G. E. Sterility and fertility in women with pelvic endometriosis. *Clin. Obstet. Gynecol.* 3:456, 1960.
19. Rubin, I. C. Sterility. *Obstet. Gynecol.* 3:161, 1933.
20. Spangler, D. B., Jones, G. S., and Jones, H. W. Infertility due to endometriosis: Conservative surgical therapy. *Am. J. Obstet. Gynecol.* 109:850, 1971.
21. Stein, I. F., and Leventhal, M. L. Amenorrhea associated with bilateral polycystic ovaries. *Am. J. Obstet. Gynecol.* 29:181, 1935.
22. Te Linde, R. W., and Mattingly, R. F. *Operative Gynecology* (4th ed.). Philadelphia: Lippincott, 1970.
23. Ulfelder, H. The treatment of endometriosis. *Med. Sci.* 8:503, 1966.

# Presacral Neurectomy and Uterine Suspension

**Presacral Neurectomy**

Subsequent to the introduction of hormonal agents for the amelioration of primary dysmenorrhea, pelvic denervation procedures have been used only rarely [1,3]. However, we feel that presacral neurectomy should be an integral part of the so-called conservative laparotomy for endometriosis.

Endometriosis is a recurrent disease whose rekindling depends on the process of ovulation [4]. Thus a conservative procedure with excision of all areas of endometriosis does not guarantee permanent control of pelvic pain. A properly performed presacral neurectomy will usually prevent recurrent discomfort. It should be pointed out, however, that this procedure does not prevent the recurrence of pain or discomfort of ovarian origin. Although transection of the infundibulopelvic ligaments has been suggested [1,3], we have not adopted this procedure in infertility surgery because of potential alteration in ovulation. Although collateral blood supply is made available from the uterus, we do not believe that compromise of ovarian function is acceptable. Removal of portions of both uterosacral ligaments has been suggested to remove both parasympathetic and sympathetic nerve fibers, thus effecting *complete pelvic denervation* [4]. We remove portions of the uterosacral ligaments only if they are involved by endometriosis. The ligaments are then sutured to the cervix and plicated as described in Chapter 8.

*Technique*

Proper exposure is essential for performance of presacral neurectomy. In order to accomplish this, Mersilene sutures are placed around the round ligaments; these sutures will be used later for the suspension. With these sutures providing traction, the uterus is held forward toward the symphysis. The adnexal structures are mobilized and freed from adhesions. They are held laterally by retractors and laparotomy pads. The retractor should be placed over the pad to prevent trauma to the undersurface of the mesosalpinx and infundibulopelvic ligament. The sigmoid colon is displaced to the left side and is held in that position by the left lateral retractor. A curved retractor holds the upper part of the incision away from the sacral promontory.

Although the exposure provided by a midline or paramedian incision is superior to that provided by a suprapubic transverse incision, the operation may be performed through the latter incision if care is taken to provide adequate exposure. If a transverse incision is utilized, the peritoneum should be opened vertically and the anterior rectus fascia opened to a point above the promontory of the sacrum. Figure 9-1 shows the technique of presacral neurectomy.

**Figure 9-1.** Technique of presacral neurectomy. **A.** The operator and his assistant elevate the posterior peritoneum with thumb forceps in the midline just below the promontory of the sacrum. A vertical incision *(broken line)* is made through the peritoneum, curving slightly to the right in order to avoid the sigmoid mesentery. The incision, however, should remain medial to the right ureter. Furthermore, the ureter is left attached to the lateral flap rather than the medial flap as is done in a radical hysterectomy. The inferior limit of the vertical incision is approximately 2 cm above the junction of the uterosacral ligaments and the cervix. The incision is then extended cephalad to a level just above the promontory of the sacrum.

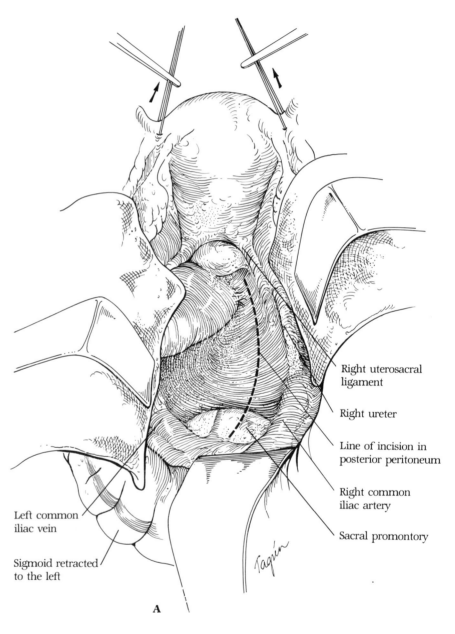

Right uterosacral ligament

Right ureter

Line of incision in posterior peritoneum

Right common iliac artery

Sacral promontory

Left common iliac vein

Sigmoid retracted to the left

**A**

**B.** Allis clamps are placed on the right lateral peritoneum, traction is exerted, and the tela subserosa is dissected from its attachment to the undersurface of the peritoneum with fine scissors. At this point the right ureter is easily visualized and it now becomes the lateral border of the dissection of the superior hypogastric plexus. The ureter is *not* dissected free but is permitted to remain attached to the lateral peritoneal flap. All tissue medial to the ureter is mobilized. After the tela subserosa has been freed, the Allis clamps are removed and the peritoneum is held laterally under the blade of a retractor.

**C.** An Allis clamp is then used to elevate the substance of the superior and middle hypogastric plexus and traction is made toward the midline so that all tissue may be mobilized.

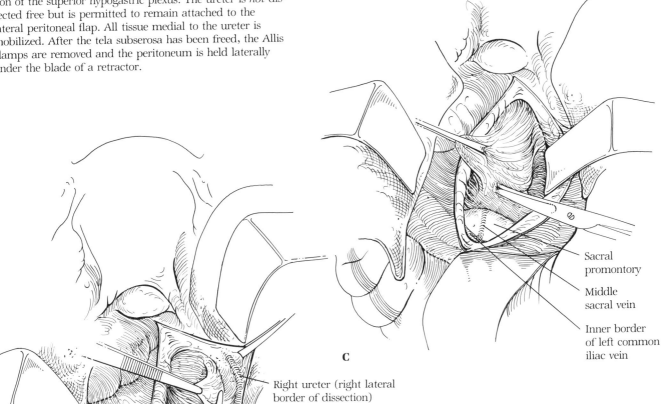

Sacral promontory

Middle sacral vein

Inner border of left common iliac vein

**C**

Right ureter (right lateral border of dissection)

**B**

9. Presacral Neurectomy and Uterine Suspension

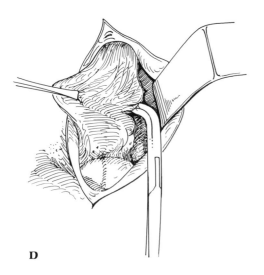

**D**

**Figure 9-1 (continued)**

**D.** A right-angle clamp is used to free the undersurface of the plexus where it is attached to the midportion of the sacrum. Care is taken to avoid laceration of the middle sacral vein and the inner border of the left common iliac vein, which is easily visualized in the upper part of the dissection. **E.** The inferior portion of the hypogastric plexus is then dissected free. This is evident by the lateral flaring of the nerve fibers and the formation of a triangle of tissue whose base is toward the cul-de-sac. **F.** Attention is then directed toward the left side and the procedure is repeated. The lateral landmarks on the left side, however, are the superior hemorrhoidal vessels situated above the left ureter. The ureter on the left side is not usually visualized as well as that on the right, but it is easily identified if the dissection is carried to a deeper level along the sigmoid mesentery. Care must be taken in the dissection along the sigmoid mesentery to stay medial to the major vessels and the smaller tributaries. An easy line of cleavage is usually obtained just below the superior hemorrhoidal vessels and the plexus is mobilized to the midline.

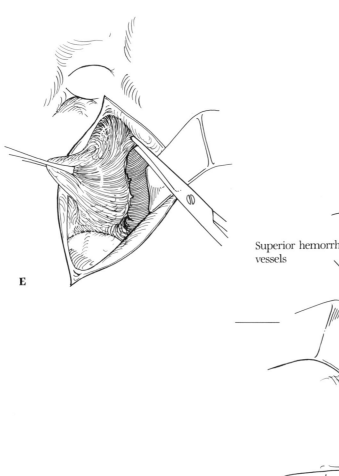

**E**

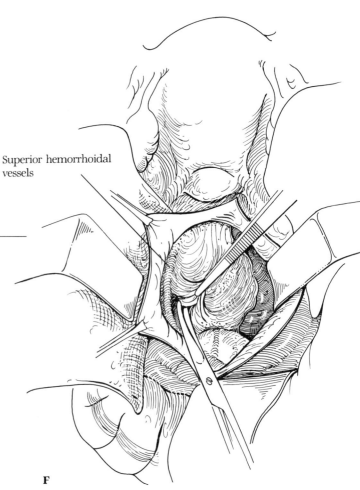

Superior hemorrhoidal vessels

**F**

**G.** After the entire plexus has been dissected free, it is tied at the level of the promontory of the sacrum and at the lowest point of the inferior dissection and then removed. **H.** Inspection is made of the presacral area to be certain of complete hemostasis. Bleeding from small veins must be carefully controlled since it may lead to large retroperitoneal hematomas. **I.** The peritoneum is then closed with a running suture of 0 chromic catgut, care being taken in placing the sutures on the right side of the peritoneal flap not to incorporate or kink the ureter. Prior to placement of the last few sutures, the peritoneum is pressed against the sacrum to expel air and eliminate dead space.

If other procedures are done in the pelvis, the retroperitoneal area should be inspected prior to closure of the abdomen to be certain that a retroperitoneal hematoma has not occurred. When extensive endometriosis involves the ovaries and cul-de-sac, closure of the peritoneum is deferred until after ovarian resection and uterosacral plication have been accomplished. This permits visualization of the lower ends of the ureters during the adnexal dissection.

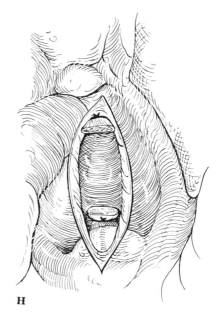

**H**

Presacral area after removal of plexus

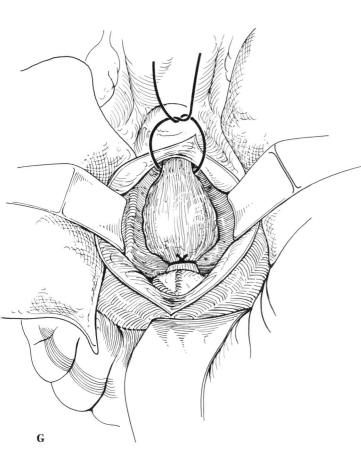

**G**

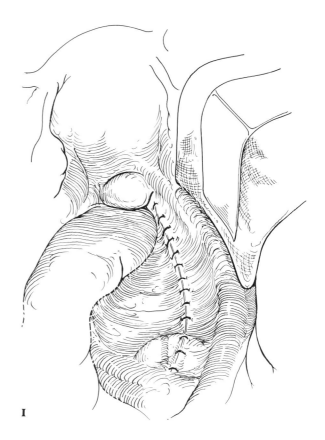

**I**

## Uterine Suspension

Suspension of the uterine fundus is one of the oldest, and perhaps one of the most maligned, gynecologic operations [2]. During the first half of this century it was performed for hypermenorrhea, backache, dyspareunia, vague pelvic pain, and habitual abortion. Gradually the operation fell into disrepute among most gynecologists because there was no clear evidence that these symptoms were related to the abnormal position of the uterus unless other pelvic disorders such as endometriosis or pelvic inflammatory disease existed simultaneously.

The major indication for uterine suspension is in the conservative surgical management of endometriosis, whether this be for infertility or for the relief of pain. It is also employed in patients found to require lysis of extensive pelvic adhesions. It is not routinely utilized in patients undergoing reversal of sterilization, salpingostomy, or fimbrioplasty. Occasionally it is performed for acquired dysmenorrhea, dyspareunia, and hypermenorrhea associated with the so-called pelvic congestion syndrome. Before the operations is carried out, however, the patient should have a trial period with anterior replacement of the uterus aided by a pessary. If this provides amelioration of symptoms, one may conclude that the retroversion is indeed the major etiologic factor. This is probably the only indication for a so-called primary uterine suspension.

### Technique

Numerous variations in surgical technique have appeared in the last half century [2,5,6], but the basic principle in most has been that of shortening the round ligaments. This combination draws the fundus of the uterus forward and the cervix posteriorly. We have used 0 Mersilene sutures for this procedure in those patient with endometriosis rather than the chromic catgut advised by some gynecologists. Chromic sutures are utilized to achieve a temporary suspension in those patients with adhesions secondary to an inflammatory process. Figure 9-2 shows the surgical technique.

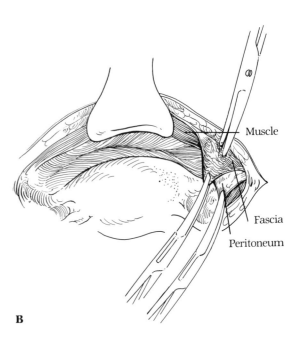

Muscle

Fascia

Peritoneum

**B**

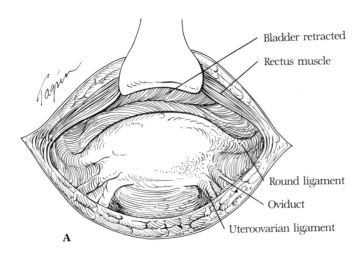

Bladder retracted

Rectus muscle

Round ligament

Oviduct

Uteroovarian ligament

**A**

**Figure 9-2.** Technique of uterine suspension. **A.** Normal anatomical relationships of the round ligaments, oviduct, and uteroovarian ligaments. **B.** A Kelly clamp is placed on the peritoneum, and a Kocher clamp is placed on the fascia just medial to the insertion of the round ligament as it curves toward the inguinal ligament. At the point selected for suspension, a small area of fascia is denuded of overlying areolar tissue and fat. **C.** The suture is actually a double strand of 0 Mersilene and is placed directly under the attachment of the round ligament to the uterine cornu, care being taken to avoid the oviduct. **D.** This needle is then directed medially through the uterine cornu for a distance of about 1.5 cm.

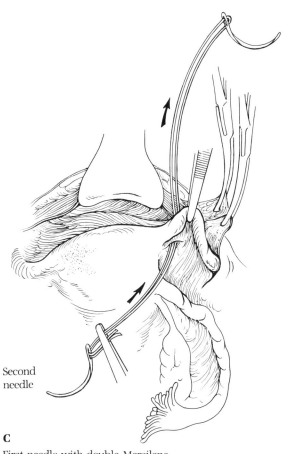

First
needle

Second
needle

**C**

First needle with double Mersilene
suture passed under round ligament

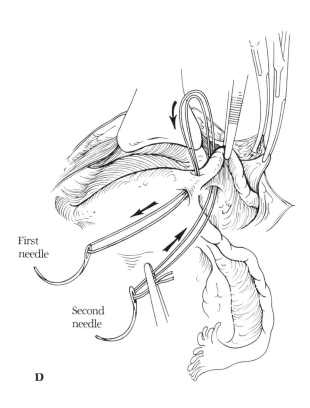

First
needle

Second
needle

**D**

**Figure 9-2 (continued)**
**E.** The first needle is directed through the peritoneum, muscle, and fascia, following the curve of the round ligament. The bladder is held out of the field with a retractor, but care must be taken not to direct the needle too close to the pubic symphysis. **F.** The second needle is directed along the same pathway about 0.5 cm. cephalad to the first suture. The double Mersilene suture is then tied snugly on top of the fascia. **G.** Because of the tendency of Mersilene to slip when tied, five knots are utilized to secure the fixation. The same steps are repeated on the opposite side. The uterus should be held forward manually from the undersurface while the sutures are being tied. **H.** The completed suspension. If a suprapubic transverse incision has been made, the same type of suspension is utilized but the sutures are brought out through the inferior flap of fascia. Occasionally, depending on the site of the incision, it is preferable to place one suture through the lower fascial flap and the second suture through the upper flap. The tie is then secured at the angle of the incision.

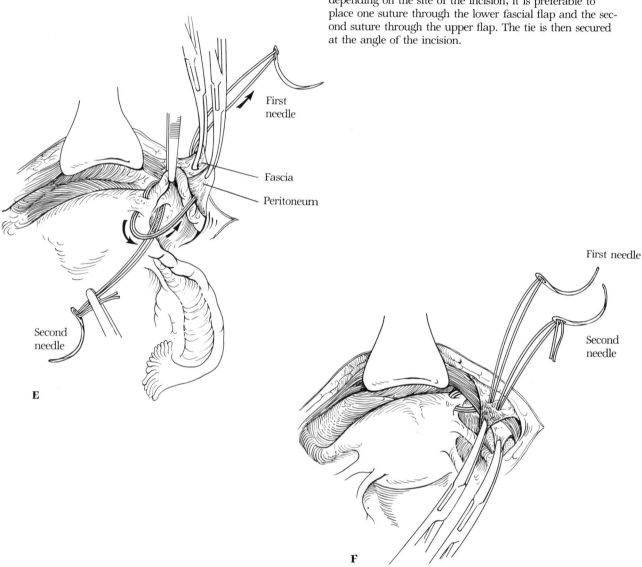

First needle

Fascia

Peritoneum

Second needle

E

First needle

Second needle

F

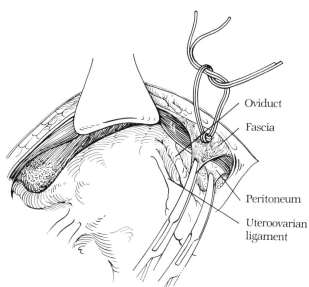

Oviduct

Fascia

Peritoneum

Uteroovarian
ligament

**G**

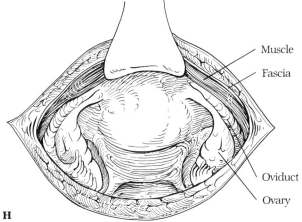

Muscle

Fascia

Oviduct

Ovary

**H**

As the illustration shows, the Mersilene sutures are placed around the round ligaments at the beginning of the operative procedure. These sutures are then used as tractors to hold the uterus forward. This obviates the need for placing a traction suture through the uterine corpus.

The placement of the suture back through the uterine cornu prevents undue tension on the round ligament and prevents avulsion when the suture is tied. Occasionally, a small rent in the uterine serosa is noted medial to the round ligament, and this is closed with interrupted sutures of 0 chromic catgut. Plication of the uterosacral ligaments is then performed as shown in Figure 8-6D.

This type of suspension has been stable and has been noted to persist after several pregnancies. No instances of small-bowel obstruction have been noted. The patient may note pain in the region of the round ligaments for 3 to 4 weeks, but this usually subsides gradually. We have had to disengage the suspension in only one patient because of pain, and this occurred during the third month of pregnancy.

## References

1. Black, W. T., Jr. Use of presacral sympathectomy in the treatment of dysmenorrhea. *Am. J. Obstet. Gynecol.* 89:16, 1964.
2. Graves, W. P. Olshausen operation for suspension of the uterus. *Surg. Gynecol. Obstet.* 52:1028, 1931.
3. Ingersoll, F. M., and Meigs, J. V. Presacral neurectomy for dysmenorrhea. *N. Engl. J. Med.* 238:357, 1935.
4. Kistner, R. W. *Principles and Practice of Gynecology* (3d ed.). Chicago: Year Book, 1979.
5. Parsons, L., and Ulfelder, H. *An Atlas of Pelvic Operations.* Philadelphia: Saunders, 1953.
6. Te Linde, R. W., and Mattingly, R. F. *Operative Gynecology* (4th ed.). Philadelphia: Lippincott, 1970.

# Index

Page numbers in *italics* indicate figures.

Transabdominal isthmic cervical cerclage, 74
Transcervical cannula, in microsurgery, *171, 172*
Transfundal hydrotubation, defined, in tubal anastomosis, 266
Transverse electromagnetic mode, in lasers, 196
*Trichomonas*
    infertility and, 6
    salpingitis and, 214
T-shaped anomaly of uterus, DES exposure and, 92, *93*
Tubal adhesions, surgical repair of. *See* Oviduct, surgery of; *see also specific procedures*
Tubal anastomosis. *See* Anastomosis, tubal and uterine
Tubal implantation. *See* Uterotubal implantation
Tubal inflammation, tubal pregnancy and, 288
Tubal lavage
    in microsurgery, special instruments for, *170*, 171–172, *171, 172*
    in tubal anastomosis, 266, *267*
Tubal ligation. *See* Tubal sterilization
Tubal phimosis, 237
Tubal pregnancy. *See* Pregnancy, tubal
Tubal sterilization
    cornual occlusion from, 279
    diathermy in, 260
    electrocoagulation techniques, 260
    Falope ring in, 259, *259*, 260
    fimbriectomy in, 260
    Hulka clip in, *259*, 259–260
    Madliner procedure, *259*, 260
    Pomeroy technique, *259*, 259–260
    procedures for, 258–261
    reversal of, 258–259
        results of, 274–276
        uterotubal implantation for, 285
    three-burn technique in, 260
Tubal surgery. *See* Oviduct, surgery of; *see also specific procedures*
Tubal transplants, 304–305
Tuboovarian distortion
    adhesions producing, 225, *226–227*. *See also* Adhesion(s), pelvic
    anatomic forms of, 225
Tuboovarian hiatus, defined, 222
Tubotubal anastomosis. *See* Anastomosis, tubal and uterine, tubotubal
Tubouterine anastomosis. *See* Anastomosis, tubal and uterine, tubouterine

Unicornuate uterus, 84, *85*, 86, *86*
Ureteric bud, 78
Urogenital system, female, embryogenesis of, 78, *79, 80, 81*, 82
Uterine anastomosis. *See* Anastomosis, tubal and uterine
Uterine suspension, 338, *338–341*, 342
Utero-isthmic anastomosis, *272–273*, 278
Uterotubal implantation
    bilateral isthmic closure and, histologic findings in, 280
    carbon dioxide laser in, 281, *283*
    cornual occlusion indicating
        diagnosis of, 280–281
        etiology of, 279–280
    history of, 278
    results of, 284, 285
    surgical approach to, 280–281, *282–283*
    technique of, *282–283*
Uterotubal junction (UTJ), function of, 262

Uterus
    anomalies of
        bicornuate uterus. *See* Uterus, bicornuate
        cervical cerclage and, 103
        cervical incompetence. *See* Cervix, incompetent
        classification of, 82–84
            clinical, 83–84, *85*
            functional, 82–83
        DES-related, 92, *93*
            surgery for, results of, 105–106
        embryologic considerations for, 78–81, *79, 80, 81*
        etiologic factors in, 97
        genetic factors in, 97
        renal anomalies associated with, 97
        segmental Müllerian agenesis/hypoplasia, 84, *85*
        septate uterus, *85*, 88, *88, 89, 90, 91*
        surgery for, urologic evaluation for, 97
        T-shaped, DES exposure and, 92, *93*
        unicornuate uterus, 84, *85*, 86, *86*
        uterus didelphys, *85*, 86, *86*
    bicornuate, *85*, 87, *87*
        cervical cerclage for, 103
        classification of, 83
        dysmenorrhea in, 94
        dyspareunia in, 95
        embryologic considerations for, 78–81, *79, 80, 81*
        fetal wastage in, hormonal therapy for, 96
        habitual abortion and, surgery indicated for, 95–96, *95*
        menometrorrhagia in, 94
        primary sterility and, surgery for, 95
        Strassman metroplasty for unification of, 94, 97, 102,
        surgery indicated for, 94–97, *95*
            results of, 104–105
            urologic evaluation for, 97
    didelphic. *See* Uterus didelphys
    double. *See* Uterus, bicornuate
    evaluation of, 11–19, *12, 13, 14, 15, 16, 18*
    leiomyomata of, pregnancy wastage and, 106, *107*, 108
    myomatous, 106–118. *See also* Myomectomy
    preoperative approach to, 109–110, *109, 110, 111*
    septate, *85*, 88, *88, 89, 90, 91*
        classification of, 83
        habitual abortion and fetal wastage in, surgery indicated for, 95–96
        unification of, 97–101, *97, 98, 99, 100, 101*, 105
    septum of, hysteroscopic resection of, 103
    subseptate, Jones procedure for unification of, *97, 98, 100–101*
    surgery of, 77–118. *See also* Myomectomy
        cervical cerclage, 103
        for DES-related anomalies, results of, 105–106
        hysteroscopic resection of uterine septum, 103
        indications for, 94–97
            dysmenorrhea, 94
            dyspareunia, 95
            habitual abortion and premature fetal loss, 95–96, *95*
            menometrorrhagia, 94
            primary sterility, 95
        metroplasty, history of, 94
        results of, 103–106
            for bicornuate uterus, 104–105
            for DES-related anomalies, 105–106
        unification of bicornuate uterus (Strassman procedure), *97*, 102, *102*
            results of, 103–104
        unification of septate uterus, 97–101, *97, 98, 99, 100, 101*, 105